BETTER THAN
MEDICINES

I hope my book
is useful & entertaining
on your path
to better health

M Cultur, MD

BETTER THAN MEDICINES

The Ten Essential Health Habits

Michael Carlston, MD

Santa Rosa, California

This book is not intended as a substitute for the medical advice of physicians. The reader should consult a physician in matters relating to his or her health and particularly with respect to any symptoms that may require diagnosis or medical attention.

This is the first book in a series called *Better Than Medicines: Getting Healthy and Feeling Better by Taking Care of the Simple Things*. For more information, see better-thanmedicines.com.

Book cover design by www.jdandj.com.

Book interior design, layout, and indexing by Marina Michaels.

First edition

ISBN 10: 1507781334

ISBN 13: 9781507781333

Library of Congress Control Number: 2015901643

LCCN Imprint Name: Santa Rosa, California

Contents

Acknowledgments............................ix

Part 1. Introduction......................1

1. Introduction...........................3

It Is Best to Dodge Magic Bullets 3
You Have the Magic 4
The Road Map 4
What This Book Is Not 6

2. How Did a Conventional, Highly Credible Minnesota Doctor Get Here?.................9

Why Should You Trust Me? 9
How I Became a Doctor......................10
My Introduction to Homeopathy..................11
In Medicine We Know Less Than We Claim to Know 13
Lessons from the Hmong People 13
Critical Thinking and Self-Criticism 14
Our Job Is to Learn........................16

3. Ways of Thinking about Health 19

A Philosophy for Life and Health..................19
Simplicity 30

Part 2. The Ten Essential Health Habits......39

4. An Introduction to the Ten Essential Health Habits........................... 41

Healthy Habits Make You Biologically Younger 42
More Powerful than Pills......................42
The Choice Is Yours 43

5. Essential Health Habit #1: Drink Enough Water 45

6. Essential Health Habit #2: Exercise Almost Every Day 49

You Are an Athlete 49

Aerobic Activity plus HIIT. 53
Strength Training. 54
Flexibility 56
Balance Training 61
Exercise Principles. 61
Building an Exercise Program 68
Good Gadgets for Exercise. 70

7. **Essential Health Habit #3: Eat Well** **75**
The American Diet Is a Problem 76
Your Food Should Be Diverse 77
Your Food Should Be Simple 79
Your Food Should Be Organic. 83
Your Food Should Be Local .91
Omega-3 Oils—On the Food/Supplement Borderline 95
Shopping and the Modern Hunter-Gatherer Society. 103
The Process of Eating 105
Diet—The Bottom Line. 107

8. **Essential Health Habit #4: Take Your
Supplements** **109**
Deficiencies Are a Problem, Really. 110
Food Fortification/Supplementation 115
Nutritional Research Confusion and Controversy 116
Testing for Vitamin Deficiencies 120
Self-Testing 126
Telomere Testing. 126
My Pragmatic Approach to Vitamins. 127
MVM Supplementation—The Bottom Line 129

9. **Essential Health Habit #5: Avoid the Things
That Make You Sick**. **133**
Environmental Chemicals .135
Air Pollution 151
Indoor Air Pollution. 152
Antibacterial Soaps. 156
Drinking Water 156
Getting the Best Water 162
Pesticides, Paints, and Cleaning Products. 165
Cookware 166
Flame Retardants. 168

Electromagnetic Radiation. 169

Food Additives 172

Cosmetics 173

Nanotechnology 174

Medications in Your Body and in the Environment. 177

Work and Play. 183

Tobacco, Alcohol, and Addiction 184

10. Essential Health Habit #6: Get Enough Sleep . 187

What *Do* We Know?. 187

Creating Good Sleep. 189

**11. Essential Health Habit #7: Be Involved in
    Your Community 191**

We Sense How Important Relationships Are. 192

Relationships Are Even More Important to Women 193

Science Supports Social Connections 193

The Downside. 194

**12. Essential Health Habit #8: Create a Healthy
    Sex Life 197**

Sex Is Natural, So What Could Go Wrong?. 197

Why Sex Is Biologically So Cool 198

What Is Healthy Sex? 198

**13. Essential Health Habit #9: Remember That
    Attitude Is Important. 201**

The Unity of Thought and Health. 201

Habits of Thought Change Brain Anatomy 202

Optimism Is Healthy 203

Coping with Life's Challenges 204

Positive Coping Skills—Recipes for Lemonade 205

It All Adds Up. 205

Where Are You Now? 206

Anticipate 206

The Challenges of Work. 207

A Specific Set of Skills 207

Forgiveness 209

Recreation Beyond Stress Management 210

Attitude Isn't Everything 211

14. Essential Health Habit #10: Develop a Purpose or Spirituality in Your Life 213

Spirituality and Psychosis. 214
A Purposeful Life Is a Healthy Life 214
Prayer for Everybody, Including Atheists 214

15. Achieving Essential Changes. 217

Self-Assessment. 217
Step 1—Set Achievable Goals. .218
Step 2—Create Specific Goals. .219
Step 3—Achieve Early Success .220
Step 4—Pay Attention to the Process 220
Step 5—Build on Your Short-term Successes 221
Failure 221

Part 3. Consider the Alternatives. 223

16. Consider the Alternatives 225

What Is Complementary and Alternative Medicine? 226
Americans and CAM 228
Who Uses CAM in America? 229
Why Do People Use CAM? 230
A Third Path—You Can All Take a Hike. 231
American CAM Usage—Patients and Physicians 233
Categories of CAM 235

17. How and When to Use CAM 239

Establish the Medical Diagnosis. 240
Understand Conventional Treatment Options. 241
Evaluate CAM Practitioners 242
What about Self-Care? 245
With Choice Comes Responsibility 246
Steps to Manage Your Health Care Responsibly. 247
When Is Which Therapy a Good Option? 248
For Physicians. 253

18. Herbal Supplements. 257

Traditional Use 258
Scientific Investigation 259
Conventional Medicine and Herbs. 260
Safety Issues 260

Herbal Safety—Solutions 265
How to Read a Label. 269
Long-Term Concerns 271

19. Homeopathy. 273

Confusion about Homeopathic Principles 274
Definitions. 275
Hahnemann's Story 275
Homeopathic Principles 279
Homeopathic View of Health and Disease 286
Homeopathic Survival. 288
What Is Homeopathy Good For?. 290
Optimal Use of Homeopathy for Self-Care 291

20. Acupuncture. 293

History 293
More Than Just Needles. 294
Acupuncture in the West 295
Adverse Effects 296
Effectiveness. 296
Growing Popularity 296
My Recommendations for Use 297

21. CAM as an Essential Health Habit. 299

22. Resources 301

Concentrated Dietary Sources of Protein 302
Concentrated Dietary Sources of Calcium 304
Essentials for Healthy Body Composition 306
Ideal Sports and Recovery Drinks 308
A Taste of Homeopathy. 310
Things to Know about Homeopathy 315
Research: Lies, Damned Lies, and Statistics 316
How to Study a Study 319

Index. 327

Acknowledgments

Acknowledging the influence of others on the creation of a book such as this is essential. As the fruit of a lifetime of experience, the only truly adequate acknowledgment would include tens of thousands of people. First place on the list, and by far the greatest number, are the patients who placed their trust in me and taught me by word or example. The debt I owe to them is immeasurable. I also must offer specific thanks where confidentiality is not an issue.

I would like to thank my professional mentors, some of them because they exemplified finding their own paths, and all of whom perceived something in me worthy of their attention and encouraged me along my path of discovery. Thank you, Donna Fasching, John Brantner, Patricia Wagner, Roger Jones, Maesimund Panos, Charles Thiesenhusen, Donald Asp, and Richard Holloway. Special thanks to Rudolph Ballentine, who provided an inspiring example of how medicine could be practiced differently, thoughtfully and scientifically.

My colleagues in practice, fellow travelers if you will, deserve recognition. In our shared interests we discovered a way forward, while at the same time our differences revealed unexpected, but vital lessons. Thank you, Richard Hruby, John Roos, Paul Erickson, Ann Barnes, Kathy Antolak, Roger Morrison, Ron Hood, Brian Karvelas, David Field, and Andrea Gordon.

The guidance of Brete Harrison was invaluable (thanks for sending him my way, Dana and Rob). The combined wisdom of Marina Michaels and Susan Bono was of great help in translating the nuts and bolts of my vision into the book format you are now reading. The designers at JD&J were patient and creative. Thanks also to Margot Comstock for some early editorial suggestions.

Friendship helps everything. The stalwart encouragement and support of Joey Brochin, Kathie Schmid, Michael Friedenberg, Betsy Stewart, and Craig Stewart convinced me of the value of this work and kept me going.

Thanks to my extended family. Just like my patients, but in a more personal way, this wildly divergent collection of humanity taught me all kinds of lessons about the realities of life, health, illness, and the varying ways we choose to respond. Special thanks to my parents and my in-laws who taught me so much about attitude, questioning, respect and exploration.

My children deserve special attention, like everyone's children, I suppose, but also for their direct contributions to this book. Rachel got the project started by collating the considerable mass of writing I had produced on relevant topics. Morgan's critical perspective was always uniquely insightful. Marissa's gentle but firm biomedical reminders kept me on track.

My deepest gratitude goes to my wife, Melanie. Her editorial skills, like her personal qualities, balance my deficiencies. Without her shared belief in this view of health as well as her personal commitment to help me educate others and treat patients, none of this would have been possible. I hope the results are worthy of her self-sacrifice. The rest goes without saying.

Michael Carlston
April 24, 2015

Part 1

Introduction

Chapter 1

Introduction

Ihave been a medical doctor, "practicing" medicine (as it is wisely described), for over thirty years. Every day new patients come to see me because they aren't well, despite carefully following the instructions they got from other health-care providers. Despite such admirable diligence, their chronic diseases are out of control, or they don't feel well, even though they have faithfully taken all the medications they have been prescribed.

Every single day I also see patients who started out just as unwell, but now feel better, and their health is better. Why? What is the difference? The key is that they made simple changes in their health habits. My impetus for writing this book is to help you see just how important these habits are, and then help you identify and implement the changes you need to make to become healthier and happier.

I'm creating this book to help you reevaluate your health care at the most fundamental level. My experience teaches me that basic, common-sense approaches should be the foundation of your efforts to maintain and improve your health. Unfortunately, common sense is woefully underappreciated. The fundamental elements of leading a healthy life seem so mundane or trivial, compared to the latest drug or diet fad, that most people overlook them.

The truth is that the *fundamental* nature of these heath habits is what also makes them *the most powerful and impactful steps you can take to improve your health and feel better.*

It Is Best to Dodge Magic Bullets

All of us—patients, health-care providers, and caring loved ones—are looking for magic bullets. This fact is just as true of alternative practitioners as it is of conventional ones. This is a huge mistake. There *is* magic, but it resides mostly in the seemingly mundane.

On the conventional side, drug companies and their representatives seduce naive physicians into prescribing drugs and devices that are exceptional only because they are new. Again, again, and again that newness conceals the bitter truth that the remarkable efficacy they promise will prove to be, at best, only a marginal improvement over the tired old drugs. Worse, the newness hides as-yet-unrevealed dangers. This is an old cycle. Those who love conventional medicine blindly throw themselves into the arms of these modern snake oil salesmen and saleswomen, while they look down their noses at those espousing herbs and natural cures.

On the alternative side, radical supplement advocates churn out the latest miracle cure, "long suppressed" by the American Medical Association (AMA). In truth, there *is* much of value in alternative therapies, and that is precisely why the concept of integrating methods of healing is so important for the health of us all. However, the issue is the same one. The more extravagant the claims, the less reality there is behind them.

You Have the Magic

I admit it. I'm a skeptic. I'm also an optimist. This could all sound quite gloomy, but there is no reason to despair. On the contrary, the truth is that you have far more power over your health than you and your doctor probably recognize. This book is about that power. It is about empowering *you* to improve your health more than about the expensive pills your doctor has for you. That's where the title *Better Than Medicines* comes from. There is a time and place for those pills, but in my experience, it is about 90 percent less than they are prescribed. Overuse of medication isn't in your best interest and really needs to change.

The Road Map

The first book in this series, *Better Than Medicines: The Ten Essential Health Habits*, is the fruit of thirty years of practicing medicine and thinking about how to boil good health down to a simple list of habits. What works? What is most essential? Accomplishing anything, including achieving excellent health, is much easier when the steps are clear. This book starts out with information about the behaviors that create or destroy your health, identifying those that are good and those that threaten your well-being. Some are extremely simple. Others are more complicated. Science and, maybe more importantly, clinical experience well support each of these habits.

In each chapter I give you specific suggestions to help you implement the most important changes. If you're already working to optimize your health in this deeply considered way, this book will add some pieces you've forgotten or didn't know about. If you haven't been tending to your own wellness in this manner, the book will give you motivation and clear steps to get you moving in the right direction.

There are a couple of organizational features in the chapters to help you most effectively absorb and apply the information there. All but the very smallest chapters include a concise bulleted summary at the end to keep you on target. The longer chapters also start with a list of the sections within the chapter so you can see what's up ahead.

Health matters are important to us all, so the media flood us with the latest discoveries and controversies. They do a very poor job of critiquing this material. Consequently, this information is more confusing than enlightening. You are a bit on your own. Chapter 3, Ways of Thinking about Health, relates my perspective on health and the basis for my critiques. Part of this analysis deals with underlying assumptions. Again, the emphasis isn't academic. It will provide you with simple questions to ask and a framework for clearer thinking about your own health.

There is a fuller, more scientifically detailed explanation in Chapter 22, which teaches you how to perform the critical assessment you need to make better health decisions. That information grows out of my experience reviewing articles for publication in some of the most important medical journals in the world; in that chapter, I guide you toward identifying the flaws and misleading presumptions in those articles.

To achieve the best health possible, you shouldn't confine the treatments you receive to conventional medicine. Conventional medicine is too limited and too obsessed with overly toxic therapies to be your only choice. In Chapter 17, How and When to Use CAM, I tell you more about complementary and alternative therapies and introduce you to some of them. Since 80 percent of the world's population uses these therapies, it would take many, many books to do them all justice. I chose the therapies featured in that chapter either because they are especially useful or because, in a couple of cases such as homeopathy and acupuncture, most are in need of explanation, since they are so different from conventional medicine. Others, like chiropractic medicine, for example, are so widespread and familiar that you probably don't need any input from me.

Following this first book, I'm planning two more books specifically focused on different parts of the human life cycle. Essential health habits are essential throughout life, but the emphasis and implementation are different. So too are the health issues. In these books I will discuss health problems common at those points of life and the best ways to both prevent and treat them. Each of them will include recommendations for the alternative or complementary therapies I have found useful for certain problems.

One book will guide parents through pregnancy, birth, and childhood. Parents have such huge responsibilities and must make decisions with lifelong repercussions. That book will help guide you through that process and, I hope, then alleviate some of the stress. The other will cover adulthood and aging. As the architects of the world, we all rely on the strength of adults. Whether you are ill and need help or just want to be stronger to feel better and do more, this book will be useful to you. Although the most profound benefits are visible over many years, even very late in life our health habits bear fruit quickly. Quality of life is more evidently important when the quantity is likely to be limited.

The fourth book is a bit different from the others. I'm pragmatic. I want to see results. My greatest passion in medicine is helping patients achieve success. Theories are fun but completely pointless if they don't lead to better health. There is way too much of that failure in medicine, in conventional as well as alternative medicine. Consequently, I'm quite excited about the *Better Than Medicines Workbook*. It will take each of the essential health habits and help you create your own plans to successfully incorporate these habits into your daily life.

What This Book Is Not

Finally, here's just a note about what this book and the others are not. They are not hammers forged to beat you into submission. They are not written to tell you how bad you or your health habits are. None of them is a dispiriting litany of woe. I'm certain you can become healthier by making changes in your life. I know your situation isn't hopeless. Even *you* can make changes. Most importantly, I know from my clinical experience that when you make these changes, the being-healthier part will be just a bonus, icing on the cake, compared to how much better you will feel. Again, based on my experience of what works, I will give you specific suggestions so you can achieve your health goals.

There is one more thing this book isn't. It isn't perfect. The idea of "practicing" medicine fits in the sense that there is always room for improvement. The same holds true of this book. While I'm confident about all I have learned and proud of so much that was evident to me long before others recognized such truths, I learn every day, and there are certainly a few minor mistakes in this book. *Always remember* that you know you, maybe not as well as you might, but no one has your experience. Seek out advice and work to apply the recommendations of experts (especially mine) but watch your reactions and apply your own growing wisdom.

I hope you will find this book and all others to be as interesting, useful, and (dare I say it?) even as fun as writing them has been for me.

Chapter 2

How Did a Conventional, Highly Credible Minnesota Doctor Get Here?

In this chapter I introduce myself and make sense of the path that led me to think the way I do. Part of that story is about the changes roiling conventional medicine, really now for generations. Asking questions leads us forward. Medicine is far less self-questioning than it should be. The "pole star" of medicine, the reliable and steady principle guiding all of us toward better health, is the experience of patients. This chapter is about my experience, based on the life experience of thousands of patients.

Why Should You Trust Me?

Before we set sail on this journey together, you might reasonably ask, "Why should I trust you?" I won't be offended. The first step in taking charge of your health and really learning about anything is to ask questions. The first question is questioning your sources of information.

Personally, I mistrust "experts" who haven't walked the walk. Some of them have done a lot of reading, but they lack the experience confirming whether something really works. They haven't seen it with their own eyes.

I'm a medical doctor, proud of medicine's tradition of caring for others to the very best of my abilities. I'm also proud of the tradition of self-examination, testing theories in the real world of clinical medicine. Therein lie medicine's greatest strengths and worst failures.

The uncertainties inherent in caring for complicated living beings have many, many times led physicians to prescribe treatments we later recognize were worse than just unhelpful. The consequences of our errors are often severe. There is nothing new about physicians making mistakes. Mistakes will persist as long as our knowledge is imperfect—in other words, forever. Consequently, critical thinking is a vital quality for any physician regardless of the prevailing dogma. Dogmatism via underexamined clinical routines or medical theories is the bane of medicine or any method of healing. Unfortunately, physicians often behave like our profession is a secret guild, reflexively rejecting criticism, especially when that criticism strikes at the most unexamined (in other words, dogmatic) beliefs. Critics are too frequently considered heretics.

For decades, I've been viewed as a heretic. Now many of my "heretical" beliefs are gaining acceptance, and some have become the new norm. I started teaching about nose rinses and mindfulness in the early 1970s. After my patients have listened to me for decades, rarely now do I ever need to tell them about probiotics or vitamin D. Thirty years ago I was breaking the cycles of antibiotic overuse, which was inflicted on so many children with ear infections. Now I treat the children of those children. My dissenting opinions have almost always been proved to be correct, probably because my views are founded on common sense and on paying attention to the lessons my patients teach me. I have learned that *good health depends on the fundamentals, the essential health habits any medicine, conventional or alternative, cannot replace.*

How I Became a Doctor

Just before graduating from high school, my girlfriend's older sister asked me what I wanted to do with my life. Adults like to do that to teenagers. Her question got me thinking about who I was and about my completely nebulous future. We were on a long car ride, so she had me cornered. After squirming a bit, I told her that I liked helping people and that I also liked science. Although she was an acutely insightful person, only a sliver of her brilliance was needed to recognize that medicine contained the balance of qualities I had described. On my own I'd read a good deal about nutrition, exercise, and some forms of alternative medicine, such as acupuncture and meditation. However, the idea of becoming a doctor had never entered my thoughts, and now that it had, I resisted it at first. On the contrary, I decided not to continue my education, at least for the time being. A "real-world" education seemed more important and more appealing than college.

Limited job opportunities quickly drew me into the world of health care. I took nursing assistant jobs, first in a nursing home and then on the general surgery ward of a large county hospital. This work experience changed my life. The gritty realities of the working world heightened my enthusiasm for going back to school and getting a university education. At the same time, I enjoyed working in the hospital, and I continued there until I completed college.

As a seventeen-year-old from the suburbs, moving to the inner city and working with the population of patients whom such facilities serviced then and now broadened my world view in unimagined ways. Our patients were "bums," prisoners, and the poor. The "bums" I saw sleeping in the public library now had names and life stories. A newspaper article or report on radio or television was often my first introduction to a patient or prisoner who was literally chained to one of the beds when I next went in to work. The medicine practiced in such settings was at its best courageous, compassionate, and skillful. Unfortunately, the worst of humanity was also on display on a daily basis—from the compromises in care that the financial constraints imposed on these institutions and their patients necessitated, to the horrific violence one person inflicted on another. Many of our patients came to the hospital as casualties of some act of violence. Both the best and worst of what I saw in this place inspired me. I wondered what I could do to make things better.

Simultaneously, I became a yoga teacher and pursued my interest in alternative forms of medicine. Acupuncture and vegetarian diets were the first areas I explored. There was no realistic way for me to seriously study acupuncture at that time. Acupuncturists were very rare, and China was still politically off limits.

My Introduction to Homeopathy

It was a revelation when I met a medical doctor practicing homeopathic medicine. Dr. Rudolph B. Ballentine was highly inspirational and possessed of a bright and broadly inquisitive mind, which he expressed in his enthusiasm for teaching. Dr. Ballentine was also an excellent and caring clinician. He modeled a highly appealing style of patient care that was both completely new and firmly rooted in ancient medical tradition. He also encouraged my own intellectual curiosity. His introduction to homeopathy and its appealing philosophy of health and medical treatment set me on the path that has defined my professional identity.

My experience as his patient was enormously important. I sought his care after first seeking help at the university health service. When that conventional treatment was simultaneously unsuccessful and mildly harmful, I was determined to take the nine-hundred-mile journey to see whether the homeopath could do any better. It turned out that the care I received was profoundly different, maybe even more than nine hundred miles distant from the conventional treatment I had gotten. The big deal was that this care actually worked. I felt better. Like any other patient, feeling better was what I cared about.

The effectiveness of his treatment was surprising and not just because it worked when the conventional treatment had not. Equally or even more surprising were the improvements in my general well-being. I clearly remember when my two roommates and I went out to play tennis a few days after my first appointment with the homeopathic medical doctor. As the odd man out, rather than waiting for my turn to play tennis, I began running around the park. I had been a distance runner as a child, but I hadn't done anything athletically for several years. I felt so energetic that I really wanted to move. Standing around, waiting, just wasn't in the cards. Just as unexpectedly, I experienced some important emotional changes. The sum of this experience was a conviction that his approach was quite valuable and in surprising ways.

Perhaps just as importantly, I later experienced his imperfection when a subsequent treatment made me worse. My most troublesome physical problem (eczema) was eventually eliminated but only after I disobeyed his instructions and stopped his treatment. The prescription drugs didn't cure me, but he hadn't managed my treatment well either. His recommendations had helped, but he hadn't known when to stop.

Clearly the homeopath possessed unique and useful knowledge. He knew things the other doctors I had seen had not. But my experience as a patient showed me that his knowledge or his clinical judgment was also imperfect. Furthermore, while the philosophy of homeopathic medicine was attractive and in many ways made a great deal of sense, its methods contradicted the scientific training I was accumulating. Despite my positive experience, I often asked the homeopathic physician to account for the scientific inconsistencies or share his most impressive successes to bolster my faith and justify my continued interest. We had some excellent conversations, but his reticence reflected his own uncertainties.

In Medicine We Know Less Than We Claim to Know

It became clear to me that homeopathic medicine poses a nearly perfect set of counterarguments to conventional medicine. We will talk about some of those specific issues later in this book. Caught in the tension between the conflicting viewpoints of conventional and homeopathic medicine, I learned to view each of them, as well as all other therapies, with a critical eye. I perceived that in medicine we often know less than we think we know. Not infrequently, what we know for certain is certainly not so. Although our work is to continually expand our knowledge, it is routine for the realities of clinical practice to force us to step beyond what has been proved to aid our patients in their distress.

My positive but scientifically perplexing experience with homeopathy and other forms of alternative medicine prepared me well for medical school and my residency in family and community medicine. I had to struggle at times during my training because I simply refused to accept what we were taught at face value. Like trying to drink from a fire hydrant, the volume of information we must absorb in medical education makes it nearly impossible to examine any of it critically. Simply swallowing it all as fast as you can is the easiest way to get through. Although this internal conflict was difficult, navigating my medical training with my eyes open to other possibilities and critical thinking was, in retrospect, a fantastic gift.

Lessons from the Hmong People

Studies of health professionals, including academics, show that individual experiences, including those of family, friends, and patients, are crucial to changes in thinking and behavior. The residency phase of medical training is the most intense time in a doctor's life. It is an immersion in the cauldron of cutting-edge medicine, intended to give us a tremendous amount of experience in a very short time. In my case, caring for many hundreds of Hmong refugees from Southeast Asia had a profound personal and professional impact.

The Hmong people I encountered were every bit as independent as one would expect to see in a community of resistance fighters forced to flee their jungle home for the unimaginably different environment of a city in Minnesota. An oppressed minority in their home country, they had for generations been fighting merely to survive. Pressures from the outside pushed them more tightly together, and they held closely to their traditions. Their healing traditions couldn't have been any more different from those we were taught in medical school and residency. That difference was a huge source of frustration for my classmates.

Personally, I loved the differences. So many times I saw how their approach was no worse than ours. When there were problems, such as the poisonings caused by the lead-based powder they sometimes used to treat infant fevers, the challenging process of communication and building trust was educational. I still don't understand all that I experienced. For example, why did I have to deliver so many babies in the backseat of cars in the hospital driveway when they didn't arrive soon enough to make it all the way into the hospital? How could it be that the young man with the abscess in his brain caused by a parasite, who refused our treatment, was healthy three years later when I finished my residency? For me, the experience of my residency was a tremendous gift. It was excellent training that taught me to think about healing in the broadest ways possible. I am deeply indebted to those patients, and to every patient since then, for the experiential instruction they have given me.

Critical Thinking and Self-Criticism

As I was an innately critical thinker, my conventional medical training also taught me how to better evaluate the claims and traditions of alternative medicine.

Prejudiced Opinions Are Common

It is also essential to comment on the intellectual narrowness I have witnessed at times in the alternative health community. While conventional medicine can be "antiscientific" in the sense that too many physicians make too many assumptions about the value of conventional drugs and the deficiencies of all other approaches, this problem is almost equally true in the alternative community. Two experiences in one week long ago cast a bright spotlight on this dogmatism in both communities.

On a Saturday I attended a meeting of a small group of researchers in my department at the University of California, San Francisco (UCSF). During a break, I had a pleasant conversation with another MD sitting next to me. Later it was my turn to present my research proposal, which was a placebo-controlled protocol studying the effect of individually selected homeopathic remedies on children with acute diarrheal illnesses. The feedback I got was that the design appeared sound to nearly everyone in the room. Nevertheless, the previously friendly MD sitting next to me nearly exploded because I had proposed studying homeopathy.

The vehemence of his response stunned the department's research chairperson (a PhD, not an MD), because it was so clearly emotional rather than scientific. Intrigued, she asked him what he would do if the study was perfectly designed and found that homeopathic treatment worked for this condition. His response was, "Design another study." He was unable to accept the results of a carefully designed scientific study if it contradicted his entrenched beliefs.

Days later I attended a study group of experienced homeopathic clinicians in the Bay Area. About half of them were medical doctors. After learning about my research work and intention to conduct homeopathic trials, the eldest MD homeopath rebelled. He exclaimed to me and to the group that homeopathy was a "spiritual" science and therefore impossible to research.

We each have our unique points of view. If a therapy can benefit human bodies, it must be measurable and open to scientific evaluation. A scientist must accept unexpected study results. *What is the point of conducting research if it doesn't unveil our ignorance?* With the passage of time we are making headway, but we delude ourselves if we think we've reached anything close to a full understanding of all the beneficial approaches to human healing. Arrogance and ignorance are a widespread and deadly duo.

To Those with the Courage to Ask Questions

I dedicated my textbook on homeopathic medicine "To those with the courage to ask questions." I have yet to fully understand why the practice of medicine is treated like a narrow religious faith, where fundamental criticism or deviance from the "usual" is marked as heretical.

In my opinion, part of every physician's responsibility to his or her patients is to ask questions, big and small, about the treatments he or she provides. Forget the history books. I remember the days when we performed circumcisions and even major surgeries on newborns without pain medications because we bizarrely thought babies didn't feel pain, or we thought pain-controlling medication was too much for them. How could anyone with open eyes not be critical?

I accept responsibility for annoying my teachers of all healing traditions. I thank those who have endured my recalcitrance and wish to honor those who have been sufficiently confident and intellectually honest to welcome my questioning.

Although I appreciate their patience, there is also no reason for me to apologize. If a treatment cannot withstand the light of critical evaluation, it is unworthy and shouldn't be used. It is such critical thinking that improves those methods and in medicine most benefits the patient. I critique my own work every day, testing and incorporating or rejecting new and old treatments.

In this manner of criticism, one of my inspirations has been the founder of homeopathic medicine, Samuel Hahnemann. In the first lines of the book he wrote, founding the "modern" systematic use of homeopathic techniques (the underlying principle had been used in various forms for two thousand years before Hahnemann), he proclaimed that the physician's duty isn't to construct systems of philosophy but to heal the sick. As he defined the system of medicine he espoused, he deflated the importance of that system as a construct. The well-being of the patient is *always* more important than any theory.

Our Job Is to Learn

Thankfully, medicine and our knowledge of human health are perpetually expanding (although typically in fits and starts). Today we look back on past mistakes with disdain or embarrassment, depending on how long ago they occurred and whether we made them ourselves. Too often we don't look back and reflect. We don't learn from our mistakes; we just turn away, pretending they never happened.

As we are still learning, it is a stone-cold guarantee that in a few years we will look back on this moment in health care—the common and perhaps even the "best" medical practices of today—and shake our heads at the errors we haven't yet recognized.

How is it that we're not outraged or at least powerfully motivated to do a better job when we do make mistakes or realize we had it wrong? Making mistakes is one thing. Not learning from our mistakes is quite another and less forgivable. Even when we have made the best judgments possible at the moment, more time and understanding hopefully increase our abilities. Each new patient and each new visit with an old patient present a unique opportunity to learn more about health and healing.

I'm a believer in both the importance and limitations of medical research. Wearing that hat, I have served on the editorial board of many peer-reviewed medical journals, reviewed articles for many others (including the *Journal of the American Medical Association*) and evaluated research grant applications for the National Institutes of Health (NIH). So in this book you will read a lot about research findings supporting the arguments I make. I will also discuss many instances where the media or medical community promoted some therapy chiefly because they overlooked or ignored errors in the design of the relevant studies.

Summary

- The basics are neglected but immensely important.
- Alternative therapies are vital counterpoints to convention.

Where have I arrived after this lengthy journey? Alternative approaches are a vital counterpoint to the accepted habits of medical treatment and thought. Alternative and conventional therapies together can help the other therapies improve and help all of us move forward. I'm disappointed that each "side" seems so compelled to demean the other. Each side has strengths and weaknesses. Neither is anything close to perfect. Like two sides of a coin, they need each other. Taking a look at things from an entirely different point of view and periodically reconsidering even the primary elements of our methods are as vital as breathing.

Summary, continued

Thirty-five years of clinical experience practicing medicine in this manner, while seeking out and applying the best of conventional medicine in combination with alternative medicine, has been enlightening. Most importantly, this method has been beneficial to my patients. It is normal for my patients to get better, even when they come to me because other treatments have failed. That process isn't really so remarkable. It is a simple matter of helping them identify and fix fundamental problems.

Most importantly, I have learned that any battles between conventional and alternative treatments are secondary. The essential health habits are precisely that: *essential*. They are better than medicines, because they do more. No ancient healing tradition or high-tech medical intervention can fix you if you don't take care of the essentials. A pill can't replace water. A supplement can't replace exercise. An alternative therapy can't replace a healthy diet.

Chapter 3

Ways of Thinking about Health

This chapter explains how I've learned to think about health. It describes the thought process and attitudes that led to my conclusions. It won't tell you what to do, but it does tell you how I have learned to think about health. It is sort of a checklist of the most useful tools in my intellectual toolbox. If you trust the experts to do all the work, you don't need these tools, but you'd be better off knowing how to use some of them yourself.

Chapter 22 includes a section, "Research: Lies, Damned Lies, and Statistics," that extends this consideration.

A Philosophy for Life and Health

A coherent and consistent approach to life can be both comforting and useful. Reliance on certain principles can help us make difficult decisions when the correct choice might not otherwise be entirely obvious. There are basic facts about the ways human beings function in the world. *Understanding those basic facts and using them to heal are the foundation of wise health care,* whether that health care comes from a physician, some other health-care professional, Dr. Mom, or your own efforts at self-care. Sometimes we learn these basic truths from scientific research. That is typically the exception rather than the rule. More often these fundamentals are so basic that they become evident through experience.

At the same time, oversimplification entails its own risks, can become dogmatic, and can lead us to make poor judgments—decisions that are "obviously" correct but—oops!—wrong. That tendency has, in fact, been a major recurrent theme in medical errors over the millennia, not just in recent times. We need to be cautious when applying broad, general principles to very specific circumstances. General principles and scientific research help us predict what might help patients, but sometimes (or even often) common sense trumps the latest scientific theory.

For over two thousand years, various oaths of practice have guided physicians. These oaths are statements of ethical principles intended to provide a stable foundation, a consensus understanding about the nature of our interactions with patients. In the past, these were truly "oaths," communally recognized commitments to a specific code of conduct. For example, the oath of Hippocrates is still recognized as a guide for modern physicians.

In college I was surprised to learn that the oath of Hippocrates was but one of several such medical oaths passed down from the ancient world. I linked my undergraduate major (South Asian Civilization) to my future medical career by writing my honors thesis on the connection between the medical oaths of ancient India and the Hippocratic Oath. My studies made it clear that other, even older, creeds had influenced the content of the Hippocratic Oath. Evidently physicians across the ancient world felt the need to define ethical principles for them to abide by. The importance of the Hippocratic Oath is still felt so strongly that, thousands of years after it first came into use, many medical schools continue to use this code of conduct as a reminder to students of our ethical heritage. Even many laypeople are aware of the existence of the Oath.

First Do No Harm, but Then Again, Why Not?

Experience is the best teacher. Just so, it is wise to use this hallowed declaration of medical ethics and practice as the starting point for our discussion of a philosophy of health. Similarly, the Oath of Hippocrates is itself founded on this primary principle, which states, "First do no harm." This is an obviously vital concept. Why should a healer endanger those who are seeking help? It's a real no-brainer, but is nowhere as easy to apply as it is self-evident.

Any healing intervention entails risk, and so it demands the responsibility of careful use. Anything with the power to heal, to change human function, must also contain the power to cause harm. Once again, this is far from a new idea.

> Within the infant rind of this small flower,
> poison hath residence and medicine power.
> —William Shakespeare, *Romeo and Juliet*

The US government has tracked adverse drug effects for many years. Recent information shows a startling increase and change in the pattern of adverse drug reactions. Over a seven-year period (1998–2005), the rate of serious and fatal drug reactions nearly tripled in the United States.[1] In 1998, nearly thirty-five thousand Americans experienced an adverse reaction to a drug that caused a birth defect, created disability, or required medical intervention either to save the person's life or to prevent further harm. By 2005, that number jumped to nearly ninety thousand. The number of Americans losing their lives to these adverse reactions nearly tripled, increasing from fifty-five hundred to fifteen thousand. Figures show these numbers are still rising. Again, proving just how serious this problem is, bad reactions to drugs are the fourth leading cause of death in the USA, ahead of diabetes, automobile accidents, and lung disease.

Advertising to consumers has changed the practice of medicine and increased physician prescribing (as well as markedly increasing drug costs for everyone). During that 1998–2005 interval, the total number of prescriptions increased by 50 percent (from 2.7 to 3.8 billion). That 50 percent increase doesn't mathematically account for the even more dramatic rise in the number of adverse drug reactions.

While the increased number of prescriptions doesn't solely account for the rise in adverse reactions, the more medicines one person takes, the greater is the likelihood of an adverse interaction between the drugs. How are we doing on that score? Not so good. Over 20 percent of us have taken three or more prescription drugs in the last month, and a shocking 11 percent have taken *five or more*!

Drugs that were withdrawn for safety reasons also didn't fully account for the rise. Of nearly fifteen hundred drugs faulted in these case reports, only fifty-one of them accounted for over 40 percent of all seriously adverse drug events (nearly two hundred four thousand reports). Medications for pain and immune-modifying drugs were the biggest problems. Problems with immune-modifying medication aren't at all surprising. They are very powerful drugs, and the people who use them are quite ill.

Prescriptions for painkilling medication have doubled every seven to ten years in the United States. This is a very big part of the problem. Prescriptions for the most notorious of these medications, OxyContin,

---

1   Moore, Cohen, and Furberg, "Serious Adverse Drug Events Reported to the Food and Drug Administration, 1998-2005," *Arch Intern Med* 167 (2007): 1752-9.

increased six fold. *In 2010, when a patient saw a physician and left his or her office with a prescription in hand, on its label was most likely written hydrocodone/acetaminophen (Vicodin).* There were over 130 million prescriptions that year for Vicodin. The second most common prescription (the cholesterol-lowering drug Lipitor) was way behind at 94 million. The CDC reported that in 2012 there were over 259 million prescriptions for painkillers in the United States.[2] Adverse effects from painkilling drugs are common and range from fatalities caused by acute overdoses (fifteen thousand per year) to kidney failure caused from years of low-dose usage. People tend to forget that a little bit over a long time can cause just as much harm as a huge amount all at once.

When patients come to me for treatment, they tell me they want to feel better, but they also want to avoid the use of conventional prescription medication. Sometimes they figured out that the prescription medication they were taking to improve their health was the reason they didn't feel well. They don't think that conventional medicine is evil, just a bit riskier than they would like. While they certainly wouldn't want to see an ancient Greek physician, they want to live in accord with the first precept of the Hippocratic Oath, avoiding needless harm to themselves. They are willing to take prescription drugs only if there is no other option. They hope that in their circumstance, prescription medication is unnecessary, or at least maybe they can use less than they have been using. It turns out that they are usually correct; better still, they don't have to trade worsened medication-free health for feeling better.

Why is that? One answer is that there are *many effective healing options other than prescription medications, but these interventions are either undervalued or less well known.* For many health problems, these other treatments are actually better than prescription medications. They are better because, while they relieve the problem, they do so with less in the way of adverse effects. In fact, the "side effects" of these treatments are often improvements of other aspects of the person's health. Also, these interventions usually cost much less than prescription medication. Simple things like exercising, eating reasonably, drinking enough water, and getting enough sleep can be extremely powerful treatments for problems usually treated with prescription medication. Decades of

---

2 "Opioid Painkiller Prescribing," http://www.cdc.gov/vitalsigns/opioid-prescribing/

experience have taught me that these simpler lifestyle habits are *more powerful* than conventional medicine.

Another answer is even more elementary: many health problems will go away without active medical intervention. This wonderful ability of the body to heal itself has often ironically led us to believe that something we did made the difference. Of course, we did "do" it, but not consciously.

For example, for fifty years the medical establishment believed that antibiotics cured almost all ear infections, and such prescriptions were the well-established norm. When investigators finally got around to performing careful studies, they learned (drum roll please) that antibiotics helped only a small percentage of children to get better. At the same time, the prescribed antibiotics exposed all the patients to a significant risk of adverse effects. As these studies were confirmed again and again over decades, very slowly clinical medicine changed. Today many millions of children no longer receive needless antibiotics for ear infections, and we're all better off because lowering antibiotic use lowers the risk of more serious antibiotic-resistant bacterial infections.

As Shakespeare observed, any healing intervention conveys its own risk. Consequently, if a patient would get better without any help, *we must be very careful not to "help" in some manner likely to cause harm.* Doing nothing is the simplest approach.

Learning the natural history of disease, the behavior of health problems over time, is necessary for optimal care. That understanding tells us when to be patient and when rapid response is essential. It takes time for physicians to learn patience, to develop the confidence to "first do no harm," as Hippocrates admonished. Many of the most experienced and skillful clinicians will intervene the least, understanding that more is often not better. It also takes time for a doctor to explain to patients why it is better not to use the latest expensive drug advertised on TV, on the radio, on the Internet, and in the newspaper. Although giving every patient a prescription is easier than educating the patient, waiting can be best. Doing simple things to help can be the best approach of all.

If It Is Safe, Then Why Not Take a Chance? (Risk-Benefit Ratio)

In medicine we frequently make treatment decisions based on a concept we call the *risk-benefit ratio*. The risk-benefit ratio is an analysis of the likelihood of good or bad effects resulting from some intervention. This concept is exceptionally useful and should be the measuring stick for any therapeutic intervention of any sort, not just prescription medication. *If the risk of harm is low, then why not try it?* Conversely, if the treatment is dangerous, we should avoid it unless the need is more extreme than the risk.

Often the more immediately powerful the treatment is, the greater is the likelihood of serious ill effects. For example, steroids are strong drugs that mimic powerful hormones our bodies produce. Steroids usually cause powerful adverse effects. Long-term use is associated with suppression of adrenal function, bone destruction, and a long list of other problems. Even short-term use can make patients jittery, anxious, or depressed with the abrupt rise and fall of blood levels. At the same time, steroid medications are lifesaving for other patients. It is best then to use steroids only when patients suffer from very serious problems. Steroids shouldn't be used for lesser problems. Unfortunately, because steroids are so powerful, physicians are tempted to use them more often than is wise.

At the other end of the spectrum are interventions that are very safe but might not help so much. Then again, they might actually help a great deal, but usually there has been little careful scientific study of these approaches. The tendency in medicine is to assume that these treatments won't work, passing judgment in ignorance. *Why are these other treatments neglected?*

Sometimes physicians and patients are simply unaware of treatment options. New ideas and treatments are waiting to be discovered, confirmed, and applied. How can we not expect the future to hold great advances in human health care? However, "we" honestly don't even know what some others know now. Some of those great "future" treatments are undoubtedly already in use, but they are unknown to, or unexamined by, the conventional medical community. Some surveys tell us that 30 percent of conventional medications, which conventional physicians currently prescribe, are derived from herbs. In fact, roughly 20 percent of those prescription medications are manufactured by processing the raw plants. Despite their too-common discomfort with, or even antipathy toward, herbal medicines, conventional physicians *are* practicing herbal medicine. We need to thoroughly investigate traditional, non-Western medical practices to learn what conventional medicine is missing. We medical doctors need to recognize the limitations of our knowledge, acknowledge that there may be better treatments already out there, and then, fulfilling our moral obligation to our patients, set aside prejudices and consider those other possibilities.

Sometimes we medical doctors overlook safer treatments because *we're biased in favor of conventional prescription drugs.* Our bias is that prescription drugs must work better. The fact that they are available only by prescription makes them appear innately more powerful. The accouterments of seriousness and responsibility surround these drugs, heightening that impression of efficacy, as does their familiarity. That familiarity can be scientific or simply come from advertising. Even if the only appearance of a drug in a medical journal is among the advertisements, not in the research articles, those ads are created to make the drugs look effective and scientific. Truthfully, even the mere visibility of a drug in a medical journal lends an aura of credibility that is too often unwarranted or even contradicted by medical research.

The bottom line is that we medical doctors should be critical. We think we are. But studies show that we really aren't. We're less critical than we believe, especially when it comes to prescription drugs.

The pharmaceutical industry invests billions of dollars every year to shape our opinions. In a more skeptical view of that industry, *shaping* is too kind of a word. The word *deceiving* is more accurate. In a world where drug companies block publication of data showing the lack of effectiveness of their drugs and the existence of serious adverse effects, medical doctors must be more critical. If drug companies had only once or twice behaved unethically, we might be forgiven our naïveté. That would be overgenerous. We're far past that time of forgivable innocence. The problem has gotten so bad that editors of three of the four most highly regarded medical journals have each made comments to the effect that their journals have become publicity arms of the big drug manufacturers. Drug companies are now budgeting for criminal penalties, not just civil penalties, resulting from their miscreant activities. *In 2011 alone, one company paid $3 billion to settle criminal and civil penalties.*[3]

In medicine, the big four-letter word is *fear.* Patients are afraid of losing their health. They want to be well, and many will do just about

---

3   Hawkes, "GlaxoSmithKline Pays $3bn to Settle Dispute Over Rosiglitazone and Other Drugs," *BMJ* 343 (2011): d7234, doi: http://dx.doi.org/10.1136/bmj.d7234.

anything doctors or the media tell them so they will live longer. Fear is totally not limited to patients. We're all, physicians and the public at large, too easily manipulated by fear-generating health headlines and our own nightmares.

Caution is reasonable and prudent. However, irrational fear leads to bad decisions. Fear and suspicion make it hard for doctors to drop dangerous but familiar treatments while simultaneously assuming that an herb, used for the same problem for generations, might turn out to be deadly. Any medical doctor can tell you stories of patients he or she had to hospitalize due to serious drug reactions. Physicians are overly comfortable with medications we all know can be risky while simultaneously getting nervous about other healing methods that have been used for far longer.

Medical bias against unfamiliar treatments is an insidious obstacle. In addition to hypocritical acceptance of prescription medication, physicians are hypercritical of unfamiliar treatments. A great deal of research tells us that medical doctors make treatment decisions at best only loosely related to scientific evidence of efficacy. The great majority of conventional medical interventions (80 percent, according to a World Health Organization estimate) are not supported by research evidence. At the same time, physicians often drag their feet about using dietary supplements, herbs, and vitamins, even in the face of research demonstrating efficacy. While leaping onto the latest bandwagon without thinking a bit is unwise, it is easy to argue that it is irresponsible not to give therapy a try when the likelihood of harm is small (in other words, a good risk-benefit ratio).

All these factors make it far easier to simply toe the party line, prescribing the latest and greatest prescription drug, rather than asking questions. We should ask why this new drug is better. Isn't it more expensive? What about the adverse effects? So many new drugs are eventually taken off the market as wider use of the drugs uncovers very serious unwanted effects. Is it worth the risk? Why not recommend an inexpensive dietary supplement that appears both effective and safe? Why not take the time to explain to patients why they really don't need prescription drug X and why it isn't worth the risk for them to take it?

What about actually helping patients change? Why not put out the energy to coach patients through the process of developing better health habits? We give prescriptions with very specific instructions on how to take the medication. Even when a good doctor tells patients to reduce stress, get more exercise, or eat better, why does he or she stop there? Why don't we give patients specific steps to take and then follow up to make sure they achieve their goals, and offer problem solving when they fall short? Is it physician laziness, lack of confidence, the fact that insurers would rather pay for procedures, or something else? Isn't it our responsibility regardless of the obstacles?

Skepticism—We *All* Need to Ask Questions

In my opinion the lack of appropriately directed skepticism among physicians is a serious problem. We think of ourselves as scientists, critically examining our work in a never-ending process and striving to better our care of patients. There is some truth in that belief but, in my experience, far, far less than there should be.

The most telling examples of this dysfunctional behavior in my training came in the month I spent working in a large and highly regarded neonatal intensive care unit. The two neonatologists who ran the unit were very intelligent physicians, skilled clinicians, and more than decent human beings. My experiences in that short month occasionally verged on the bizarre, largely because almost no one was willing to question what we were doing.

There were typically twenty to forty infant patients in this Neonatal Intensive Care Unit (NICU). The NICU environment was, like any intensive care unit, filled with machines, light, noise, and tense activity. I found the environment disorienting, partly because even just seeing our very, very small patients in the midst of such a buzzing mass of medical devices and expert caregivers was hard. It was further disorienting when the group of medical residents, staff physicians, nurses, and other therapists would make our rounds and move from patient to patient, discussing each case in detail and quite often talking about "she" when, restrained and naked, the patient was obviously a "he." Just as often, a female would be discussed as "he." This lack of respectful individual attention to gender was emblematic of an extensive, deeply rooted pattern of unthinking, uncritical behavior pervading the otherwise skillful, brilliant, and caring medical staff.

One day the team of NICU residents on duty was called to attend the birth of twins (one male, one female) with a hereditary bleeding disorder. The birth went well, so our expertise was thankfully not needed. Three days later, however, we were called to the normal newborn nursery to care for the boy because he couldn't stop bleeding after the attending obstetrician had circumcised him. As you know, performing an elective surgery on a child with a bleeding disorder was obviously foolish. Tragically, the only means of stopping the bleeding was to give the boy a transfusion of the rare clotting factor genetically absent from his blood. To obtain one unit of this factor required pooling the blood of hundreds of donors. HIV was in the US blood supply but not as yet recognized. This transfusion almost certainly exposed this newborn infant to HIV and, given the lack of effective treatment at that time, quite possibly led to his death years later.

Many of these premature infants needed surgery for one reason or another. Often the surgery was major, such as fixing a damaged heart valve, for example. At that time it was common practice to avoid using anesthesia in the belief that these children didn't experience pain as we do and that the drugs used for anesthesia could be harmful to them. Although several years later the American Academy of Pediatrics issued a policy statement that such anesthesia was safe and encouraged its routine use, changing the norm and allowing premature infants the same pain control you and I would have received took decades.

Adult medicine is no different. For decades, the tradition was to tell patients with heart disease to rest as much as possible, fearing further injury to their vulnerable hearts. Now we put heart attack survivors on a treadmill ASAP. Physicians have always told women suffering from lymphedema, one of the most common adverse effects of breast cancer treatment, that they must avoid lifting heavy objects with the affected arm. New evidence tells us that such a recommendation is entirely wrong and that strength training actually greatly reduces the risk. There are many such examples of conventional medical wisdom being not just off but 180 degrees wrong.

My point is neither that we should never make mistakes, nor that mistakes are unforgivable. On the contrary, medical errors are inevitable. We must, however, learn from our mistakes. Because physicians are certain to make mistakes, we should always ask questions, challenging the status quo. Questions should be encouraged, not suppressed. If we don't accept questioning current medical practice as an ethical responsibility, we perpetuate our mistakes and, in our willful ignorance, needlessly harm our patients. We must recognize that we're ignorant and fallible;

consequently we should ask questions of our colleagues, our teachers, and even ourselves. Such questioning is our duty. Moreover, as you have the most "skin in the game," you should be asking questions for your own sake. We *should* ask questions. You *must*.

This isn't to say that skepticism should be directed only at conventional medical approaches. Just as we must fight the tendency of conventional medicine to avoid self-examination, we must understand that *unconventional approaches must be held accountable as well.* In a perfect world of unlimited research budgets, enthusiastically brilliant researchers, and willing subjects, we would examine every healing approach to fully understand the extent of its powers and limitations. As you know, the real world demands compromise. Risk-benefit considerations are the best method to begin sorting out wise compromises. We can wait to invest the huge sums of money, time, and effort required to evaluate the long-term health effects of good hydration—for example, simply choosing the "why not" approach. However, potentially toxic alternative treatments for life-threatening disease should be scientifically studied before we use them with patients.

Like I mentioned in the introduction, many years ago an elderly homeopathic MD told me that I was wasting my time working on homeopathic research, because "homeopathy is a spiritual science." It was and is clear to me that the effects of any treatment that can help people physically *must* be physically measurable. With all due respect, my colleague was wrong. Even if homeopathy or some other treatment was "spiritual," if the treatment can affect a living body, the impact must be measurable. Otherwise, we're just making up excuses to hide its ineffectiveness from ourselves.

As in conventional medicine, alternative therapies can become rigid, with practitioners unthinkingly hanging onto every word of authority figures. "X" must be so because the tradition says so. Wrong. This sort of attitude is extremely unhealthy. As a practicing physician or as a patient, each of us must take what he or she is taught and test it out. If we simply march ahead together in lockstep, following the lead of the past, we're likely to plunge over the same cliff, one after the other. Course corrections are part of life, including the life of a healthy profession.

Conventional medical practitioners and alternative healers are usually very good at criticizing each other's methods. *We're less vigorous, however, in our self-criticism.* We must be strong enough and wise enough to second-guess ourselves. We need to value the perspective of "outsiders," as they are the best at seeing our blind spots. However, the "insiders" know their own terrain the best, and so, if we're honest with ourselves, we should be able to identify innumerable weaknesses in our methods and figure out ways to improve those methods.

The third side to this dynamic is the most interesting one. It has also been relatively invisible. When David Eisenberg's surveys of alternative medical usage in the United States exposed the popularity of other approaches to health care, most observers overlooked what was to me the most fascinating finding. That was that one-third of those surveyed, those believing they had a "significant health problem," *didn't see either a conventional physician or alternative health-care provider.* While access and cost must have partially explained this pattern, unfortunately it is likely that this one-third lacked respect for both conventional medicine and alternative therapies. Health-care professionals of all allegiances should remember that none of us "own" this debate. We don't own the health of our patients. Patients and healers must remember that healers work for the patients, not the other way around. Certainly patients come to see us because of our expertise, and we shouldn't shirk our ethical responsibility by prescribing a dangerous treatment just because a patient requests that treatment. At the same time, cultivating humility about our limited knowledge and our roles as helpers rather than dictators will be healthy for us all.

As local health experts, it is the responsibility of all physicians to think deeply and carefully about health. No other group of individuals is so well trained to identify the weaknesses in our health care. No other group is so capable of balancing the hysteria too often generated by underinformed media articles and the self-serving marketing apparatus of the pharmaceutical industry. While you should take responsibility for your own health-care decisions, we physicians must do a better job fulfilling our responsibility to you, pushing past our own biases and limited understanding.

Simplicity

We live in a time of rapid change. The word *revolution* seems dramatic, but might be an understatement, because there are revolutions every way you turn. Technology, information, global politics, and our environment are all in the greatest flux humans have ever experienced. The bright flashing lights of change are fun and exciting, but we're at risk of losing our way in the tumult.

When we consider only medical technology, the changes in recent years are simply astonishing. Many of the tools we use in surgery have changed significantly in the last twenty years or didn't even exist two decades ago. Genetically engineered drugs are common. Medical nanotechnology is rapidly advancing. I totally love the fact that I can carry dozens of medical books worth of information around in my pocket. Better still, I can search through all of them to find what I need in just seconds. If the answers aren't there, I can dive into the unfathomable depths of the Internet from that same device almost wherever I am. It would be difficult to find any sane person who really wants to turn back the clock.

At the same time, we haven't changed. Our surroundings, daily activities, eating habits, and expectations have changed dramatically, but our bodies are still version 1.0 or perhaps 1.1. The circumstances in which human beings developed over millennia are gone or nearly so. Our lives have changed rapidly in ways that don't suit our bodies so well. Again, very few of us would honestly want to live as our ancestors did. At the same time, to be healthy we should consider how our place in the world has changed and how to best adjust to these changes.

We are who and what we are. We have to live our lives within certain constraints to be healthy and feel well. Humans are athletic-endurance animals needing a variety of fresh nutritious foods, lots of physical activity, water, sleep, and sunlight. Our brainpower may be our most unique characteristic. We should use our intelligence to avoid things that harm us and to make life better for us all, learning from our missteps. We're communal creatures, so we have to work out how to get along and enjoy each other. Our diets have always been diverse and change with the seasonal availability of foods. Although we have long worked to change our living conditions to our advantage, adapting to our environment is mostly what we have had to do and is still demanded of us.

Basic human needs haven't changed. Ignoring those basics inevitably keeps us from achieving optimal health, and, worse still, just as inevitably it eventually makes us seriously ill. In most people's minds, basic is boring. In a world where things are changing so rapidly in such exciting ways, too often we undervalue the old and familiar. We can delude ourselves when we think we can pick and choose among the health basics because some new drug or supplement will rid us of any health problem. *It simply isn't so.*

After many long years of studying the powerful interventions of conventional medicine and learning how to best use them to help my patients, I didn't expect the lessons that were to come. Clinical practice taught me the power of simple things, such as drinking more fluids, allowing enough time for sleep, eating better, cultivating healthier relationships, and establishing a good exercise routine. These have cured more of my patients than any prescription or alternative medicine. Quite often patients come in suffering from some problem or other that conventional medicine hasn't relieved, only to be cured after I persuade them to attend to one or more of these basics. It's easy to get fancy and complicated. *It is impossible to be really, truly well if you don't take care of the fundamentals.* If you want to feel your best, you have to do your best.

The biggest and most common mistake patients and their physicians make is to take a pill when a simple life-enhancing behavioral change is what is needed. For example, I have treated hundreds of women for osteoporosis; other physicians didn't address these patients' poor calcium intake, low vitamin D, and lack of bone-building exercise. They did prescribe medication that was likely to cause adverse effects, some severe.

This next point is colossal, maybe even the sum of this entire book.

While the strength of prescription medication makes adverse effects nearly inevitable, *the "side effects" of basic interventions are usually beneficial.* Taking calcium not only helps bone density but also relieves insomnia for many people, reduces colon cancer risk, and helps muscles, blood vessels, and nerves function properly. Using a pill while neglecting a basic need is what foolish patients and bad doctors do.

What Is Your Health Worth?

Probably ever since our caveman ancestor across the valley found a better rock to use as a weapon, humans have coveted "stuff"—the newer and cooler, the better. I see patients who say they don't have the money to buy better food, purchase supplements, join a gym, or see some therapist I recommended; but they spend thousands of dollars on the latest HD flat-screen TV. Huh?

What is good health worth? Ask anyone who is wealthy and unhealthy. When we're very ill, health care can be incredibly expensive. Most figures show that 90 percent of lifetime health expenditures come in the last months of life. Investing modestly in the years before has a much greater impact in terms of feeling better and living healthier for a long time. *We know that people who do the right stuff health wise live longer and shorten the time they are incapacitated just before death.*

Fortunately most of the fundamentals cost very little. You can put on a pair of shorts and run around your neighborhood for free. If you want to spend more, you could invest in a good pair of running shoes. Eating a healthy, diverse diet with lots of vegetables is great. If your veggies are local and organic, you will probably pay more, but you are likely to get more nutrients from them and fewer harmful chemicals.

Another cost that bothers people is the time spent taking care of themselves. These days we rush around trying to pack each day with so much more than even our parents could have imagined, mostly just because we can. Traffic might slow down, but we can still use our phones to conduct business or make personal plans, jamming up our time. A car passenger (no drivers, please!) can use a smartphone to make airplane reservations, buy concert tickets, or text some thoughts that really could have waited. We expect our food to be instantaneous. We wonder why we can't relax, why we have indigestion, and why Americans get fatter and fatter. All day long we make compromises in the interest of speed, shortchanging our health and our happiness, if not our souls, in the process. What is that worth to you?

The bottom line is more about commitment than money. Monetary wealth increases your choices, but if you are determined to take care of yourself, willing to put out the effort to be as healthy, happy, and strong as possible, you can make it so. It is up to you.

Thoughts on Prevention—A Stitch in Time Saves Nine, or Not

Good health habits help you feel better right away. They are also the best long-term investment you can make for your future wellbeing. Everyone knows that it is easier and healthier to prevent a problem than it is to cure that same problem. Week after week evidence piles up that eating right, exercising, and taking care of the other elements of a healthy lifestyle discussed in this book lead to a long-term payoff. Mark Twain commented that a vice-free life might just seem longer because it is tedious. With all due respect to Dr. Twain, if you live your life well, it can be both longer *and* more pleasurable.

The positive effects of living well accumulate over time, so the longer you have led a healthy life, the longer you will continue to lead a healthy life. Changing your habits even a little now leads to big effects down the road. Sometimes bigger lifestyle changes are actually easier because bigger changes have more dramatic immediate effects; you feel better, and then you naturally want to keep it going.

It is never too late to start your own prevention strategy. Regardless of past failings, making positive changes at any time still helps. *These changes will help you feel better right away* and reduce the likelihood of serious health problems returning or being as bad as they might otherwise be. For example, there is good evidence that men with prostate cancer increase their chances of slowing their cancer and feeling better if they shift to a more plant-based diet, exercise regularly, and meditate.

In medicine we use the term "secondary prevention" when discussing measures to prevent the return of an old problem or the appearance of one for which a patient already has the risk factors. Often secondary prevention looks a lot like primary prevention—in other words, better late than never. Exercise reduces the risk of a first heart attack and helps strengthen the heart, lowering the risk of a second or third. Smoking increases the risk of many illnesses. Stopping smoking allows the body to begin healing the damage and reduces the risk of those illnesses returning.

Screening procedures have been a big part of preventive medical practice for decades. These screening examinations have become more and more controversial over the years as we have examined them scientifically. It turns out that often the risks outweigh the benefits. Medical opinions favoring interventional screening such as x-rays and blood tests have often turned out to be wrong. Cancer screening is especially confusing at this point in time.

When I was a young athlete, I often saw public service announcements on television recommending exercise but cautioning that adults over thirty-five should first see a doctor for a checkup and a cardiac stress test. That announcement seemed reasonable, but it was misguided. Those commercials disappeared after a Stanford pathologist and runner did some simple math, calculating that the number of healthy young adults who would die from the seemingly rare complications of the testing process was more than the total number of adults who had undiscovered heart disease. In addition, the cost of the testing would ruin the American economy.

In the past many Americans got a chest x-ray every year to screen for lung cancer. Not any more. The risk of radiation outweighed the benefit. Simply asking patients whether they smoke and then helping smokers stop is more effective.

Prostate cancer is very common (the second leading cancer killer in the United States) and extremely variable. Most elderly men have prostate cancer, but not the sort that will kill them or even give them any symptoms. A huge recent study of Norwegian women found mammogram associated with a substantially increased (22 percent) risk of invasive breast cancer.[4] A few years earlier, a study of over one-quarter million Chinese women showed that breast self-examination didn't reduce deaths from breast cancer.[5] A study published in the *New England Journal of Medicine* found that 2 percent of healthy adults over age forty-five had primary brain tumors (cancer) and that over 7 percent had suffered strokes.[6] More information sometimes creates confusion.

In the past, finding a cancer meant we automatically treated it, unless it was so bad that treatment would be ineffective and it would only make the patient sicker. As our technology has improved, we have reached a point where our ability to find diseases, especially cancer, has overreached our knowledge about the behavior of these diseases. There is a very big gulf between finding a cancer and knowing what to do about it and when.

We now find ourselves in an increasingly uncomfortable position. Screening for any disease that kills people over years seems like it might be a pretty good idea. If we believe that we can do something to treat that disease early, keeping those people alive and improving their health, screening seems even more obviously attractive. On the other hand, when careful scientific studies show that our assumptions may be entirely wrong, we have to rethink our obvious conclusions. Even more challenging is the realization that if an obvious conclusion is wrong, we

---

4   Zahl, Maehlen, and Welch, "The Natural History of Invasive Breast Cancers Detected by Screening Mammography," *Arch Intern Med* 168 (2008): 2311- 6. doi: 10.1001/archinte.168.21.2311.

5   Thomas et al., "Randomized Trial of Breast Self-examination in Shanghai: Final Results," *J Natl Cancer Inst* 94 (2002): 1445-57.

6   Vernooij et al., "Incidental Findings on Brain MRI in the General Population," *N Eng J Med* 357 (2007): 1821-8. DOI: 10.1056/NEJMoa070972.

have a fundamental misunderstanding about human health. It is quite unsettling to discover that we were ignorant at such a basic level on such important matters. (See Gilbert Welch's book *Should I Be Tested for Cancer?: Maybe Not and Here's Why* for further discussion).

Medicinal versus Lifestyle Prevention

Americans are increasingly overweight, inactive, stressed, and suffering the consequences. Some physicians believe the solution is to take a "polypill," including three blood pressure medications, aspirin, folic acid, and a cholesterol-lowering statin medication, to make us all healthier. Many people, including other physicians, believe this sort of approach is entirely wrongheaded for a host of reasons. Among those reasons are cost, adverse effects, and the problem of effectively telling everyone over age fifty-five that they are diseased.[7]

A Dutch researcher decided to calculate the effect of eating more almonds, garlic, and other research-proven heart-healthy foods (dark chocolate, the recommended amount of fruits and vegetables, fish). It turns out that men aged fifty and older would add six years to their life expectancy, and women of the same age would add five years.[8] This "polymeal" had a greater effect than expected from the "polypill." The "side effects" of this nonmedicinal lifestyle intervention would be a tastier diet and a clear message to the fast-food industry.

Other simple preventive activities are also underappreciated. Accidents cause more damage to the health of Americans under age forty than any other factor. Paying sufficient attention to child safety in the home and adult driving safety (using seat belts, not using a cell phone, not drinking alcohol) has a dramatic impact. Eating breakfast is strongly associated with improved health. Avoiding tobacco and being cautious about the use of alcohol and other mind-altering drugs and medications have obvious benefits.

Clearly, leading a healthy lifestyle is a good idea. The evidence is that *people with good health habits live longer and happier lives.* Leading a healthy life is wise. It is less clear which medical screening procedures

---

7   Wald and Law, "A Strategy to Reduce Cardiovascular Disease by More than 80%." *BMJ* 326 (2003):1419-24. doi: 10.1136/bmj.326.7404.1419.

8   Franco, et al., "The Polymeal: A More Natural, Safer and Probably Tastier (than the polypill)" *BMJ* 329 (2004): 1447-50. doi: 10.1136/bmj.329.7480.1447.

or preventive interventions are useful. We will discuss much more about the specifics—the good, the bad, and the dubious—later on.

Being Perfect Isn't

It is fantastic to create a plan for a healthy life and stick to it. However, don't go crazy with it. It isn't healthy to be inflexible, to never bend the rules just a little. There are times when you really should take a day off from exercising, stay out late with friends, or taste that special (but maybe not so healthy) dish your mom made just for you. A balanced life is a healthy life, especially when it wobbles just a bit.

The truth is that we don't know everything we think we do. Our knowledge is imperfect, and we have so very much to learn about individual differences. Consequently, a little bit of deviation might even be good for you. Even if we did know precisely what your individual ideal should be, one strong characteristic of human physiology and psychology is that some variation is a healthy necessity.

Summary

- How likely is it to help?
- What are the risks if you try it?
- You need to think critically—it's your health.
- Keep it simple.
- Improving your health is doable and well worth the effort.
- Going faster won't get you to a good place.
- Errors are inevitable, so being perfect isn't.
- *Change is possible, and it feels good.*

Part 2
The Ten Essential Health Habits

Chapter 4

An Introduction to the Ten Essential Health Habits

Several habits are fundamental to good health. Each has its own benefits. Skip any of them, and you will suffer the consequences. Ignoring the fundamentals won't kill you today, but years down the road your poor choices will come home to roost. Forget those long-term benefits and nagging do-it-because-it-is-good-for-you reminders. Don't do the right thing just because I say you should. *Do it to help yourself feel better.* If you make poor choices right now, today, you will certainly not feel as well as you would if you did the right things. That is hard to argue against.

Admittedly, no matter how hard you and your health-care providers work, you will eventually die. Most likely you will get sick sometime before reaching whatever end awaits you. We know now that if you follow these habits, you will live longer and spend less time in poor health before your final end. While we cannot choose to live forever, we can choose to live as healthily and happily as possible. Our lifestyle choices largely determine the diseases we suffer and, maybe more importantly, how much we can enjoy each day to the fullest. The impact of prevention is obvious. If you follow good health habits, you will keep a long list of diseases from becoming part of your health history. Prevention does work. You will also feel better and enjoy your life more. What's not to like about that?

Healthy Habits Make You Biologically Younger

On the topic of longevity, I should say just a little bit more. Like so many others, I've noticed that people who are dedicated to living well often look much younger than their age. In recent years, we have learned that youthful appearance of these health enthusiasts is a biological reality. The essential health habits make you younger. These habits change your genes. They turn off genes that make you sick and shorten your life, while turning on the good genes. These essential health habits also lengthen your telomeres, the caps on the end of your genes that determine how many more times your genes can be copied, in other words, how much longer you can live. Telomeres are so important that the 2009 Nobel Prize in Physiology or Medicine was awarded to scientists who figured out how they protect our cells. (See Chapter 8 to learn about testing telomeres.)

More Powerful than Pills

I want you to understand that taking care of fundamentals is way more powerful than you probably think. As an advocate for "natural healing" and excellent health habits, I took longer than I want to admit to grasp this truth. These essential health habits not only prevent serious diseases, *they also treat diseases*, often more effectively than prescription drugs. It is very common for me to see patients suffering from a long list of medical conditions, all of which they can cure themselves, without medical help of any sort. All they need to do is to start making better health choices.

For example, recently a middle-aged man with elevated cholesterol, high blood pressure, borderline diabetes, an early cataract, and obesity came to see me. His cataract was largely a consequence of his uncontrolled blood sugar. He was on medication for elevated cholesterol and high blood pressure, but neither was horribly elevated. His diet wasn't so good. He didn't exercise regularly. He felt stressed and complained that he didn't have the energy he used to have. His mood was down, as he felt hopeless. He felt bad, and his health was getting worse and worse.

After treating hundreds of patients with problems like his, I confidently told him that if he established a regular exercise program and improved his diet, he would no longer need cholesterol or blood pressure medications. His blood sugar problems would go away. As he improved his body composition, building muscle and reducing body fat, his metabolic rate would increase, lowering his weight and making his body more sensitive to its own insulin. His energy level and physical strength would also increase, while he could expect improvement in his emotional outlook and mental sharpness. He had been in a vicious cycle of weight gain and physical inactivity, leading to insulin resistance, elevated cholesterol, and high blood pressure. He could *reverse the vicious cycle*, transforming it into a healing cycle by changing how he lived. By that effort he could then cure his diabetes, elevated cholesterol, hypertension, and obesity. Despite his lengthy and potentially disheartening list of serious medical diagnoses, he had the ability to cure them all. And he did.

I'm not making this up. Not only does a mountain of medical research prove it, but I have seen it again and again in my practice. Like so many others, this gentleman could choose to take prescription drugs that would entail significant risks of adverse effects, or he could change his health habits. He could invest in actions leading him to a healthier life, or he could fork over serious dollars for pills that just might poison him. Either way, the numbers on his laboratory tests would look better. The most common side effects of medications needed for this patient's problems include fatigue, dizziness, digestive problems, sexual dysfunction, rashes, liver damage, and muscle damage. In the interest of full disclosure, I must mention that study after study shows that achieving good numbers by taking medication isn't as good as achieving the identical numbers by living healthily. The most common side effects of changing his bad health habits include having more energy and feeling better.

The Choice Is Yours

Which would you choose? You are already making choices. Which are you choosing right now every day? I encourage you to recognize that you are making choices and to make the best ones you can—not only so you live longer but because you will feel better, often nearly right away, if you make better choices.

Procrastination—putting off those positive changes and delaying for the dawn of some easier day—comes with a price tag and makes it harder to achieve your goals. It isn't impossible, but it is much more difficult, to get an exercise program going when you are seventy years old and one hundred pounds overweight, with two knee replacements, than it is when you are thirty and carrying only an extra thirty pounds. If you've already had a heart attack, making changes *will* make you stronger and lengthen your life, but you cannot erase the scar on your heart. If you are disease-free but not feeling well, your body is sending you warning signals that sickness is coming your way. Fix the problems to feel better and prevent disease. Don't wait. Do it now!

You don't need a doctor to improve your health habits and your life. It is painful to admit it, but honestly, we docs don't do a good job helping with that. Medical education teaches us what to tell patients but precious little about how to help them implement our recommendations. One without the other is useless. Physicians really need to learn how to better help you make the healthy changes you need. In fairness to you, if your physician can't help, you need to find such practical assistance somewhere else.

I'm grateful that I do have the practical knowledge needed to guide my patients through the most effective ways to make changes. I gathered those insights mostly from other patients and my own life. I learned more about getting patients to change from my training for a national-level soccer coach's license than I did from my medical training. My most effective work with patients, the work that has the greatest impact on their health and longevity, is more as a coach or cheerleader than as a pill pusher.

The reason something is *fundamental* is that it is *essential*. Often fundamentals seem boring and not so important, especially when they are obvious. Believing that fundamentals have only a weak influence on health is seriously wrong thinking. Fundamentals are irreplaceable. Fundamentals are just like the solid foundation of a house. I don't care how big or nice your upstairs bedroom is if the foundation is poor. All your pretty things are going to come crashing down with the first stiff breeze. Fundamentals are far more important, with much more impact on your health, than the latest and greatest prescription drug.

Chapter 5

Essential Health Habit #1: Drink Enough Water

Like big salty water balloons, our bodies are comprised mostly of water. While ancient life lived in the salty sea, we carry our ocean around inside us. Some believe water is an essential ingredient for all life, at least on this planet. Others go so far as to say that "water *is* life." No one doubts that life without water can't last very long and that we feel very badly when we desperately need it. Many though are blind to the obvious truth that between death and well-being, there is a range where too little water makes people feel unwell. Their thinking runs, "Unless I'm thirsty, I'm totally fine." It turns out that thirst isn't a trivial reminder. It is a warning that a crisis is imminent.

The number of studies published on the quantity of water humans consume and the effects on our health is an amazingly small figure. Then again, maybe the absence of research on something so important isn't really surprising. Although each of us needs a steady supply of clean water to survive and be healthy, why would anyone waste any money to learn more about such a fundamental and nearly free health habit? There is no significant financial incentive, and there are no obvious ill effects of minor errors in our water consumption. That doesn't mean we know otherwise. We really don't know that much, scientifically anyway.

It is widely assumed that drinking enough clean water is just a matter of getting a drink from the water tap when you feel thirsty. Assumptions, however, can be foolish, especially when "everybody knows that."

The published research isn't much help at all if we want to consideration the possible consequences of drinking too little or too much water. In 2008, a study was published reviewing medical research on the general health effects of water consumption.[5] The authors looked for

---

5   Negoianu and Goldfarb, "Just Add Water," *J Am Soc Nephrol* 19 (2008):1041-

evidence that drinking a certain amount of water would treat or prevent problems which they assumed might be influenced by how much water people drank.

Their review found that there was very little published data on this topic. Unfortunately, particularly in interviews, the authors overstated the meaning of their nonfindings, suggesting that lack of evidence meant there was no effect. No evidence means, well, that there isn't any evidence. Nothing more. Nothing less. Like nineteenth-century doctors who "knew" exercise was harmful or twentieth-century physicians who recommended mentholated cigarettes to asthma patients; their conclusions betrayed their bias. They were uninfluenced by mere facts, or more precisely, the absence of facts.

Ignorance isn't the same thing as being right. It just means we don't know. The media magnified the author's careless statements, presenting this review as definitive proof that drinking more water was useless.

This sort of simplistic rush to judgment is bad science and contrary to both common sense and a significant amount of data in the sports medicine literature. If we can die from lack of water, there must be a gray zone, short of lethality, where our health or functioning is compromised. There must also be levels that are relatively healthy or healthier. We can't possibly move from the edge of death to perfect wellness with just one sip, can we?

We do have evidence about the effects of hydration on healthy individuals from sports medicine. While I will discuss fluid needs for athletes in greater depth later in this book, a few simple points here will illuminate the discussion.

The first bit of evidence is that athletic performance declines once an individual loses 1 to 2 percent of his or her body weight due to dehydration. If you weigh one hundred pounds, that means one to two pounds lost; and since one quart of water weighs two pounds, you can easily translate pounds lost to how far down your fluid level is. That's not quite like your car's oil dipstick, but close. If you weigh two hundred pounds and want to figure out your percent depletion, just double the number. If you pass 3 percent, you are at risk of serious problems such as heat exhaustion or heat stroke.

Second, *we don't usually get thirsty until we're 2 percent or more dehydrated.* So we know that our physical abilities are usually compromised

---

3. doi: 10.1681/ASN.2008030274.

before we become thirsty. If you are thirsty, you have a considerable fluid deficit to overcome (one quart for a one-hundred-pound individual), and your body is warning you that you are endangering your health.

Your need for fluids varies a lot based on environmental conditions (temperature, humidity), your activity level, and your health. You get a certain amount of fluid in your diet, but you need to drink water as well. How much?

The guideline of eight glasses a day has been floating around for decades. While that goal maybe useful for some, we can refine and individualize the target. It is more than enough for some people sometimes, way too little for the same people at other times, and just about always not enough for others. We know that athletes competing in warm weather often lose more than a gallon of fluid in just one hour. Eight glasses of water is way not enough for them (and also unsafe since plain water lacks the salty electrolytes lost in sweat).

Studies show that each person has his or her own visual water gauge that is quite accurate but usually ignored. Your kidneys produce urine by filtering your blood. If our kidneys become clogged or stop working for some reason, we die. Research on athletic performance and heat illness shows that *the color of urine is a very good gauge of hydration.* Excepting an hour or so after taking a vitamin pill, your urine should be very close to clear when it is mixed into the water of your toilet. So get used to taking a look before you flush away the evidence.

Studies are great, but real-world, clinical experience has really impressed me with the importance of hydration for well-being as well as disease prevention. In truth, many patients come to see me with one problem or another that is solved simply by drinking more water. Chronic cough, fatigue, dry eyes, and headaches are quite often merely symptoms of dehydration.

The first case that really convinced me of the unrecognized consequences of chronic dehydration was a vigorously healthy man in his thirties who had a difficult heart problem. Although he was very active physically, emotionally balanced, and remarkably successful financially, he had developed a persistent heart irregularity. He had undergone extensive testing to confirm that he didn't have any underlying health conditions leading to the irregularity. The best cardiologists at the University of California, San Francisco, also did a very thorough cardiac workup for him. The cardiologists had tried medication after medication and were then suggesting an experimental drug. He was wary, so he decided to see what I could do.

The heart muscle contracts partly in response to getting filled by blood. If it is incompletely filled, it contracts weakly, and the rhythm can be disturbed. In addition to a few other recommendations, I gave him hydration goals.

When he returned four weeks later, the eighteen months of heart irregularity had ended. By self-experimentation, he had learned that the key was that if he fell below a certain amount of daily fluid intake, the irregularities would return. As long as he drank enough water, he had no problem. He didn't need any medication or, for that matter, any supplement either.

Inevitably, there are special circumstances. People with heart failure or kidney failure need to be careful about drinking too much. Also, athletes participating in endurance events stress their bodies so severely that their kidneys slow down, forcing them to walk (or run?) a narrow line between too much and too little fluid.

Remember, water is life.

Summary

- We're mostly water.
- Chronic dehydration is the norm.
- Dehydration makes you unwell before it kills you.
- Checking urine color (it should be clear) is the best way to confirm whether you are drinking enough.

Chapter 6
Essential Health Habit #2:
Exercise Almost Every Day

It has been pummeled into your head that exercise is good for you. Despite that onslaught, exercise is still probably more important to your health than you know. It lowers the risk of nearly every disease human bodies and minds suffer. Exercise doesn't just prevent disease; it is also an effective treatment of many of those diseases. Exercise also treats just about every infirmity Father Time inflicts on us. It turns back the clock more than anything else you can do. Not exercising and perfecting your couch-potato training regimen are as devastating to your body as smoking two packs of cigarettes a day or developing diabetes. Even athletes who sit around all day after their hard workouts put themselves at risk. If someone could discover a way to put the benefits of exercise in a pill and sell that miraculous medication, that person would certainly collect the Nobel Prize and more money than he or she could ever dream of. Why is exercise so magical? The answer is as simple as exercise is powerful.

- You are an athlete.
- The essential elements of a good exercise program
- Exercise principles
- Building an exercise program
- Good gadgets for exercise
- Summary

You Are an Athlete

In fact, you are a member of the greatest team of land-endurance animals the world has ever seen. Seriously.

Have you ever heard the phrases "running to ground" or "I'll run that down for you"? They grew out of one of humankind's most unique abilities. We humans have a greater capacity for running than any other land animal. That is how our ancestors got their meat, and some rare tribal peoples still do so today. Their strategy was to find and pursue a large animal all day, staying close enough to keep it in sight. By the end of the day, the animal could run no longer. They would then skewer it with a spear. Those animals are faster than we are in a sprint, but they can't keep going all day like we can. Humans are special.

So, when I tell you that the official recommendation that you need to exercise for one and a half hours a day is unrealistic, I mean that one and a half hours are way less than what our bodies and brains are designed for. Truthfully, to be fully healthy, we need to be very active, almost certainly more so than we are now.

Some believe humans developed as we did (upright posture, ability to cool ourselves in hot weather by sweating and mouth breathing, big ligament to hold our heads upright, big buttock muscles) because of running. Others take the idea still further, proposing that our exceptional endurance abilities led to the development of our exceptional brains. This view, in essence, credits our physical endurance as the key factor transforming us from simple primates into human beings. (For more discussion, also see the 2004 article in *Nature* by Bramble and Lieberman).[6] Even if these surprisingly well-reasoned theories are disproved, the effects of exercise on our brains and thought processes are powerful and now incontestable.

Until quite recently, neuroscientists believed our brains stopped developing around age twenty. It was all downhill from there. Sure, we knew it was possible to learn a few new things (despite what teenagers think of old folks), but we thought that every day we lost more and more brain cells. That concept took a while to die (perhaps proving those old brain cells are especially long lived?). It turns out that we can make new brain cells throughout our lives. Interestingly, physical activity more powerfully stimulates the growth of new brain cells than anything else we know of. Exercise not only makes children, with their rapidly growing intellects, smarter but also helps the rest of us.[7]

---

6   Bramble and Lieberman, "Endurance Running and the Evolution of Homo" *Nature* 432 (2004): 345–352. doi:10.1038/nature03052.

7   "The Association Between School-Based Physical Activity, Including Physical Education, and Academic Performance" CDC website http://www.cdc.gov/healthyyouth/health_and_academics/pdf/pa-pe_paper.pdf

Our brainpower is more than the sum of how many brain cells we have. It is determined more by the links between the brain cells. In a process very much akin to a chemical spark leaping from cell to cell across a gap, a brain cell sends a message, a thought, and another cell receives it. The cellular physiology of learning is all about making connections between cells and reinforcing those connections. Of course, you have to have brain cells, but nothing happens without the spark of thought that connects them. When you learn anything—a language, a dance move, the appearance of your friend's face—those chemicals jump across the void, establishing the connection. Then when you repeat the thought, the link gets stronger and faster. It becomes a more deeply ingrained part of you incorporated into your mental data bank, into your memories. You also get better at that specific process of thought.

Exercise stimulates the birth of new brain cells, but they will die unless you use them by learning something. The new mental muscles must be used, or they will wither away. Both sides of the process are essential. These elements combine to make us smarter—and smarter in a very practical way.

The back and forth between sprouting new brain cells with activity and integrating those cells into our brain activity by learning something new neatly matches the life pattern of our hunter-gatherer ancestors, who had to learn "on the fly." As they covered great distances to find food, either they learned what worked and what didn't, or they starved to death. This adaptation, reinforced by life or death, the most pragmatic outcome of all, gave a powerful advantage to those who were not only fast but also learning the most during their travels.

Anyone who exercises with any regularity soon discovers the problem-solving insight physical activity grants us. We find that as our thoughts wander during exercise, obvious solutions to previously challenging problems just seem to pop into our minds. Is this from some new brain cell or synapse sparking unexpectedly? Is it a consequence of achieving a different perspective from stepping away from the problem and seeing it in a new light? If so, maybe that "new perspective" reflects a change in brain functioning at that moment. Whatever the explanation, the experience is a common one and an underappreciated benefit of exercise.

So, our brains are brilliant, and exercise makes our brains work even better. Ironically, our brains really excel at devising ways to be more efficient, to not work so hard, or they simply enable us to be as lazy as can be. Exercise makes our brains smart enough to figure out how best to avoid exercise. The wonderful labor-saving achievements of our brains have transformed daily human life so extremely that we must now invent ways to get the exercise we got simply by finding our food. This perversion of human life is a very recent phenomenon. The average daily physical activity of human beings has dropped rapidly, even in the last 50 to 150 years.

Many medical organizations recommend that we target ten thousand steps a day as the minimally essential level of physical activity. The average American presently covers three thousand steps a day. Investigators affiliated with the American College of Sports Medicine decided to see how much activity individuals leading a less technologically supported life engaged in. Studying Old Order Amish in the United States, they found that Old Order Amish housewives averaged sixteen thousand steps and that their husbands averaged much more. Those sixteen thousand steps equate to roughly eight miles! One man averaged fifty thousand steps a day, mostly because he was plowing his farm fields and walking behind his horse during the study interval.

You should understand that healthy physical activity isn't only a matter of whether you exercise. Huh? Well, we now know that even if you work out intensely almost every day, sitting still the rest of the time still hurts you. We're starting to call people who maintain a concerted exercise program but then sit all day at work or in front of a video screen "sedentary athletes." Our bodies don't like to be still for too long. You might have heard that long airplane flights put travelers at risk of blood clots. That's because even our blood needs to constantly move, or it gets thick and dangerously sluggish. If you sit for even just one hour, your heart output drops by 50 percent! It doesn't take a lot of exercise to fix this problem. Some dedicated folks get a standing desk or even a treadmill desk. That is good but probably more than you really need to do. The science is still in its infancy, but so far it appears that simply getting up and moving around for five minutes out of every hour will counteract the stagnating effects of immobility.

On the other hand, some of us lead unusually active work (for example, carpenters and professional athletes) or personal (those living "off the grid") lives. I find that even those active individuals usually miss one or another important element of a good exercise program. The rest of us are, of course, basket cases by comparison. We all need to put some conscious effort into designing a healthy exercise program and creating the exercise habit.

The Essential Elements of a Good Exercise Program
- Aerobic activity plus HIIT
- Strength training
- Stretching
- Balance

Aerobic Activity plus HIIT

Air Force surgeon Kenneth Cooper coined the word aerobics ("with oxygen") and made aerobic physical activity popular with his 1968 book of the same name. Like so many others, he set my feet on the road to good health. The term aerobics describes physical activity that requires moderately increased oxygen consumption and subsequently strengthens the heart and lungs. The exertion intensity of an aerobic activity is sustainable for long periods of time, because the body can obtain enough oxygen through breathing to go on and on. We call other more strenuous physical activities like sprinting "anaerobic," because the effort they require cannot be sustained and leads the athlete to build up an "oxygen debt." That debt soon forces the athlete to slow down or even stop.

As is usually the case, such a simple description isn't entirely accurate. Athletes engaging in aerobic activities can exert themselves beyond their oxygen-utilizing capacity; and, in fact, most competitors in aerobic sports build up significant oxygen debts. Also, recent studies show that high-intensity interval training (HIIT), though anaerobic, is an extremely efficient means of building aerobic capacity.

Because this is a recent discovery, we have a great deal to learn about HIIT. The core principle of HIIT is to go almost as hard as you can for a short interval, go easy, and then go hard again. We aren't clear yet on how short these intervals can be, although recent evidence (and my experience with patients) shows that even five cycles of thirty seconds hard and thirty seconds easy lead to significant fitness improvements. So far, we know that HIIT should be performed no more than two or three times a week. A routine of more than that seems to backfire.

These discoveries are largely the consequence of the enthusiasm Dr. Cooper inspired. His advocacy of aerobics inspired the most important exercise-related public health movement in modern America. Dr. Cooper's work triggered the running boom of the 1970s, fathered the modern fitness movement, and released a flood of exercise books that followed his Aerobics. Directly or indirectly, his work has impacted just about anyone who exercises today.

We all need aerobic activity, and it is the base of the athletic activity pyramid. You should participate in some sort of aerobic activity almost every day. Examples of aerobic activity include brisk walking, running, cycling, swimming, using elliptical machines, cross-country skiing, soccer, basketball, and tennis. Any physical activity that gets you breathing heavily and which you can sustain for a while is aerobic.

Patients frequently ask me what the best form of aerobic exercise is. My answer is always, "Whatever you will do." You don't get any extra benefit doing something you don't like doing. Also, if you enjoy an activity, you are more likely to do it. That's what really counts. Find some exercise you like.

Strength Training

When I was running marathons in the 1970s, many of my friends were exceptional endurance runners; some were among the very best in the world. They could run fast and, to those of us less gifted, seemingly forever. Their legs were as strong as their hearts and their wills. However, many of them would have struggled to carry a bag of groceries home from the store. Something was missing.

Another clue in my intellectual puzzling about physical activity appeared when I spent a month simultaneously studying for my first vitally important national medical exam and training for my first marathon. During that time, I didn't have any soccer games. At the end of that month, I played a little soccer with some friends and was very surprised when, after just a half hour, my endurance-trained legs cramped up. How could that possibly be? I was running for hours every day, but long and slow distances make different demands on our bodies than the mix of sprints and endurance soccer or similar sports require.

Although humans are remarkable endurance athletes, we sometimes need explosive muscle strength as well. For that matter, even endurance itself comes in different varieties. The big lesson is that there are many kinds of fitness.

Besides moving our bodies around, we use our bodies to move other things. Both activities demand work from our muscles. We have different types of muscle fibers, which help us with different kinds of tasks. While my endurance-athlete friends could run and run, most of them would have been useless helping me move furniture. None of them would have been welcome additions to my soccer team. Aerobic exercise trains the heart muscle, but we have to train our skeletal muscles as well. Of course, aerobic exercise also trains our skeletal muscles to a certain degree, and strength training can also strengthen our hearts, but these activities are fundamentally different and complement each other.

Strength training has suffered from a poor image for too long. Jack LaLanne, like Charles Atlas before him, did his best as a strength-training evangelist. But for whatever reason (I think it was the organ music and jumpsuit combo), strength training didn't catch on like aerobics did. As unappealing as it was to nonathletes, even most athletes at that time didn't incorporate strength training into their exercise regimens. The infamous extremes of Arnold Schwarzenegger and other bodybuilders put off many people and eclipsed much of the positive regard for strength training LaLanne created. Many people still have the feeling that strength training is for self-obsessed freaks.

The truth is that we all need to train our muscles, and those who stay the farthest away from gyms are the same people who must urgently need to be there. Fortunately, these days strength training is increasingly popular. Most gyms, though, are filled with healthy young adults, most often male. Healthy young adults do need strength training. However, unhealthy young adults and all older adults need it much more. Men certainly benefit from strength training, but women have much more to gain. Carefully supervised strength training should also be a significant component of fitness programs for children.

Studies show that you get a big payout for just about any effort. Even very modest strength training generates more weight loss than a program of moderate aerobic exercise. Strength training builds healthy bone and gives elderly individuals the strength they need to catch themselves, keeping a stumble from turning into a head injury or a broken hip, wrist, or shoulder. A well-designed strength-training regimen reduces the incidence of athletic injuries and improves sports performance, whether the sport is football, tennis, soccer, basketball, or (as my old friends didn't yet know) even distance running.

Adding to the pile of positive research on the specific health effects of strength training is a study of over eight thousand men between the ages of twenty and eighty.[8] It showed that strength training markedly lowered death rates. The weakest men had a death rate that was one and a half times greater than the strongest men. Their risk of dying from cancer increased one and one-quarter times. The biggest difference was in risk of death from cardiovascular disease, which was 1.6 times greater.

Flexibility

Just as general public opinion has been biased against strength training, it has been strongly biased in favor of flexibility. This belief is also uninformed and at least partly wrong. When I speak to the public about exercise, people get really upset when I challenge conventional misconceptions about stretching and flexibility—it's like I'm putting down motherhood, babies, or flowers. The audience just "knows" stretching is good. This combination of intensely held opinion and lack of understanding isn't at all good and must be corrected.

"Everyone knows" that we all should be more flexible. That just simply isn't true. Too much flexibility equals instability. Other tissues, especially muscles, tendons, and ligaments, hold your bones together. If those tissues, including muscle, become too weak—in other words, too loose (a.k.a. too flexible)—you will be more prone to injury. When joints are too loose, they bang around, injuring the tissues lining the joints. For example, I have many times seen middle-aged women develop back problems because the muscles supporting their spines have become too weak. With the best of intentions, these women, by working to increase the flexibility of their already unstable back, have aggravated their problem, leading to more pain and disability. We aren't only talking about the backs of middle-aged women. No matter what your age, your knees are probably the joints most vulnerable to injury if your leg muscles are too weak. Good muscle tone (in other words, inflexible tightness) protects your joints.

As our bodies adapt to a specific activity, the most-used muscles tighten up. People think this tightening is bad. It can be. Mostly, though, this tightness is helpful. When a muscle is very loose, a lot of energy and force

---

8   Ruiz, et al., "Association Between Muscular Strength and Mortality in Men: Prospective Cohort Study," BMJ 337 (2008): a439. doi: 10.1136/bmj.a439

are lost just by starting to contract those relaxed muscles. It's like trying to pound in a nail using a sponge instead of a hammer. Have you ever seen a cat preparing to pounce or watched sprinters race? The sprinters start in the blocks with their muscles tensed up, primed to explode into action. The cat is coiled, quivering with the just-barely restrained muscle explosion to come. When the muscles are already partially contracted, that muscle tension is stored energy, ready to be used. To prove this to yourself, try jumping as high as you can. First, jump up from a hard floor. Next, try jumping up from a pillow. The difference is clear.

Before you get upset, tense your muscles, jump up, and burn this book, let me say that being too stiff also isn't good. Being too tight is also inefficient and often leads to injuries.

You need to figure out whether you are too loose or too tight. How should you get loose enough? Things you might not think about, such as diet and drinking enough water, have a big impact on flexibility. Stretching also has a part to play. All of us need to stretch from time to time. Some of us are innately more flexible than others, who need to work hard to combat getting too tight.

Stretching Is Bad or Good

The obvious way to increase flexibility is by stretching. Not so fast. Not quite so simple. Stretching is bad for you. Wait! I just wrote that stretching is good for you. Huh? Does it seem like I can't make up my mind here? That's because stretching is complicated. There is stretching, and then there is stretching. There is also a good time to stretch and a bad time to stretch.

Many think that standing still while grabbing your ankles for thirty seconds or more is the only way to stretch. Some of you might have had a gym teacher who made you stretch by bending forward and bouncing up and down as you reached for your toes. Both of these activities are called "stretching," but they are quite different. Some of you might understand that these are only two of the many different forms of stretching and that they all have different effects.

If you just look at research, you will learn that most of it shows that stretching is harmful, since it increases injury rates and decreases strength. Unfortunately, nearly all those studies have been designed and conducted with too little understanding or thought. Researchers have generally failed to consider the type of stretch or the timing of the stretching.

Their carelessness has led most of them to conclusions that are exactly the opposite from what everybody knows. I think they are just as wrong for the same reasons.

Like almost everyone, I do believe that stretching is good for us. However, that is true only if you stretch in the right way at the correct time. The type of athletic activity an individual is engaged in is another important factor to consider and is relevant to stretching habits. A stretch that is good to do before a long, slow run isn't a good stretch to do before sprinting or strength training. A stretch that is good in the morning is great after strength training, but it's a bad idea before lifting weights.

The two most familiar and entirely different forms of stretching are static (i.e., not moving) and ballistic (i.e., explosive). A static stretch is the one you see runners do out in the park before they go on a long, slow run. Typically you bend a joint far enough that you just start to feel a pleasant stretch in the muscles on the lengthening side (for example, the backs of your legs if you are bending forward). You then hold that position for a number of seconds (usually somewhere around thirty) without moving much, if at all. If, instead of slowly going to that point and holding it, you bounced in and out of the stretch, you would be doing what is called a ballistic stretch of those same muscles.

We have learned that static stretches appear to make muscles weaker and mess up our ability to sense the position of our body parts (proprioception). Those effects last for about an hour. Making your body weaker right before you engage in a physical challenge has some obvious problems. Also, you can imagine that losing some of your capability to know where your foot is and tilting your ankle slightly as you run, especially across an uneven surface, could make you more likely to stumble. Certainly, these research findings could explain why studies have shown increased injury rates when static stretching is used before explosive athletic activities (for example, soccer or weight training). On the other hand, static stretching feels good and does improve flexibility.

In my opinion, static stretching in the morning and after explosive muscular activities is a good idea. I think your stretch then should be like that of those gorgeously flexible and athletic felines, shorter and more fluid than the stretching you see in the park on Saturdays. Prolonged static stretching is most useful for a stiff person who has trouble in some area caused by that lack of flexibility. I strongly advise against static stretching before weight training or sprinting.

If you have tightness in some area of your body, remember that tendons, the tissues attaching those tight muscles to bones, can get irritated from muscle tightness, but tendons don't stretch. So, in this circumstance, static stretching can be harmful or helpful—plus or minus coming from what tissue you stretch. Stretch so you feel the pleasant pulling sensation in the muscle, not near the joint (which won't tend to feel so good either). That's because tendons attach near the joints. Tugging there, on the unstretchable tendon, will only injure the tendon more.

It's time now for a brief side trip. Conventional medical wisdom has long held that tendonitis is the consequence of chronic inflammation in a tendon caused by a tight muscle pulling on it. The conclusion was that flexibility is good, muscle strength is bad, and loading up on anti-inflammatory drugs is the way to go. However, all those years of telling patients to just stretch more didn't help as had been expected. We were wrong in more than one way. It is now clear that we shouldn't call this problem tendonitis, since the primary problem isn't inflammation. As we think about the problem in a different way, we should drop the routine dash to anti-inflammatory medications. The damage to the involved tendon is of a different sort, and the term tendinosis is more accurate. It is best to think of the problem as a biological vulnerability (largely nutritional) manifesting as an injury. In my experience it is most effectively cured by fixing the systemic biological issues (most commonly deficiencies or excessive inflammation) combined with the right kind of exercises.

It turns out that strengthening muscles near the painful tendon can actually cure the tendinosis if performed correctly. Stranger still, the best kind of muscle strengthening (eccentric) is the kind thought to be most stressful to muscle tissue.

Muscles work when we move. When we shorten our muscles, like when we pick something up, that is called concentric strengthening. The work muscles have to do when we put something down (eccentric strengthening) is good for the tendons but harder for the muscles. That hard work is why so many misguided gym rats drop the weights. They would get more out of their workouts and avoid injury if they carefully put the weights down. The other gym customers would be happier too.

One of the first clinical studies of the eccentric training approach showed that 80 percent of patients with more than two years of chronic tennis elbow (one form of tendinosis) were cured after two weeks of eccentric strengthening of their forearm muscles. That study, along with many more studies since then and now years of collective sports medicine experience, adds up impressively and convincingly. Eccentric strengthening might be the single most important treatment component. Again, for each of us, flexibility and strengthening are both important, sometimes for reasons in defiance of common understanding.

Ballistic stretching doesn't lead to flexibility. Instead, ballistic stretching mostly tightens muscles. Every muscle in your body has at least one other muscle working against it. Otherwise if you scratched your ear, you'd never be able to bring your arm back down again. That's not so good. It is also obvious that when muscles tighten up to move your body one way, the muscles that move you the other way had better loosen up. Ballistic stretching has a deservedly bad reputation these days because it manages to tighten both sets of muscles involved in the ballistic stretch. Again, think back to the cat or the sprinter priming muscles for the pounce by slightly bouncing in preparation. Ballistic "stretching," then, performed properly, can be an excellent method of preparation for explosive physical activity, precisely because it doesn't make you more flexible.

There is a form of stretching, called "dynamic stretching," that looks similar to ballistic stretching. Dynamic stretching is another excellent way to prepare muscles for explosive activity. This is the kind of stretching one should use before strength training and other sudden forceful activities like sprinting. Dynamic stretching looks a lot like what most of us are familiar with as "warming up." All muscles work better after they are warmed and flooded with oxygen by getting the blood flowing through them. A dynamic stretch moves a muscle through its motion and progressively increasing speeds. An excellent image of dynamic stretching is a baseball player waiting his turn to bat in the "on deck circle." Holding one or more bats, he swings his arms around in a variety of motions, gradually speeding up and becoming more and more like how he will use his muscles when he steps up to the plate for his turn.

Speaking of warming up, one mistake associated with stretching is stretching aggressively before warming up. A little bit of a gentle stretch isn't going to hurt you if you haven't warmed up, but vigorously stretching cold, stiff muscles isn't a good idea. Another way to look at it is that stretching properly is part of a good warm-up.

Stretching is way more complicated than even this complicated summary. There are active and passive stretches involving purposefully tensing certain muscles by yourself or with a partner and all sorts of combinations and gradations of these elements. In my experience, understanding the basics of static and dynamic stretches, including how and when to apply them, will meet the needs of the great majority of us in almost all situations.

Balance Training

Balance is, hands down, the single most neglected aspect of fitness, even more neglected than strength training. That is surprising to me. No matter how overweight you are, you are taller than you are wide. Any movement requires balance. The more vigorous or complex the movement is, the more difficult balance is. Many sporting activities are contests to determine how good a person's balance is. Think of it. In some cases, such as skiing, balance is obvious. But in just about every sport, falling to the ground or out of the field of play means you lose.

As we age, losing our balance is a very serious health threat. Health-care data shows that after age sixty, four to five times as many Americans die from falling compared to dying in automobile accidents. On average every year, one out of every three elderly Americans suffers a serious fall.

Practicing balance is easy and can be fun. Little girls play hopscotch. Older folk dance. Driving through Golden Gate Park on Sunday mornings, I loved watching elderly Chinese Americans gracefully practicing tai chi movements. All you have to do to improve your balance is to leave the stability of the couch, get up off your backside, and move a little. Maybe stand on one leg while watching TV or working at your computer. You can make the movement tougher by using a BOSU ball or just an old pillow. Use a jump rope. Put on some music. Have fun!

Exercise Principles

Like any other healing modality, exercise can hurt or help. You don't want to do it wrong. There are three principles to keep in mind. It is surprising to me that just about every one of us, including professional athletes, either ignores or is unaware of at least one or two of these fundamentals.

These three principles are
- Overload
- Variability
- Recovery

Overload

Working harder than the requirements of your usual activity is how you get stronger. We call this practice "overload" in sports medicine. I don't like the term. Exceeding our usual capacity is uncomfortable, so it sounds off putting for that reason alone. But my dislike isn't just because so many of us hate pushing ourselves physically and because it reminds us of that aversion. I really don't like the term overload because it implies going so far that you will hurt yourself; being almost like that is the goal. No, you shouldn't hurt yourself. You don't have to, and you really don't want to. Getting injured sinks your exercise program faster than anything else.

When I encourage patients to create an exercise program, I work very hard to get them to understand that they will get stronger faster by going slow. Too many patients embark on a new exercise regimen, determined to achieve what should be long-term goals practically overnight. That admirable but foolish determination leads to injuries. By the time that person recovers from the injury, he or she is in worse condition than the person was before he or she dived into the new exercise program.

You must work a bit harder to get stronger, but putting that simple idea into practice calls for some thought and self-awareness. When you consider how hard you are working, using a scale of relative effort can help keep you from going overboard. In sports medicine research, a scale called Rating of Perceived Exertion (RPE) is often used as a measurement. You can use it to adjust your workouts. Don't worry about how formal or scientific it sounds. It is actually quite simple. This scale is simply an objectification of your sense of effort and quite useful each day you exercise (see also the CDC's "Perceived Exertion"[9]).

During aerobic activities such as running, cycling, basketball, soccer, tennis, and swimming, "physical effort" is closely connected to how hard your heart and lungs are working. Measurements of your ability

---

9   "Perceived Exertion (Borg Rating of Perceived Exertion Scale), " CDC Website, http://www.cdc.gov/physicalactivity/everyone/measuring/exertion.html

to breathe or your heart rate are then a precise and useful gauge of how hard you are exerting yourself.

The "talk test" is a simple way to objectively confirm whether you are working hard enough to become short of breath. Being short of breath means you are stressing your cardiovascular system enough to create a training effect. The target is to be able to speak during exercising while still feeling that you are breathing harder than you did before you began to exercise.

The point where speaking becomes difficult is the threshold where your body is working so hard that the effort cannot be sustained for a long time. Another way to target this range is to exercise at an intensity level where you can talk but not sing. Athletes who want to spend a fraction of their training at a higher level can tell they have reached that intensity level when they have to chop up their sentences.

When you cannot talk at all, you are training at a high intensity. Although there are advantages to some training at this level, it is very challenging, not sustainable for an extended period, and increases the possibility of injury. To put it simply, this intensity is unsustainable, because you are using more oxygen than you can take in. Before too long, your tank will be empty, and you won't be able to continue. You will have to slow down or stop. (See the CDC website for more about measuring physical activity intensity.[10])

The most precise method of determining how much an exercise, any exercise, increases the work of your heart is to measure your heart rate. Taking your pulse while you are bounding along through the woods or lifting a barbell isn't realistic, so electronic heart rate monitors were developed. You can spend a great deal of money on all varieties of training technology, but even a very inexpensive heart rate monitor can be a uniquely useful exercise tool.

Somewhere in just about every gym you walk into is a chart showing how heart rate is linked to exercise intensity. Wall charts and exercise machines show training zones determined by combining your age and heart rate. Although those charts are not very accurate, they are somewhat useful. They overlook important individual differences, but the science on which they are based is sound. You can do much better if you devote a bit of effort to tracking your resting heart rate. Once you have established

10 "Measuring Physical Activity Intensity," CDC Website, http://www.cdc.gov/physicalactivity/everyone/measuring/index.html

even a rough estimate of your maximal heart rate, you can use that and your resting heart rate to very accurately determine your own heart rate ranges. You can then use them in your training. These individualized numbers, your numbers, transform the crude chart estimates into very accurate and reliable personalized information for you.

Considering a few factors will help you learn the information you need to optimize heart rate training for your use.

Determining your resting heart rate is quite simple. Measure your heart rate in the morning in bed, right when you wake up. If you are sick or training too hard, your resting heart rate will usually be higher than normal. You want to collect this information when you are well. When you get in the habit of checking your resting heart rate in the morning, you can use it to adjust your plans for the day, cutting back a bit if you are overtraining or starting to get sick. Very generally, unless you have heart disease, lowering your resting heart rate indicates that your heart and lungs are healthier than they were before. Comparing your resting heart rate to that of someone else won't tell you whether you are healthier than that person.

Illness, dehydration, and hot weather will change your maximal heart rate. Aging lowers maximal heart rate, and resting pulse also changes throughout our lives with fitness levels, age, and other factors. Just as we must adjust to our changing circumstances and capacities, we should adjust our ranges from time to time. Maximal heart rates for females are lower than for males. Measuring maximal heart rate is challenging, in part because you have to work as hard as you can to get there. Your cardiovascular system has a reserve of energy, so you cannot just warm up and then immediately sprint to reach your maximal heart rate. Most people will hit their maximal heart rate after running for ten minutes and sprinting as hard as they can during the last quarter mile or so. That isn't fun.

Trying to reach your absolute limit is risky. I don't recommend trying to push yourself that hard unless you are in excellent health and your physician tells you he or she thinks it is okay for you to test yourself in this way. Instead, after you grow accustomed to using a heart rate monitor, you can use the highest heart rate you achieve when you really worked hard on some day. You can also forget all this and use some of the various formulas scattered across the Internet. (For example, check these out.[11])

---

11 http://www.brianmac.co.uk/maxhr.htm

The muscles you use and the nature of activity affect your heart rate. Runners move their entire bodies, and generally speaking, running leads to the highest heart rates during exercise. The legs of cyclists perform almost all the muscular work. Because less of their body is utilized during activity, cyclists tend to have slightly lower heart rates during exercise than runners do when they are pushing themselves just as hard. Although swimmers use more muscles vigorously than either cyclists or runners, their prone position and gravity-free suspension in water give swimmers heart rates averaging about twelve beats a minute lower than those of runners (nine less than cyclists).

The demands you place on your body differ at different heart rates. Because of this, people speak of heart rate training zones. These zones are expressed in percentages of maximal heart rate. At the lowest ranges, there is no significant training effect.

According to the American College of Sports Medicine's book *Exercise Is Medicine*, from 55 percent to 65 percent of maximal heart rate, you are in a range of light intensity training. From 65 to 75 percent, you are in a moderate intensity range, and above 75 percent you are in a high intensity range. Most well-trained athletes find these ranges overly conservative. Highly trained endurance athletes can maintain an 80 percent-plus level for hours.

In my own training, I have developed my own sense of how hard I'm working and adapted the numbers accordingly. I prefer to use 65 to 75 percent as my light training range, 75 to 85 percent as my moderate range, and over 85 percent as my heavy range, spending very little time over 85 percent. I split most of my time between 65 to 75 percent and 75 to 85 percent, depending on my goals at the time. When I run, my heart rate is usually right about 85 percent. Probably because I have been running since childhood, I don't feel like I'm crushing myself at that level. When I'm doing HIIT, I push myself closer to 90 percent. As you become accustomed to using a heart rate monitor, you can individualize your heart rate ranges to your own training goals and fitness.

As you get stronger and fitter, you will need to work more intensely or longer to overload and benefit from the exercise. Your heart rate can help you recognize when it is time to pump it up. As you get stronger, your heart won't have to work as hard to accomplish a task, so it will beat more slowly than it used to during the same exercise. That is the

---

http://www.sarkproducts.com/targetzonecalculator.htm

counterpart to the "slow it down" warning of an elevated heart rate, either at rest or while you are exerting yourself.

Just as the physiologic demands are different at different heart rate intensities, so are the fuels your body uses. Consequently, your heart rate during physical activity is closely tied to the fuel you are burning. Understanding this can be useful as you try to meet certain goals. For example, for weight loss and body sculpting, maximizing fat burning is important. Marathon runners are fueled almost entirely by carbohydrates, so for them, paying attention to carbohydrate consumption is helpful. The body stores only so much carbohydrate (about 1,800 g for a 150 lb male). Unless you are really small, you will burn over 100 calories per mile. After not so long, you simply can't just burn carbohydrates. Those whose sporting activity is prolonged need to store and burn fat efficiently. That is one reason English Channel swimmers look like seals in contrast to the greyhound look of marathon runners.

In addition to telling you how hard you should exercise, a heart rate monitor is great at telling you to take it easy and back off. That leads us to the next fundamental principle of exercise.

Variability

Human bodies get bored just like human minds do. They don't like to do exactly the same thing all the time. Performing the same workout day after day is bad for you. Exercise very quickly becomes tedious, and getting stuck in an exercise rut significantly increases your chance of injury. That monotonous regimen will cause your athletic performance to plateau or even decline, no matter how hard you push yourself to get stronger. Worst of all, you will almost certainly grow to hate your workouts. You don't earn any extra points for hating exercise, and you aren't going to want to keep at it if you do. You must change your physical activity from day to day and ideally over the long term as well.

Your brain needs new challenges to develop greater capacity. So does your body. One change is to work harder some days than others. Another kind of change is varying the intensity within one workout. Working more or less intensely is part of the idea, but the underlying concept is different work. Different can refer to intensity. It can also mean doing a different kind of exercise. For sure, changing the intensity of your exercise from day to day and week to week is essential. So too is just doing something different. For instance, many people lift weights two or three days a week and then do some sort of aerobic activity on the other days. Some people swim a couple of days a week and then play tennis on other days. You have so many choices!

Over the course of a week, an optimal exercise habit will include a variety of aerobic activities as the foundation, with strength training at least twice a week, daily stretching and some balance training thrown in occasionally. On some days you will perform a certain exercise at a greater intensity than on other days. You can also change the activity in other ways such as lifting heavier weights less often or performing the movements more slowly. If you are a runner, on some days challenge yourself with a hilly route, a longer run, or (if you don't have any hills nearby), a sprint every once in while during the run. Don't forget that dialing it down, easing up on some days, is an essential part of a healthily variable exercise regimen. Your routine should never become, well, routine. Our ancestors survived by being versatile and adaptable. Your exercise patterns should reflect that variability.

Recovery

One of the great gifts of experience is making lots of mistakes. William Blake, the famous English author, artist, and mystic, wrote, "The road of excess leads to the palace of wisdom." Of course, the point is learning from mistakes so you make fewer mistakes (or at least different ones) in the future. Considering my own mistakes in a positive way, I've created many opportunities for learning (and enriched many orthopedic surgeons in the process). I have learned a lot from my athletic life, some of it quite surprising. Running a marathon wasn't so hard; the key was just going slower to be able to run longer. Running as hard as I could run every time out was actually hurting my performance; learning this lesson was maybe the most welcome surprise. Most of us think that to become stronger, pushing ourselves as hard as possible day after day is the key. That thinking is very wrong.

What you do the day after an intense workout day is just as important as the intensity on that day. On the hard day, you press beyond your comfort level, challenging yourself and your muscles. At a microscopic level, that activity actually damages your muscles a bit. This micro damage leads to restoration and improvement. Your body doesn't just make repairs; it rebuilds, becoming stronger and more efficient by virtue of that process. If you cause too much damage or don't give your body the time to rebuild and make the improvements, you won't benefit from the physical training as you should. Working out hard, day after day, will backfire, destroying the gains of your determined efforts. A day of rest that allows recovery is good for you. A day of gentle activity that encourages rebuilding as well as recovery is even better. In fact, recovery is one of the most important facets of a well-designed exercise program.

What does a good recovery day look like? The simplest example is to follow a day of high-pace endurance running or interval work (for example, sprint intervals) with a day of easy, slow running. You can use a heart rate monitor to hold yourself back, keeping below a certain intensity level. Often the recovery workout is a shorter one. This approach accelerates the rebuilding partly by increasing blood and nutrient flow to the very same muscles without putting a huge demand on those tired muscles.

Inevitably, we cannot fully consider any one aspect of health without considering others. Every piece fits together as part of a greater whole. Psychological aspects are also important. Nutritional considerations are vital.

In recent years, we have learned that from twenty to forty minutes after exercise, the body cranks up its nutrient-absorbing operations. Consuming a recovery drink containing protein and an appropriate amount of carbohydrates during that time window greatly accelerates recovery and boosts muscle building in response to the exercise. We now have evidence that without this nutritional support, your body will break down its own protein (in other words, muscle), rearranging your muscle mass rather than increasing it. We can prevent many exercise-related challenges, such as muscle soreness and end the pattern of getting sick after intense workouts, through good sports nutrition, especially a good recovery drink. Although milk is sometimes touted as the ideal recovery drink, you can do better. Many of us are sensitive to the lactose in milk, and milk lacks other components that appear to optimize recovery.

(See "Ideal Sports and Recovery Drinks" in Chapter 22.)

Building an Exercise Program

It is wise to consider your goals and then create your exercise program to meet those goals. We all come from different places with different limitations, abilities, injuries, and experiences. Our individuality means we will be at our happiest and healthiest if we exercise in our own way.

Our bodies adapt to our activity patterns. We get better at doing what we have been doing. For example, if you want to complete a triathlon and you aren't a good swimmer, you need to work on that. If you want to improve your performance in a certain sport, you need to learn about it and apply sport-specific training.

Sometimes the path to achieving your goals might not be quite so obvious. While we all need aerobic conditioning as well as strength, balance, and flexibility training, one size doesn't fit all. If you are a middle-aged individual with knee problems, you must select aerobic activities that are less stressful to your knees. You also need strength-training exercises that stabilize your knees and, at the same time, are ones that don't increase your risk of more serious knee injury. If you are elderly and want to build your muscle strength so you are less likely to fall, super-slow muscle training isn't going to protect you as well as strength training involving quicker motions. Those quicker motions are more like what happens when you stumble and have to catch yourself quickly. If you are already quite fit but your aim is to become a competitive bodybuilder, perhaps surprisingly some of the things you need to do are exactly the same as an obese person who needs to lose weight, because you are both trying to drop body fat. Understanding your circumstances, learning about exercise, and making a sensible plan will lead to success.

Sometimes people fail before they even begin. If you weigh 600 pounds and your goal is to run a marathon next month, I love your desire, but you need to walk before you can learn to fly. Your immediate goal should be to get some physical activity six days a week. You could also set a long-term goal to complete a marathon in the next five to ten years. With that kind of approach, your feet are on the road to success.

A patient came to see me once because he knew he'd been working too hard, neglecting his diet and his exercise; he was now overweight and out of shape. He had moved to our beautiful semirural area from a big eastern city, partly to lead a healthier life. We created some long-term goals, and I asked him to come back in a month to assess his progress and help him move forward. Instead, he came back in two weeks. He had decided to push himself just as he had in his professional life. After spending a long day riding a mountain bike over very rugged terrain, he had hurt his back. Just about every other part of his body hurt as well. He had done too much too fast. By the time he was able to resume his exercise program, he was in worse shape than before he'd started out.

Increasing your physical activity gradually is crucial. If you overdo it, you will get injured and waste time recovering from your injuries. Just like this overzealous patient, by the time you get back into your exercise program, you will be in worse shape than before you began. I often tell patients that the fastest way to get stronger is by going slowly.

One reasonable guideline for increasing your physical activity is to target a 10 percent increase every week until you reach your goal. That means you first have to assess just how active you are now. For walking, running, and just generally moving around, using a pedometer is a great way to assess your activity level and then increase it in a controlled way.

In essence, a pedometer measures your motion. Other activity tracking devices (Fitbit, Fuelband, Jawbone, Apple Watch) use the same concept with greater accuracy and consequently sometimes greater utility. Runners were the first to discover that using GPS watches helped them track their workouts better and allowed electronic sharing of favorite routes with friends and strangers. There are now many devices one can wear that measure even subtle movements such as when you turn over in sleep, helping you learn more about the quality of your sleep, for example. You can use these devices to keep more accurate tabs on your physical training. You can also learn about your sleep cycles and other habits, especially if you are willing to upload diet logs and personal information. Since smartphones use GPS and motion detectors, you might find simple apps that are even cheaper and more useful that an inexpensive pedometer.

Alternatively, if you are not ill or disabled, you can start with fifteen to twenty minutes every other day. See how you feel the next day and over a week. If the effort doesn't seem like much, boost it up. If it's too much, back down.

Remember to have fun with it!

Good Gadgets for Exercise

Creating better lifestyle habits doesn't require going high tech. "Just do it," as Nike says, forgetting perhaps that the slogan should remind us that we also don't then need Nike. While it is important not to let consumerism clutter our lives or obstruct the pathway to better health, there are a few simple bits of exercise equipment that can be very helpful while sometimes making exercise more fun.

Pedometer

You can pick up a pedometer for five to ten dollars, and it can become the most useful piece of exercise equipment you own. If you wear it every day, you will learn how much you are moving around (almost always less than you think). Remember, ten thousand steps a day is a reasonable long-term goal for almost everyone.

How to Use a Pedometer/Activity Tracker

Wear it for one week to learn about your current activity level. At the end of the week, divide the total number of steps by seven to determine your daily average.

Your target is to average ten thousand steps a day.

If you aren't there yet, increase your activity by 10 percent every week.

For example: If you reach thirty-five thousand steps in a week, your average is five thousand steps per day. The next week, increase your activity so that you average fifty-five hundred steps per day. Then, the following week, move up to six thousand-plus steps a day.

Increasing gradually will help you get stronger while avoiding injuries caused by doing too much too soon.

Heart Rate Monitor

These gadgets have become quite inexpensive and more easily linked to activity tracking devices. While a pedometer tells you how much you move, heart rate monitors are the best way to learn how much effort you are putting into your exercise. They can be very helpful on recovery days when you should be working significantly less than on intensive training days. That monitor will scold you to slow down with its beeping. If you really want to maximize your use of a heart rate monitor, get in a habit of checking your morning resting heart rate and learn to use the Karvonen (Heart Rate Reserve) formula to establish your training zones.

MP3 Player/Smart Phone

Yes, I love my iPod, but I use it only for exercise. I never wear it when I run or walk, much preferring to enjoy the sounds of the outdoor world (and hoping not to miss hearing that car coming up behind me!). When I lift weights at the gym, my iPod keeps me going and limits social distractions. Many people love their MP3 players for exercise. They help them work harder and enjoy their exercise time or make it pass more quickly.

Good Shoes

Okay, maybe Nike knows this one is inevitable. We wear shoes all the time. Athletic shoes have become quite specialized and very expensive. As athletic shoes have become more sophisticated, they are tailored more and more to individual needs. I think this individualization of shoes has created a situation where you can easily buy a high-quality shoe that is really bad for you. Ironically, the more expensive and well cushioned the shoe, the more likely this is. There are websites that help you get an idea of which shoes might be better for you, and many good running shoe stores will let you try out their shoes. Better still, you could start exploring barefoot running. Well, not actually barefoot but nearly barefoot, minimalist shoes. I'm convinced that, over the years, the athletic shoe manufacturers have created more problems than they solved with "the latest and greatest" shoes. Don't forget that your feet have muscles. Walk around your house barefoot to strengthen the muscles in your feet.

Trekking Poles

Trekking poles are more popular in Europe than in the United States. If you like to hike or even just walk a lot, trekking poles can be a nice addition to your exercise equipment. Those who use trekking poles activate their upper body and core, making walking and hiking more complete exercises. Because four-legged creatures are more stable than two-legged ones, trekking poles are really good if you have any joint problems.

Your Own Special Equipment

Just as each of us is an individual in other ways, there might be some piece of exercise equipment that really "changes the game" for you, enhancing your physical activity. Most exercise equipment is special to the activity. Besides helmets, mirrors, and other safety gear, cyclists often prefer special clothing for comfort. Swimming is much the same, with all sorts of float belts, webbed gloves, goggles, and so forth.

Your special equipment doesn't even have to improve your performance. Some hikers hike because they are birders and carry a good pair of binoculars. Others carry a great big bag of sticks and balls over great distances (a.k.a. golf). It's all up to you.

Sometimes the equipment is useful because of our limitations. While free weights are more like real-world activities, well-designed weight machines can help prevent injuries.

Recently I fell in love with the ElliptiGO. I saw the company's star spokesman (Meb Keflezighi) unexpectedly win both the 2012 USA Olympic Marathon Trials and the 2014 Boston Marathon while I worked in the finish line medical tent. I figured that maybe I was good luck for him, so maybe the ElliptiGO would be good luck for me. Truthfully, my knees demanded some other form of aerobic activity, and (cross my fingers) this is working well for me.

Final point: Avoid equipment that hurts you, no matter how convinced someone else is that it's "perfect" for you. Everyone is different. The "best" shoes or "best" weight lifting book might be bad for you. Learn from your mistakes.

Summary

- Exercise is magic for our bodies and our brains.
- You are one of Earth's elite athletes.
- Exercise every day.
- Move every hour.
- Change it up.
- Choose exercise you like.
- Don't forget balance and strength training.

Chapter 7

Essential Health Habit #3: Eat Well

Everyone needs to eat. Sometimes it seems that that is as much as we can agree on. Fat is bad. Sugar is bad. Protein is bad. Fat is essential. Carbohydrates, including some simple sugars in fresh fruits, are still important in our diets. Protein is the key to maintaining muscle strength and the raw material for powerful peptide hormones, hormones that regulate how our cells function. Vitamins are great. Vitamins cause cancer. We need minerals for every important bodily function. Minerals can kill you.

Every major and minor component of the diet has been touted as miraculous or evil. If we get more complicated, if we start to move past the already-controversial fundamental elements of the diet, it only gets more confusing. Dietary crazes are guaranteed to make you crazy.

Admittedly, sorting the wheat from the chaff, determining what really is a healthy way to eat, can be absolutely mystifying. It certainly doesn't have to be. Thinking about diet is a fantastic opportunity to use common sense to your advantage. Although we must allow for individual variation, meaning some of us have somewhat differing needs for certain nutrients because of our genetics or current health conditions, 99 percent of what defines a healthy diet is the same for all of us. Understanding the basics makes the process much simpler and helps you navigate around concerns with food sensitivities, likes, and dislikes.

- The American diet (probably even yours) is a problem
- Your food should be
  - Diverse
  - Simple
  - Organic
  - Local
- On the food/supplement borderline: Omega-3 oils

- Food behaviors
  - Shopping and the modern hunter-gatherer society
  - The process of eating
- Summary

The American Diet Is a Problem

The average American eats way too much "junk food." A 2004 study found that 30 percent of all calories Americans consumed was officially "junk," with almost all of those calories coming from sweets, desserts, and soft drinks.[12] Sodas alone represented 7 percent of the calories in the American diet. A 2007 survey found that less than 10 percent of American high school students ate the recommended daily intake of vegetables (three servings) and fruit (two servings). An American Heart Association survey found that the average American ate twenty-two teaspoons (nearly one-half cup) of added sugar *every day*! Teenage boys led the way with thirty-four teaspoons each day.

How could these numbers be so high and be getting even higher? Eighty percent of all the food sold in a typical American grocery store includes added sugar. In other words, that's extra sweetening in nearly every food. Even if *you* don't put sugar in your coffee, the food industry puts it in everything—your beans, bread, ketchup, salad dressing, granola, yogurt, and so forth.

Sugar is disguised through the use of different names. If the words *sugar* or *syrup* are listed among the ingredients on the label, there are sugars no matter how earthy they sound. The word *sweetener* also means sugar, except when it is an artificial sweetener. That isn't better. Artificial sweeteners are just a more complex problem. "Nectar" sounds healthy, but *nectar* is just another word for sugar. Fruit juice is sugary. Fruit juice concentrates are concentrated sugars and are unhealthy for you. The hardest sugars to identify on label lists hide because of their chemical names. The way to spot them is to remember that they end in "ose." Examples are glucose, fructose, sucrose, dextrose, maltose, and so forth. Many of us believe that high-fructose corn syrup (HFCS), a recently created sweetener, is the worst of the worst. It doesn't stand alone, though, so don't fixate just on avoiding HFCS.

---

12 Block, "Foods contributing to energy intake in the US: data from NHANES III and NHANES 1999–2000," *J Food Compost Anal* 17 (2004): 439-47.

The consequence of this disordered eating is that we're starving and overeating at the same time. We consume more calories than we need but not enough essential nutrients. National health surveys show that the majority of Americans eat diets that are deficient in vitamin C and the minerals magnesium, calcium, and iron. Deficiencies of vitamins A and E, as well as the minerals zinc and selenium, are common. Although vitamin D comes from sunlight more than from our diet, I'm among those who feel that vitamin D deficiency is so widespread and medically important that it represents a worldwide health crisis. We will talk more about that later.

There are literally thousands of studies examining the consequences of these dietary deficiencies. Let me sum up the research: we're fatter, unhealthier, and dumber than we would otherwise be. We know without any doubt whatsoever that eating a healthy diet reduces our chances of getting sick, improves how we feel, and raises our life expectancy.

We also eat the *wrong kind of calories.* Fearing fat, people load up on carbs. Many rich protein sources also contain a good deal of fat, so, by avoiding fat, many people have compromised their protein intake. The result of this pattern is to make people fat, tired, and unhealthy.

For over twenty-five years, I have been reviewing the diets of every patient I see. Since I began seeing patients who are more conscious about their health, honestly some of the biggest problems I have seen have been in the diets of those trying to manipulate their diets too precisely. Those patients carefully follow a plan that is too narrowly conceived, and because they follow it so exactingly, they fall into the hidden traps. Those patients usually eat very healthy food, *but their diets are still unhealthy* because they miss out on some of the nutrients essential to good human nutrition.

Your Food Should Be Diverse

One problem that should be obvious from the conflicting information you read is that we don't know everything, even about the basics. Every year we continue to learn more about vitamins and minerals, discovering that they are more complex than we thought and interact in many ways.

During the past decade, antioxidants were all the rage. We're learning that there are other, previously unknown or underappreciated components in foods that have important health effects. You might have heard of resveratrol, which is one member of a class of richly colorful food chemicals called polyphenols. Despite truly excessive hype, there are reasons to feel optimistic that resveratrol might be good. Polyphenols are found in tea, berries, grapes, chocolate, and nuts. Nearly 60% of Americans' polyphenol intake comes from coffee.

We are just beginning to learn of the potent effects of polyphenols. For example, we already know that consuming high amounts of polyphenols drops cardiovascular death rates much more than lowering cholesterol. Other chemicals such as the beta-glucans in mushrooms, may prevent or treat cancer. Another class of carbohydrate saccharides, the arab-inogalactans, might be an immune stimulant. Spices like turmeric and cinnamon appear to have anticancer and antidiabetic effects.

While vitamins are "old news" relative to these other "newbies," the tidal wave of unexpected data on vitamin D is probably the biggest nutritional discovery in decades. And given our generations of neglect of vitamin D, it is much akin to discovering that the cleaning girl is actually Cinderella.

All these dietary components have multiple effects (for example, polyphenols and vitamins also have antioxidant effects). Consequently, it is evident that we need to think a bit more holistically about food to avoid the arrogant and mistaken belief that we can cook up a healthy diet in a chemistry lab.

As we *do* know that we have holes in our knowledge, our best insurance to cover the gaps is to *eat a variety of foods*. While we may not know what we're missing, it is absolutely clear that if we eat the same thing all the time, we are certainly missing something. No matter how good a food is, we shouldn't eat it during every meal, day after day.

What does a diverse diet look like? It is beautiful. It *looks* good. The food constituting a healthy diet is colorful. Colors are often created by specific nutrients, especially the polyphenols I mentioned.

Maybe the most useful tip I can make is also the least well known—that is, *eat some bitter-tasting plants every day*. The reason for such seemingly inconsiderate advice is that bitterness equals biological strength. The most potent and wholesome chemicals in plants have strong tastes.

Many of us overlook the importance of fermented foods in our diet. Throughout history and in essentially every culture, human beings have traditionally eaten at least one variety of fermented food. We have been fermenting beverages, including alcohol, for millennia, and TV ads tell me they remain quite popular. There are many fermented food products, including bread, cheese, yogurt, sauerkraut, soured milks, miso, soy sauce, tofu, pickles, and olives; they are so common that just about everyone eats something off that list every day. Ever since humans discovered it, chocolate has been fermented as a key part of its processing for consumption. Traditionally these foods were locally made with local, living bacteria.

That last bit might sound horrible, but our bodies are filled with bacteria; by one measure we "humans" are 95 percent intestinal bacteria and only 5 percent human. Those bacteria make us healthier by manufacturing vitamins we absorb from our digestive tracts and regulating our immune systems. Because they are good for us they are called *pro–biotic*, meaning "in favor of life." (Recently scientists discovered that our bodies have one hundred times as many viruses as bacteria and just *one species of virus accounts for 40 percent of all the viral DNA.* The implications of that are stunning.) Eating fermented foods, replenishing those health-creating organisms, is a fundamental part of a complete diet. In our society the fermented foods we eat are usually pasteurized, so the bacteria have been killed. Also, the specific species of bacteria in the food were chosen because they work well in the factory, maybe not so much in our bodies. Taking a probiotic can help address this dietary deficiency, but again, due to our still-limited understanding, choosing fermented foods with living bacteria is a smart move.

Your Food Should Be Simple

Reading ingredient labels is good. Even just taking a glance and ignoring exactly what the label says can still be informative. Simply noticing that the list is long is a hint that you might be better off putting the package back on the shelf. The most complicated gourmet recipes never come close to the number of ingredients you can find on way too many labels at the grocery stores. I bet your grandmother's kitchen didn't look like a science lab, and she didn't use dozens of ingredients with unpronounceable chemical names in the food she made for the family. The food industry recognizes this tendency. When Pillsbury came out with Häagen-Dazs FIVE ice cream, the company showed that they had learned to use a short list of ingredients as an indicator of premium quality and a marketing tool.

It is very important to remember that *the food industry exists to make money, not to make you healthy.* Consequently manufacturers produce food they can sell to you at a maximum profit. Making it taste good helps make a product more sellable. A corporation's duty to its stockholders is to boost their profits. Creating food products that are more desirable to consumers because the food is healthier allows manufacturers to charge more. This is one way for industrial food manufacturers to achieve their financial targets. One reason so many Americans are so badly overweight is because healthy unprocessed foods, such as vegetables and fruit, now cost much more than the highly processed or highly profitable junk industrial food manufacturers favor.

One characteristic of what I mean by simple is *eating low on the food chain.* The largest animal ever to live on earth, the blue whale, eats plankton and krill, some of the smallest living animals in the ocean. When one creature eats another, that creature also eats the environmental toxins accumulated in the body of its victim throughout its life. Over its own lifetime, this creature collects the toxins in all the food it has eaten. Predators like sharks and birds of prey accumulate huge concentrations of stuff we didn't eat ourselves and wouldn't have chosen to eat in the first place. In essence, you eat *everything* your food ate. The lower you eat on the food chain, the lower your exposure levels are.

Vegetarian Diets

Vegetarian diets are naturally low on the food chain, as you skip eating the animals that ate the plants. You take that herbivore role instead, dropping down closer to the roots of the food chain. A vegan diet, excluding milk products and anything else derived from animals, is the lowest on the food chain. Since plants absorb undesirable environmental chemicals, even a vegan diet isn't risk free. There are other advantages and disadvantages to vegetarian diets. Some of those have become clear to me from my medical practice and some from my personal experience following various vegetarian diets for almost forty years.

The advantages of vegetarian diets are considerable. Eating a vegetarian diet lessens the risks of developing cancer, heart disease, high blood pressure, diabetes, and obesity, all of the most common health problems of our modern, industrialized world. A British study, published in 2009, found that overall death rates were cut by one-half among adult vegetarians.[13] Concentrations of vitamins (except B12) are quite high in vegetarian diets. With careful attention, people of any age can meet their nutritional needs on a vegetarian diet.

Although this sounds fantastic—and it is—there are problems. The simplest way to understand the most common problems is what I call "healthy, unhealthy diets." I see many patients who are meticulous about choosing healthy foods. Everything they eat is organic and of excellent quality. Unfortunately, the great majority of these patients are missing out on at least one or two major dietary elements.

My own dietary history is an informative example. In 1971, at age seventeen, I joined an organic food cooperative and became an ovo-lacto vegetarian (meaning I ate dairy products and eggs as well as veggies). Although I was relatively healthy, I did have some health problems that turned out to be caused by an undiagnosed egg allergy and lactose intolerance. After I figured this out myself and excluded those foods from my diet, I developed an odd skin rash and found it difficult to rebound from my customary athletic activities.

The rash was odd, so I saw a dermatologist who was just as perplexed. He took a biopsy, which clarified nothing. Finally I got the answer from my soccer teammates, almost all of whom were migrant farm workers. They could see the rash on my arms. They told me I needed to eat meat. While I didn't entirely accept their advice, I did realize that in a way they could be right. My protein intake was too low, and correcting it resolved my symptoms. The rash went away, and my typically excellent energy bounced back.

Consuming sufficient protein was a challenge, though. In addition to the egg allergy and lactose intolerance, I have never digested beans well. I liberalized my diet and began eating fish. Dietary flexibility (a.k.a. omnivorousness or diversity) is healthy.

I got another lesson years later when my vision began to annoy me. It seemed like I had something in my eye but couldn't get it out. "Something in my eye" was the right diagnosis, but the "thing" was a cataract. Now that seemed entirely impossible. I had worn ultraviolet light-blocking sunglasses and eaten a low-fat diet rich in antioxidants since age seventeen. No one in my family had developed a cataract at my relatively "young" age of fifty-seven. Then I guiltily remembered that thirty-five

13 Key et al., "Mortality of British Vegetarians," *Am J Clinical Nutrition* 89 (2009):1613S-1619S . doi: 10.3945/ajcn.2009.26736L.

years before, I recognized that I'd probably needed to supplement my diet with zinc because the fibrous plants in vegetarian diets, like mine, impair zinc absorption. One consequence of that relative zinc deficiency can be cataracts. Why the guilt? I hadn't acted on my knowledge by either changing my diet or supplementing it. Now, when I do take supplements, the cataracts are usually not a problem. I will probably need surgery at some point, but I should have done something about this before—way before.

Certain nutrients are less concentrated in vegetarian diets, creating the need for special awareness. Dietary nutrients we need in big quantities are called macronutrients. These include carbohydrates, fats, and proteins. Macronutrient issues common among vegetarians are protein and the omega-3 fatty acids subset of fats. Micronutrient deficiencies are minerals such as calcium, zinc, iron, and iodine as well as vitamin B12 and (like every one else) vitamin D.

Diets Impaired by Allergy, Intolerance, or Illness

When an individual has a food allergy or intolerance, the likelihood of a deficiency increases. That increase can be a consequence of recognizing the problem and restricting the diet to avoid the offending food. An individual who chooses to restrict his or her diet by becoming a vegetarian and then must further limit food choices due to a sensitivity must work hard to avoid nutritional deficiencies.

Deficiencies also frequently occur because a stressed digestive system doesn't do its job absorbing nutrients very well. For example, if a male patient comes to me with mild digestive symptoms and his blood shows low iron and maybe an elevated liver enzyme or low thyroid, I know he is likely to be sensitive to gluten.

Processed Food—NOT

Processed foods in the United States are among the greatest dietary "evils." These products are laden with harmful ingredients, and much of the good stuff, the vitamins, minerals, and polyphenols, are destroyed in the processing. The resulting products are convenient but just barely qualify as food. While many people in the developed world have high blood pressure, in part due to consuming too much salt, they get almost all that salt from processed foods and bread. My patients who eat a healthy diet, avoiding processed foods, rarely need to cut their salt intake. In fact, I need to encourage a significant number of them to allow themselves to eat a bit more salty food, because they are suffering symptoms caused by their blood pressure being too low. The US public health campaign against salt consumption is misdirected. Our efforts should be focused on reducing our consumption of processed foods. That is the real source of the salt problem and so many others. For a long list of reasons, avoiding highly processed foods is wise.

Raw Food

Eating some raw food is also wise. Eating only raw food is too extreme. The human digestive tract isn't built to break down raw foods like cows. We have one stomach. They have four. We can't extract the nutrients from some foods, so we need to cook them. Cooking (in other words, in-home food processing) also reduces the risk of most food-borne infectious diseases. Many foods (nuts, fruits, and some vegetables) are most nutritious when eaten raw. With age, we lose stomach acid, and other health issues can compromise digestion, so individual needs vary. Cook your food just as much, and no more, as needed.

Your Food Should Be Organic

When we look at the issue in the broadest way, we see that those who favor organic food are really hunting for quality. Our bodies use food as fuel and building blocks. So choosing the best food available to make yourself as strong and healthy as possible is a no-brainer. As we discussed earlier, studies have shown that nearly half of the food we eat is "junk." Over 25 percent of all the calories we eat come from sweets, desserts, and soft drinks. Not good. As our expanding waistlines attest, we eat too much junk food. While we gorge on empty calories, the average American eats less-than-recommended levels of many vitamins and minerals. Think about how many Americans have their backsides glued to the couch in front of the TV; we seem a bit like confined and force-fed veal calves or foie gras ducks, only we do it to ourselves.

It is good to eat real food and "dump the junk" is good. Generally speaking, organic food is even better.

Chemicals in Food

The reason most people think organic is better is because they want to avoid chemicals farmers and manufacturers use. They are concerned about the effects of these chemicals. Unfortunately such concerns are well warranted.

Since Rachel Carson first rang the alarm bell sixty years ago with her book *Silent Spring*, the evidence has piled higher and higher that commonly used pesticides, herbicides, and fertilizers damage the environment and those who eat the food produced in that environment.

Just as the human body is packed with other living organisms that create nutrients and influence our health favorably and unfavorably, the same is true of the soil. Adding chemicals changes the character and health of the soil. While the potential harm of chemicals that kill organisms in the soil (herbicides and pesticides) is easier to recognize, fertilizers also have a big impact.

Dr. Fritz Haber won the Nobel Prize for his development of nitrogen fertilizer because it dramatically increased plant yields. Dr. Haber also infamously developed poisonous chlorine gas as a weapon in World War I. After his death, the Nazis used a pesticide he'd developed, Zyklon B, as the favored means of killing the Jews and unwanted minorities of Europe. Dr. Haber was himself Jewish. Just as Dr. Haber's work wasn't always beneficial to humanity, the unbound nitrogen in synthesized fertilizers washes into lakes, rivers, and oceans, creating "dead zones" where aquatic plants flourish but fish die.

Nitrogen is a simple, familiar chemical that turned out to have unanticipated ill effects. There are thousands of other, much less well known chemicals in widespread use. Must of them are just too new to know everything, or even very much, about them. Very few have been thoroughly tested on humans, and we know even less about their effects on other living organisms. Just as it took decades to discover that artificial fertilizers were feeding algae and killing fish, the health and environmental consequences of other chemicals are slowly becoming evident, though much is still unknown.

When the infamous pesticide DDT (dichlorodiphenyltrichloroethane) was introduced, it earned its inventor the Nobel Prize. At the time, it was believed to be harmless to humans. After we learned otherwise, most dramatically when it pushed many species of predator birds to the very brink of extinction, it was banned from much of the world. Now, decades after it was banned, DDT lingers in the environment, because it breaks down so very slowly. DDT is very inexpensive. So, despite the damage it inflicts and the growing resistance to DDT in malaria-carrying mosquitoes, DDT is still used in the third world in attempts to control malaria.

The history of food additives is similar. A few crazies thought they were risky and should be avoided, while most believed additives were a safe way to make food taste better and last longer without spoiling. This dispute reached its controversial peak in children with attention-deficit/hyperactivity disorder (ADHD). Parents and some clinicians claimed that artificial food additives and colors were causing behavioral problems in children. As is often the case, the "crazies" turned out to be prophets. Not long ago, staid medical authorities of the British government ran their own study. Their study confirmed that avoiding artificial food additives and colors reduced behavioral problems in children with ADHD.[14]

These are not isolated, "cherry-picked" examples. Numerous other chemicals used in the environment and food production have later proved to be hazardous. The obvious conclusion is that it is naive to assume that artificial chemicals are safe and devoid of unintended effects. The evidence tells us that every chemical has many actions other than the first one that comes to our attention. It is far wiser to start from the assumption that using a foreign substance will cause problems. The burden of proof should be on the manufacturer, providing conclusive and comprehensive data on all the short- and long-term effects of these additives before millions of us become involuntary and unwitting test subjects. (See more about food additives in Chapter 9).

Weak Plants Equal Weak People

Ironically, it appears that making life easier for plants by using artificial fertilizers, pesticides, and herbicides makes the plants less nutritious for us. Plants produce nutrients, such as antioxidants, polyphenols, and resveratrol, when they are stressed by environmental factors, especially when insects, fungi, and bacteria attack them. The chemicals plants produce to strengthen themselves are good for the plant eaters as well. Organic foods are then healthier for you.

---

14   Pelsser et al., "Effects of a Restricted Elimination Diet on the Behavior of Children with ADHD," *Lancet* 377 (2011):494-503. doi: 10.1016/S0140-6736(10)62227-1.

As I mentioned earlier, I've been a big believer in organic food for over forty years, but the assumption that organic food is healthier is open to question. A label that reads "organic" is great, but don't stop there. We still need to think critically.

Let's assume that the goal is higher quality. Is organic food, flown in from another continent, healthier to eat than nonorganic food produced locally? The assumption that all organic food is even truly organic is also presumptuous.

Organic Food Often Isn't

Another excellent reason for going organic isn't what is in the food but what isn't—for example, pesticides and herbicides. Unfortunately, that is often not the case.

For example, a study of organic greens sold in the San Francisco Bay Area discovered that nearly all the samples were contaminated by toxic perchlorates. Although the greens were farmed organically, perchlorates in rocket fuel, which leaked from storage tanks at Edwards Air Force Base, had contaminated the water in that part of California. Testing irrigation water isn't part of organic certification. Ideally foods should be tested after they are produced to achieve organic certification. Although unrecognized until the late 1990s, perchlorate water contamination has been discovered in twenty-six states and in just over 4 percent of water samples the EPA has analyzed nationwide.[15]

The possibility that organic foods are not as pure as those labels suggest isn't an argument against going organic. Instead, that is an argument in favor of selecting such foods. My goal is to reduce my intake of inferior quality foods. If we might unintentionally consume nonorganic or genetically modified food, then it is even more important to try to limit our exposures. Just giving up or burying your heads in the sand isn't a smart decision, and doing whatever we can will help.

Recently we learned about a class of cancer-causing chemicals that are produced when we cook starchy foods at high temperature. Heating an amino acid (protein) called asparagine to high temperatures in the presence of certain sugars leads to the formation of acrylamides. Frying or baking carbohydrates at high temperature appears to be the key. The process of browning these foods seems to create the acrylamide.

---

15 "Perchlorate," EPA Website, http://water.epa.gov/drink/contaminants/unregulated/perchlorate.cfm

Breads, potato products, and some breakfast cereals all contain this nasty chemical. It has probably been in foods ever since our ancestors began cooking food. This is a big surprise, as we had no idea this chemical was in food, and, given these new data, estimates are that each year this chemical causes several hundred cases of human cancer in the United States. Efforts are underway to determine how concerned we should be about acrylamides and what action we might take. Even if our concerns prove to be overblown, this unexpected discovery is a further reminder that, given our always-limited knowledge, minimizing exposure to unhealthy foods is smart.

Organic Is Good, but Wild Is Better

Another exception to eating organically is that wild is often better than organic, especially when the food is another animal. Just like people, inactive animals are less healthy. Wild game has high levels of healthy unsaturated fats, unlike feedlot animals, which are laden with oxidizing saturated fats. The same is true of fish. The tilapia sold in the United States is almost always farm raised. Despite the rosy expectations we tend to have about high levels of protective omega-3 oils in fish, farm-raised tilapia contains as much or more saturated fat than a fast-food double cheeseburger. Farm-raised salmon carries high levels of polychlorinated biphenyls (PCBs are used as industrial coolants; see more in Chapter 9). Farmed salmon also contain much less omega-3 oils than their wild cousins. Certainly when we compare two feedlot-raised cows, we see that the one fed organically is going to have a smaller accumulation of toxins in its flesh. However, if you are going to eat meat, wild game may be healthier still (if you can avoid parasites in the wild meat).

When considering man-made alterations in our food, we need to include genetically modified food (GMOs, which stands for "genetically modified organisms") in the discussion. Many of us worry about the potential problems with genetically modified foods.

Just for fun, I will begin with a rather extreme example. To help increase rice output, scientists are genetically engineering rice to be more resistant to herbicides. That way they can use lots of it, kill the competing plants, and leave the rice free to flourish. Disgustingly (my apologies for the editorialization, but I'm appalled), Japanese scientists, at their National Institute of Agrobiological Sciences, inserted a human gene into rice to achieve this end. I find this idea frightening, not to mention seriously weird and certainly (sorry again) hard to "swallow."

The issues surrounding GMOs are emblematic and typical of many of the complex health considerations we face. We all know there will be consequences of our choices. However, we're scientifically ignorant of the full extent of those consequences. While this is common in medical practice and the real world of complex biological systems, we still have to make decisions and take action now. When certainty is out of reach, we just have to get by with our best guesses. No one really likes guessing, no matter how educated that guess may be. We all want results, results that are both consistent and predictable. Things just aren't so tidy. Life and living organisms are innately no more than semipredictable. In truth, we seldom know enough to understand the full consequences of our actions. We can't sit on our hands, waiting for certainty. We have to make decisions and move forward.

When semi-informed decisions are required, I find that following a certain process of consideration leads to pretty good choices. The process is innately moderating. Granting undue importance to small sprigs of data or wild speculation is likely to lead you far out onto some thin limb, leaving you in a tenuous position.

How to Make Informed Decisions—First

I gather information about what is known. Then look for the part that doesn't make obvious sense. That element is the keystone.

One example is that we know that increased levels of many vitamins are associated with lowered rates of certain diseases. At the same time, supplementation with the very same vitamins is sometimes associated with increased risk of the same diseases.

Another example is that, by definition, genetically modified foods contain amino acid or proteins from other living organisms. That modification fundamentally alters the biological activity of the organism in the environment (allergenicity, toxicity, ability to spread, and so forth). Biological modification is the point behind its creation, after all. Since we created it to be different, it must be different. It is irrational to assume that a GMO wouldn't behave differently in some still-unappreciated manner, because we *know* it does in some other ways. That is the whole point of making it in the first place.

There is a history of genetic modification causing trouble, most notably the horrendous problem with a rare disease called eosinophilic myalgia that resulted from genetic modification of the supplement L-tryptophan (which was used mostly as a sleep aid). An animal study claiming ill effects from the herbicide Roundup[16] created such a stir that it came to be known as "The Seralini Affair" after the principal author of the study. We don't yet have significant confirmed reports of ill health effects from GMO foods. It is highly likely that that will change, but how serious will the ill effects be?

To support your own considerations, one of the best sources of information on the interface between foods, industry, and politics is Marion Nestle, PhD. I highly recommend her books *Safe Food: Bacteria, Biotechnology, and Bioterrorism* and *Food Politics: How the Food Industry Influences Nutrition and Health*. Although I don't entirely agree with all she writes, her books are interesting and clearly written.

How to Make Informed Decisions—Next

Next comes critically analyzing that information to sort out the deeper meanings, the clues about what that information is really telling us. In the case of vitamins, synthetic vitamins are different from natural forms taken in food, along with other nutrients. In many instances we know *wild foods contain dramatically higher levels* of vitamins and minerals than domesticated versions. So we need to consider the forms of the vitamin, attend to a balanced overall diet, and continue to learn about varying individual needs.

In the case of GMO foods, the same old issue, an incomplete study of the problem, looms large. In other words, an inadequate research base prevents full understanding of the problem, let alone drawing conclusions. If you haven't yet looked carefully for a snake in the grass, you might not know it is there until it bites you. If you know nothing at all about snakes, you are in for a big surprise.

Other factors come into play when industrial technology or big financial interests or both are involved. In my years in medicine, I have seen many, many strongly advocated, "safe" treatments later proved to be ineffective or dangerous. That makes me skeptical of the latest advances,

---

16   Seralini et al., "Long Term Toxicity of a Roundup Herbicide and a Roundup-Tolerant Genetically Modified Maize," *Food Chem Toxicol* 50 (2012):4221-31. doi: 10.1016/j.fct.2012.08.005.

particularly when the corporations or physicians with something to gain tout the product. In the case of genetically modified organisms, the economic stakes are very high.

How to Make Informed Decisions—Finally

We move on to consider the repercussions, the consequences of action and inaction. In medicine we call this the risk-benefit ratio. If the intervention isn't likely to cause harm, the need for convincing proof of efficacy is trivial compared to its importance in a high-risk procedure. With vitamins, the risk-benefit formula is largely an individual matter. A patient who has heart disease, has never taken vitamin E, and wants to start taking a large dose is in a completely different circumstance than some other person taking vitamin E or another vitamin, mineral, or nutritional supplement. Blanket condemnation or advocacy is beyond simplistic.

The development and use of GMO includes an additional risk. That risk follows from the reality that they aren't containable. For years now, the majority of non-GMO corn and soy sold in the United States has already been contaminated by genetically modified corn and soy. Rain, wind, birds, and bugs don't respect property lines, so crops get mingled. In the 2002 "ProdiGene Incident," a corn that had been genetically modified to produce a vaccine for pigs was inadvertently released to human corn suppliers. Emergency intervention by the US Department of Agriculture might have prevented human consumption of this food/drug intended for pigs. I wrote "might" because we really don't know whether all the pig-vaccine corn was taken out of the human food supply, and no one knows the health effects (if any) of human exposure to that pig vaccine.

Following three years of deliberations, the National Research Council (the research arm of the Institute of Medicine, the National Academy of Sciences, and the National Academy of Engineering) issued a report criticizing the US government's oversight of GMOs and warned that the consequences could be severe. My summation of their report is, "We possess the technology to create unforeseen problems that could wreak havoc, but we don't yet possess the capability to confine or even safely test that technology."

Even if GMOs create problems, they might also become a useful means of improving human health. Besides the possibility of greater yields, we could incorporate medicinal substances into food crops. This could include vitamins, medications, or proteins to reduce allergies. Since my patients are very selective about their use of medication, I have difficulty imagining any of them deferring such health choices to the government or an agribusiness company. I wouldn't.

Another aspect of the process of making wise decisions applies to the GMO issue. That is to consider the timing and urgency of the decision. There are situations in which the penalty for inaction is so much less than the risks of a rash decision. Do we have to go ahead right now? The wisest decision is to go slow until more is known.

My bottom-line assessment of GMOs is that, for now at least, the risks outweigh their potential benefits. With uncertain scientific data and the potential for extreme and entirely unforeseen consequences, the risk is too great at this time. (For more consideration, see the Organic Consumers Association website.[17])

Your Food Should Be Local

Supporting local farmers and food producers is healthy for you and your community. Local food is also part of your community, your bio-community perhaps. It is healthier because it is fresher and because you also possess some "inside knowledge" about the area where the food is grown and the people involved. As small family farms die out and our food comes increasingly from industrial farming, there are many unfortunate consequences.

Farming at any size, crop, or method is a business, but *industrial farming is all about output.* The more food is produced at the cheapest cost, the better that is for the corporate bottom line. Food quality is secondary and mostly important for marketability. "Buy our food because it's cheap and maybe even good for you!" Certain varieties of plants are favored because they work better with harvesting machines, fit better into packing boxes, or survive days of shipping better than more nutritious or appealing varieties of the same plant. We lose the genetic diversity of plants with this industrial homogenization, making our food supply increasingly vulnerable to pests and climate stresses. Consequently, farmers have to use even more chemicals to support these less resilient plants.

For a long time, industrialized meat production in America has created serious problems, going far beyond mere matters of quality. One

---

17   http://www.organicconsumers.org

hundred years ago, Upton Sinclair's *The Jungle* exposed horrific practices in Chicago's meatpacking plants, including fecal matter in the meat. That isn't just old news or a historical footnote about the bad old days. A recent University of Minnesota study found that *70 to 90 percent of meat sold at supermarkets was contaminated with Escherichia coli (E. coli) stool bacteria.*

As time marches on, the old problems persist, and we have added some new, and even more dangerous, ones. No one thinks that is progress.

The worst issues arise from growing animals in industrially optimized conditions. Confining large numbers of animals into relatively small spaces makes feeding, watering, and managing them more convenient. This efficiency also damages the animals' health, makes them more vulnerable to disease, and, like we saw with plants, requires heavy use of chemicals, particularly antibiotics, to overcome the problems caused by our advanced technology. Adding growth hormones to feed to shorten the time from birth to market is widespread, with documented health effects including premature puberty in little girls.

Overuse of Antibiotics on the Farm

The overuse of antibiotics in American farm animals demands special comment. At this point, the great majority of antibiotics used in the United States go to farm animals. Every year, tens of thousands of Americans die from infections caused by bacteria resistant to antibiotics, and the numbers are rising rapidly. Infectious disease used to be the leading cause of death among Americans. It had dropped as low as number ten. *Death from infectious disease has bounced back up to number three,* and many believe it is only a matter of time before infectious disease reclaims the top spot. Those facts are inextricably linked. It isn't an overstatement to say that we're creating a nightmare for our children; because it is coming at us so fast, it is our own nightmare as well.

The great majority of pig farms, over 80 percent according to US Department of Agriculture studies, give antibiotics to their animals *when they are healthy,* hoping to prevent health problems and accelerate the growth of their animals. One estimate is that over 70 percent of the antibiotics produced in the United States are administered to *healthy* farm animals, increasing the likelihood of problems for humans. These are not "animal" antibiotics. Almost all the antibiotics given to animals are the very same ones you buy at the pharmacy. The casual overuse of antibiotics in factory farming is a dangerous practice and the major cause of what is quite probably the most serious health threat facing us in the coming decade.

Any time bacteria are exposed to antibiotics, some of the bacteria will survive the exposure. Sometimes the surviving bacteria are not the kind that caused the initial problem. Sometimes the surviving bacteria are a rare form of the troublesome ones, carrying a mutation which allows them to resist the antibiotic. At other times, the previously vulnerable bacteria themselves mutate to survive the antibiotics. Like any other living organism, they want to keep living. No matter the details, once the vulnerable common bacteria are killed off, the resistant bacteria survive with lots of nutrients and no competition. In short order, these rare bacteria then become dominant, and antibiotics no longer work.

Animal Antibiotics Cause Human Diseases

Bacterial contamination of food, even the simple kind caused by common nonresistant bacteria, is an enormous and frightening problem, rapidly growing to crisis proportions. It leads to over three hundred thousand hospitalizations and five thousand deaths in the United States each year. Estimates are that one-third of Americans suffer from food poisoning annually. Contaminated chicken is the biggest source of food poisoning, but it appears that the effects of bacterial food contamination go beyond what we have thought of as food-related illness. For example, in January 2010, Canadian researchers published their findings, linking bacteria-contaminated chickens with urinary tract infections in women.[18]

As recalls of peanut butter, hazelnuts, salsa, sprouts, lettuce, and pistachios have demonstrated in recent years, *nasty bacteria contaminate plants as well as meats*. In the setting of industrial agriculture, even the bacteria contaminating plants are often deadly mutated forms. Water running off industrial animal feedlots spreads bacteria to plant crops grown nearby.

For example, all our bodies carry *E. coli* bacteria. It doesn't bother us when it stays in our intestines, but it is the most common cause of bladder infections. It has caused some trouble from time to time, but it really wasn't too bad. Then a new and very deadly mutant form of *E. coli* (specifically *E. coli* O157:H7) arose in animal factory feedlots and spread

---

18   Vincent et al., "Food Reservoir for *Escherichia coli* Causing Urinary Tract Infections," *Emerg Infect Dis* 3 (2010):415-21. doi: 10.3201/eid1601.091118

out from there. Like the other *E. coli,* this one, the most common cause of acute kidney failure in the United States today, lives in animal waste.

In 1994, the USDA found that one cow out of every two thousand slaughtered in the United States carried this deadly form of *E. coli.* By late 2009, the USDA found this deadly *E. coli* in *one-half of the cattle they tested.* Water contaminated with animal waste and this deadly perversion of a common bacteria species commonly leaks into neighboring fields. The plants growing in those nearby fields are, in turn, contaminated before they are shipped to your dinner table. Wash your veggies, okay?

Adding to our worries, besides the nightmarish O157:H7 form, are other toxic species of *E. coli* that are starting to appear. They can be every bit as nasty as O157:H7. Earthbound Farm, the largest US producer of organic greens, voluntarily tests for all known toxic strains of *E. coli.* In a recent year, they found that one out of every one thousand samples was contaminated with one of these dangerous bacteria.

Antibiotics are wonderful and can save many lives. Precisely because they can be so useful and important, *we absolutely* must *stop using them so much.* Our overuse makes them ineffective because we are forcing bacteria to become resistant. Bacteria somehow recognize how vital bacterial resistance is to their survival. They will drop some of the genes they need to digest their food so they can hang on to the genes they picked up that allow them to survive antibiotics. Different kinds of bacteria can pass these immune genes to each other just by living nearby. Maybe the worst news in this nightmare story is that there is evidence that some bacteria retain this immunity through *fifty generations or more* without even one single additional exposure to the antibiotic. They don't even need a reminder about how important antibiotic resistance is to their survival. It seems instead that we're the ones in need of a reminder.

There is also evidence that an individual who uses an antibiotic will then grow bacteria resistant to that antibiotic in his or her own body. When you use antibiotics, you increase the risk for your neighbors, but even more, *you increase your own risk of acquiring a lethal bacterial infection.* We used to think the bacteria in your gut was messed up while you were taking antibiotics, but then your good bacteria bounced back after a few weeks. Studies as long as two years in length contradict that rosy outlook. Don't use antibiotics unless you really need them, because when you really need an antibiotic, it won't work. Buying food irresponsibly, produced with needless antibiotics, is short sighted and not in your best interests.

The prices we pay at stores for factory-farmed foods are falsely low. These prices are low because government funds support corn growers and overprocessed foods. The prices of fresh fruits and produce, not propped up by government funding, are then relatively higher to consumers. This is a deceit. Industrial farming might sometimes give us cheaper food, but at what cost? It is unhealthy, unsustainable, and potentially dangerous. When agricultural practices create deadly bacteria, what is the true cost to an infected individual and society at large?

Local Food—Summary

Local food is fresher. Local food then has higher levels of nutrients and less spoilage (in other words, less bacterial contamination). Eating locally is better for the environment. Transporting food across great distances to your table burns energy and produces greenhouse gasses. Eating locally is good for your local economy because it keeps your money circulating in your community, paying your neighbor for your food instead of some distant multinational corporation.

Omega-3 Oils—On the Food/Supplement Borderline

I rarely see a patient whose diet isn't deficient of some essential component. Although deficiencies of calcium, other minerals, certain vitamins, and even protein are common, the diet of very nearly every one of my patients and, as research confirms, every modern human being is low in omega-3 fatty acids. This is an unhappy fact because there is a great deal of evidence that these oils reduce the risk of many diseases and health problems that develop throughout the life cycle.

Omega-3 fatty acids are vital for healthy growth and reduce the risk of premature birth. They improve brain function, reducing attention deficit disorder among children. Elderly adults with the highest blood levels of omega-3 oils, achieved either by dietary intake or supplementation, were found to be 39 to 47 percent less likely to develop dementia and 47 to 59 percent less likely to develop Alzheimer's disease. Research shows that omega-3 oils accelerate wound healing and treat many skin rashes, asthma, some kinds of kidney disease, and many diseases of the eye. The anti-inflammatory actions of omega-3 oils are probably a major cause of their benefits as we see with reduced joint pain in rheumatoid arthritis patients. When they take fish oil supplements, diabetic patients experience improved blood sugar control and lessened mortality, particularly when they have elevated triglyceride levels (triglycerides are a fat in your blood, like cholesterol).

The most widely studied impact of omega-3 fatty acids on human health has been on vascular disease, especially the heart. Eating fish twice a week lowers the risk of stroke by 45 to 50 percent and fatal heart attack by 38 to 67 percent. One form of heart disease, sudden cardiac death (SCD), kills hundreds of thousands of Americans each year, usually without warning. Omega-3 oils lower the risk of SCD by 38 to 50 percent. These risk reductions are every bit as good or better than those we see from using statin drugs, the most widely used medications for preventing heart disease. Omega-3 oils also lower the risk of developing heart irregularities, as well as the likelihood of ill effects from such irregularities.

Among the most impressive effects of omega-3 oils is what they do to our brains. Many studies have found that depression is alleviated by omega-3 supplementation. Some of those studies even show that these supplements are just as efficacious or *better than prescription antidepressants.* Research has shown that when schizophrenic patients are given fish oil supplementation in addition to their medication, their psychiatric condition improves and they are less likely to experience adverse effects from their schizophrenia medications. In my clinical practice, I have also found that patients with very low omega-3 oil consumption often feel irritable or anxious, apparently demonstrating more subtle mental health benefits of omega-3 oils.

In addition to previous studies on depression, anxiety, and ADD, a Dutch study found that supplementation with essential fatty acids and vitamins reduced violent behavior by 34 percent among adult male prisoners.[19] Although I would expect positive effects from all the previous research, the magnitude of this effect, with such a large decrease in such dramatic, undesirable behavior, is quite impressive. Most impressively, the prisoners were treated only for one to three months. In

---

19   Zaalberg et al., "Effects of Nutritional Supplements on Aggression, Rule-Breaking, and Psychopathology Among Young Adult Prisoners" *Aggress Behav* 36 (2010):117-26. doi: 10.1002/ab.20335.l

my experience, it takes more time to see the greatest impact. This study was inspired by a British prison study several years earlier that found that supplementation reduced rule violations by 26 percent and violent outbursts by 37 percent.[20]

I hope this scan of the highlights is as impressive to you as it is to me. However, because omega-3 fatty acids are involved in nearly every function of every cell in our bodies, the list is certainly incomplete.

Getting Omega-3 Oils in the Diet

Our bodies use several kinds of oils (fatty acids). Most of those our cells can make from our food. Our bodies cannot make omega-3 fatty acids and can make only some kinds of omega-6. Even making the omega-6 oils that we can depends on consuming sufficient omega-3 oils. That is because we use omega-3 fatty acids to make omega-6 fatty acids. In addition, omega-6 oils compete with omega-3 oils, blocking the body from using them to create other needed fatty acids and leading to an omega-6 fatty acid excess. Understanding that our bodies use omega-3, omega-6, and omega-9 oils, some people mistakenly supplement all of them. Since we can make omega-9 oils, already get a lot of the good omega-6 oils, and can make most of those if we get enough omega-3 fatty acids, getting enough omega-3 is the key.

Women are better than men at converting the basic form of omega-3 oils (alpha-linolenic acid—ALA) to the most important and biologically active omega-3 fatty acids (eicosapentaenoic acid—EPA and docosahexaenoic acid—DHA). However, neither men nor women do very well at this conversion. Women can convert roughly 20 percent of the ALA they consume, while men can convert less than half of that. Both men and women are highly likely to benefit from EPA and DHA supplementation, to get past their limited ability to create these vital fatty acids from ALA, and to get past the metabolic blockage caused by omega-6 competition.

Ancient humans ate roughly equal amounts of omega-3 and omega-6 oils. Presently, the average person eats roughly ten times more omega-6 fatty acids than omega-3 fatty acids. The bottom line is that we need omega-3 oils because our diets are deficient and because many chronic diseases we suffer have been associated with omega-3 deficiency.

---

20   Desch et al., "Influence of Supplementary Vitamins, Minerals and Essential Fatty Acids on the Antisocial Behaviour of Young Adult Prisoners," *Br J Psychiatry* 181 (2002):22-8. doi: 10.1192/bjp.181.1.22.

Seeds (especially flax seeds) and nuts (especially walnuts and macadamia nuts) are good dietary sources of ALA, the chemical "founder" of the omega-3 family. Some seeds and nuts (most notably flax seeds) contain high concentrations of plant estrogens and phytosterols, which have other health benefits such as helping to reduce the risk of certain cancers (breast and prostate).

Wild game and grass-fed cows can be good sources of ALA; they have relatively higher levels of ALA in their tissues than their domesticated cousins. Unfortunately, as explained above, our bodies have a limited ability to convert ALA to the EPA and DHA we so badly need.

One solution can be eating fish, especially salmon, herring, and anchovies, since they are excellent sources of EPA and DHA. The oils in farm-raised fish, like domesticated land animals, are not as good for you. Studies show that the balance of oils in farm-raised tilapia is worse than what you get eating a fast-food double cheeseburger.

You also run some risks from eating fish. However, if you choose the right kind of fish, the balance of risk will still be in your favor.

Although seafood can carry toxins (especially mercury), the most worrisome problem is with freshwater fish, which have been shown to contain high concentrations of PCBs, dioxin, DDT, chlordane, mercury, and other heavy metals on testing throughout the United States. Dishearteningly, in the last decade, 28 percent of the lake surface area in the USA, 14 percent of river miles, 100 percent of the Gulf Coast, 92 percent of the Atlantic Coast, and several areas of the Pacific Coast were at some time under fish-consumption advisories from the Food and Drug Administration (FDA) due to concerns about toxins.

Studies have shown that a significant percentage of San Francisco Bay Area residents who eat a lot of fish have been accumulating high levels of mercury in their bodies. A survey by Greenpeace of nearly seven thousand Americans found that over 20 percent of women of childbearing age were above safe levels of methyl mercury, as established by the US Environmental Protection Agency (EPA). Men of the same age and both men and women past childbearing years had even higher mercury levels, with nearly 30 percent of all males past age sixteen above the EPA safe level. Over 30 percent of those tested in California, Colorado, Florida, and New York had levels above the EPA's recommended safe level, including nearly 50 percent of those living in New York City.

Mercury exposure comes not only from fish. Industrial air pollution, vaccinations, and dental amalgam are all significant sources of exposure. These figures justify our concern about environmental mercury exposures and our desire to limit them whenever possible.

What does mercury toxicity look like? The symptoms of mercury toxicity look like attention deficit disorder or Alzheimer's disease. Fatigue, hair loss, headaches, loss of fine muscle coordination, muscle pains, difficulty with concentration, and compromised language skills are all symptoms of mercury poisoning.

The FDA has issued guidelines recommending limitations to the amount of fish young children and child-bearing women should eat. The smaller fish, including the tuna that are generally canned (the big ones are saved for sushi or fillets), have less mercury than larger fish.

Mercury and Fish—FDA Dietary Guidelines

Pregnant women and nursing mothers

- Consume eight to twelve ounces of low-mercury fish a week.
- Consume no more than the following:
  - One fillet of shark, swordfish, tile fish (golden snapper), or tuna per month
  - Six to eight ounces of freshwater fish (two six-ounce cans of tuna per week)

Young children

- Consume low-mercury fish ("smaller servings than mothers").

These guidelines represent an attempt to help reduce American exposure to methyl mercury, but the effort to make the guidelines easy to follow confuses as much as it helps. Although concerns about toxicity are justified, fish and the omega-3 oils they contain have many extremely powerful beneficial health effects, and our diets are generally quite deficient. Some fish have high levels of mercury and other contaminants, but others have little or none. Dropping all fish indiscriminately would be foolish.

The following few simple guidelines will help you make good fish choices.

My Guidelines—Fishy Advice

Most important:

- Limit consumption of freshwater fish, especially from the northeastern United States.
- Avoid big fish.
- Compulsively avoid big fish that eats lots of smaller fish.
- Eat low on the food chain.
- Select seafood that is low in mercury but high in omega-3 oils.
- Farmed fish (except catfish) is generally less healthy.

This is a challenge for all of us. If you choose not to eat fish, it is important to work on achieving high intakes (well over two grams per day) of dietary ALA.

Getting Omega-3 Oils through Supplementation

What about supplements? I have found it very difficult for patients to get enough omega-3 oils without taking supplements. Most omega-3 supplements are made from fish. The process of extracting nutrients is a process of concentration. Concentrating nutrients can also concentrate toxins. Independent testing of fish oil supplements, looking for expected toxins, has been reassuring, because of the fish generally used. Manufacturers most commonly use anchovies, sardines, and mackerel. These fish feed on plankton. They are small fish, low on the food chain, so they are less contaminated than other fish.

Be very careful about using salmon oil if it is extracted from farm-raised salmon. That is because farm-raised salmon are too often loaded with toxins. Wild Atlantic salmon from the Baltic are especially likely to be contaminated. Farm-raised salmon are almost invariably the Atlantic salmon species, because this species grows much more rapidly than Pacific salmon. If it is difficult for you to find out for sure about toxicity, simply avoiding Atlantic salmon is likely to be a safe bet.

A lawsuit filed by an Oregon environmental group highlights some fish oil toxicity issues. The lawsuit alleged that some of the most widely sold fish oil supplements were contaminated with PCBs. In light of previous testing by reliable and independent groups, this seeming contradiction warranted more careful consideration. The contaminated samples were almost all fish liver oils. Those are quite different from other fish oils. Liver oils are more likely to be contaminated and often contain unhealthy levels of vitamin A. This finding supported my recommendation that patients limit or avoid cod liver oil despite its long-standing reputation as a healthy product. Even very small doses of vitamin A may interfere with vitamin D, one more reason to reconsider fish liver oils. One tested salmon oil was also contaminated, as I have long feared. The bottom line is that fish oil is generally safe, but avoiding fish liver oils and salmon oil is a good idea. Buying oils tested by outside agencies to ensure purity is wise.

There are vegetarian omega-3 supplements. They are derived from algae and are very high in DHA, but low in EPA. While DHA is helpful for many conditions, EPA may be most often the more important omega-3 fatty acid. This fact poses a challenge for vegetarians.

As with any healing intervention, fish oil supplements can cause adverse effects. The most common problem for people is heartburn "fish burps." You can avoid this unpleasantness by purchasing enteric-coated fish oil capsules. Sadly, many enteric-coated fish oil supplements, even from reputable companies, contain hormone-mimicking chemicals called phthalates to soften the coating. Although banned from many consumer items in many countries, including the USA, enteric coatings for prescription medications and supplements usually contain phthalates. Ironically, then, while ingesting something to make you healthier, you may be unwittingly increasing your risk for other health problems. If you cannot learn whether a certain brand of enteric-coated fish oil is phthalate free, you can create a do-it-yourself version of enteric-coated fish oil from a regular fish oil capsule by putting it in the freezer.

Very high-dose omega-3 supplementation might make some people more likely to have problems with easy bleeding. This problem is very rare and has been seen only in individuals consuming more than 6.5 grams (6,500 mg) of fish oil a day.

I should also mention a concern with the omega-6 oil GLA (gamma linolenic acid). This oil is commonly used as evening primrose oil (EPO). In the 1980s there were two reports that GLA could promote seizures. Despite a 2007 review disproving the connection, the warning has persisted. There was one report of seizures in a patient taking borage oil, which has a much higher concentration of GLA than is found in EPO. This patient was also taking a long list of other supplements. Caution is always prudent. However, with so very few case reports, and with all those subject to serious doubt as to the cause of the seizures, there is little justification for avoiding EPO based on this concern.

Measuring Your Omega-3 Blood Levels

There are two good reasons to check your blood's fatty acid levels, your diet, and supplementation habits. Is your dietary intake sufficient? Are you supplementing enough or more than you need?

Various governmental agencies and institutions recommend eating fish twice a week to achieve optimal omega-3 levels. My clinical experience from reviewing patient' diet records and testing their blood shows this is enough for only a small group of people.

Just like cholesterol, even if you carefully calculate your intake from supplements and your diet, you cannot predict your blood levels of fatty acids with any accuracy. Any one person is different from every other. It is very well established that consuming omega-3-rich foods and taking omega-3 supplements reduce our risk of many diseases and health problems. We have suspicions that other as-yet-unstudied health concerns are linked to omega-3 fatty acids as well. We have learned from dozens of studies that blood levels of omega-3 fatty acids are closely correlated with, and apparently predictive of, disease risk.

Testing for omega-3 blood levels has been limited to research investigations, but is now becoming available to all of us. In my practice, the degree of variability from patient to patient has been impressive and dismaying.

Some patients have been diligently taking fish oil supplements and eating fish for years, but their blood shows ample room for improvement. Others with relatively low omega-3 oil dietary intake and no supplementation have very good blood levels. After years of guessing, I'm very pleased to now be able to give patients more reliable recommendations based on their own test results.

Another concern is toxicity, with methyl mercury as the principal threat. If you are concerned, consider getting your hair analyzed. Blood levels are precise, but they change over the course of days, reflecting your immediate exposure. Although this is not so useful for other purposes, hair analysis of mercury levels gives a good estimate of your exposure over recent weeks and months.

Shopping and the Modern Hunter-Gatherer Society

The process of finding food has made us who we are. Do I really mean that shopping makes us human? In a way, yes, I do. In ancient times, hunting animal prey and learning how to make certain desirable plants grow fed our bodies and developed our brains. As we have changed, so has that process, seemingly much to our detriment.

Food is now presented to us in an increasingly passive encounter. We don't walk miles through the grasslands and woods, tracking game or hunting down the plants we want to eat. We do, however, choose the best-looking fresh produce at the grocery store, but we don't work to select and develop the most promising plants for our future harvest. There are still challenges, but they are light-years away from those faced by our cave-dwelling ancestors.

Our prehunt ritual might still include adorning our bodies. However, it has changed a bit. The modern prehunt ritual of applying cologne or perfume and distinctive clothing would likely have done irreparable harm to the success and reputation of ancient hunters.

Our indispensable hunting tools are no longer sharp and heavy ones. They are now small chips of plastic. We still have to learn where to find the good stuff, but it is all collected in one spot, almost like a beauty pageant with the contestants for our dollars prettily dressed up, presented as extraordinary, even as our ideal. We call these places supermarkets. In the past we had to outfox the fox or antelope or whatever. Humans were the predators. The marketing industry has cleverly flipped the roles. Consumers, hunting the stores for food, have become the prey.

Forget about food labels for a minute. When you walk into the supermarket, you become the victim of marketing expertise refined over generations. I'm sorry to have to tell you, but the truth is that there is little hope for you to escape without spending more than you intended on food you never knew you wanted.

You are manipulated from the moment you step in the door. In truth, the manipulation begins way, way before then, with images created in the media and on the Internet, but let's not get too overwhelmed. When you walk into a store, items are strategically placed to make you notice them and buy them. Just as they pay for television commercials, manufacturers pay to have their products placed at eye level so you can't avoid seeing them. The pinnacle of supermarket advertising, the Super Bowl commercial spots, are at the ends of aisles where you cannot help but see products and fall to their charms, as they practically leap into your shopping cart. How could you resist?

How about the labels? After returning home, your shopping passions sated, if you do read the labels, it is a sobering ordeal. The box of food that looked so natural and healthy, with the dancing chickens in bright primary colors, contains a list of ingredients that would take an afternoon to recite and a PhD in biochemistry to pronounce.

The food industry exists to make a profit by selling you food. Altruism and food quality are secondary or even incidental. Can you imagine a supermarket that sold only healthy food, where profit was secondary? The reason the food industry puts up a fight every time a consumer or governmental organization pushes to improve food labels is because the imperfections of their products are then revealed. Ignorance can be blissful, but it is also foolish. *Take the time to read the labels.* Do you really want that much fat from one food item in one meal? Pay attention to the serving size. Although the government can mandate labeling, it cannot mandate a serving size. A product might look low calorie until you discover that the package supposedly contains nine servings, not one, as you assumed. So, even if you read a label, unless you read it very carefully, you might think you are eating a healthier diet than you really are.

The Process of Eating

The consequences of *how* we eat, of our eating behavior, are generally ignored. That is a mistake.

Portion Size

Portion size is literally our biggest offense, but there are many additional ways we can do better with the process of eating. Portions have grown and grown like our waistlines. It is pretty obvious that these facts aren't coincidental or by accident. With this image in mind, it is hard not to think about the meat industry fattening animals for slaughter. Obesity combined with inactivity is leading us to slaughter. Mountains of research show that without any other intervention, people who simply eat and drink their food from smaller plates, bowls, and glasses consume less and lose weight. The fast-food industry and soda manufacturers, in particular, offer us generous deals on grandiosely sized packages of extremely unhealthy food. Spending just 10 percent more to get 25 or even 50 percent more "food" is a great deal, especially if the goal is to become fat and unhealthy. The ingredients are cheap, so cheap that the food industry boosts their profits even as they appear to be cutting us a deal.

Meal Timing

Timing meals well is a good habit. Our bodies run like highly complex factories with certain biological processes running furiously at some times of the day but shut down almost entirely at other times. These internal activities are regulated in part by our external activities and environment. Digesting food is a carefully orchestrated achievement of human physiology. Eating at regular times helps your body work most efficiently at breaking down the foods you eat and then absorbing the nutrients extracted from those foods. Also the timing of your eating, relative to your activities, makes a difference as far as what your body does with that food, ranging from storing the calories you eat just before bed to using protein to make surprising amounts of muscle tissue during that golden thirty minutes after exercise (see "Ideal Sports and Recovery Drinks" in Chapter 22). Just about the worst thing you can do is starve all day and then eat a big meal before bed. In that circumstance, your metabolic rate would slow during your daytime fast and then, when it finally got some calories in the evening, it would store them while you slept (in other words, make fat) for the next fast. (To learn more, read John Ivy's *Nutrient Timing: The Future of Sports Nutrition* or *Hardwired for Fitness*.)

Living in harmony with the rhythms of the world, fasting during the dark hours, and eating during the light and around active times aren't just pretty aesthetics. We're part of the natural world, and being "out of tune" from the natural rhythms of our world inevitably have health consequences. Studies of chronobiology suggest that disordered eating patterns might increase cancer risk. Research confirming common sense has shown that nighttime shift work raises the risk of colon and breast cancer by close to 50 percent.

Eating Slowly

Enjoy your food by savoring it and eating slowly. The first step in digestion is chewing. We need to cut up and grind down our foods into small fragments so that the digestive enzymes can snuggle up as close as they need to do their job. Disgusting as it sounds, you could eat an elephant if you really wanted to by taking your time and chewing thoroughly. The enzymes and acids are the chemical part of the digestion, breaking nutrients down into even smaller bits that can be absorbed through the walls of our intestines and into our blood, where we finally put the nutrients to work. This summary overlooks the important work of helpful bacteria in our digestive tract, but you can find more about that throughout this book.

Eating Breakfast

A few comments about specific meals are warranted. Study after study for decades has found that eating breakfast is good for us and is one of the most important dietary habits. Adults who eat breakfast are much less likely (30 to 50 percent) to suffer diabetes, obesity, or heart disease; and children who eat breakfast perform better in school. Considering the relatively poor quality, sugar-laden breakfasts so many eat, these findings are quite impressive. How much more impact might there be from eating healthy breakfasts?

Admittedly, many patients tell me they just don't feel like eating in the morning. I have a hard time convincing those patients, or myself for that matter, that they should make themselves eat right away. My sense is that those individuals shouldn't eat until they feel hungry, but they must prepare for the inconvenience of their hunger arriving after they have dashed off to work or school. They need to arrange to stop and eat at that point. There is usually an underlying digestive impairment leading to their morning distaste for food. Fixing that not only restores the morning hunger but also makes the person healthier.

Although the reasons are different, the evening family meal is critical. Research solidly supports the traditional conception that family time spent eating together maintains emotional bonds and fosters better communication.

Diet—The Bottom Line

It is easy to make eating too complicated. Trying to figure out the latest, best food can really drive you crazy. Food really is simple, though, when you boil it down. Eat like people have always eaten, joining those who continue to do so. The Mediterranean Diet, with lots of freshly prepared vegetables and fruits, whole grains, nuts, seeds, and beans, with modest amounts of fish and lean meats, is the goal. Such a diet is good for just about everyone, reducing the risk of nearly every nutritionally related disease. The label "Mediterranean" is a misnomer, because the same pattern of foods is common throughout the world, not just in the Mediterranean. Asian diets and Latin American diets are parallel expressions of the same healthy archetype. Although they don't all live the fantasy of a family or group of friends sitting together for hours, savoring a fine meal and gazing on a valley of vineyards, they do tend to take their time. Eating as a slow and savory social event is good for you. When you set research proofs aside, which sounds better to you—a meal like that, or quickly gobbling some semirecognizable "food" from a container as you rush down the street?

Summary

- Food should be diverse, simple, organic, and local.
- Eating a little bit of bitter food is a good idea.
- Be sure to get your omega-3 oils.
- How you eat is important.

Chapter 8

Essential Health Habit #4: Take Your Supplements

Clinical experience is a powerful teacher. Throughout my decades in medicine, many of my elderly patients have impressed me with their healthy vitality and youthful appearance. I noticed long ago that essentially every elderly patient who seemed especially vital and energetic was a vitamin taker, while those who weren't so healthy were less likely to be vitamin takers.

The conventional presumption is that those who are most concerned about their health do the most to stay healthy, so looking at one factor, like vitamin usage, can be misleading. It is important not to jump to conclusions, but it is also important to be open minded enough to learn from clinical experience. Since I began practicing medicine many thousands of patients ago, I have asked every single new patient about his or her health habits in great detail, including smoking, exercise, drug and alcohol consumption, stress reduction, and so forth—all the way to their use of seat belts. Among those energetic elderly, *taking vitamins was, and still is, the second most frequent behavior.* Staying away from smoking tobacco is number one, but taking vitamins challenges exercise for second place.

- Deficiencies are a problem, really
- Food fortification/supplementation
- Nutritional research confusion and controversy
- Testing for vitamin deficiencies
- Self-testing
- Telomere testing
- My pragmatic approach to vitamins
- MVM supplementation—the bottom line
- Summary

Deficiencies Are a Problem, Really

In this land of plenty, there is hunger. There are also many of us among the apparently well fed who are deficient in essential nutrients. *Many* is the wrong word. *Most* is the correct one. Ongoing government surveys of American diets show that the majority of us are deficient in at least one essential nutrient and usually a few. That statistic is surprising, but we would be even worse off if the government hadn't already required food producers to add supplemental vitamins and minerals to our foods for nearly a century now.

Government and academic surveys show that most Americans consume too little magnesium, calcium, vitamin C, and vitamin A. The majority of us are deficient in vitamin D, the real sunshine vitamin, despite over eighty years of vitamin D-fortified milk. Many of us are deficient in other nutrients, such as zinc, selenium, and vitamins B12 or E. Many athletes, especially female athletes, have iron deficiencies.

Some recent publications, which the popular media have echoed, have erroneously reached the conclusion that there is no value in nutritional supplements. Although the mistakes in this argument should be obvious, medical doctors, the public, and even some scientists are apparently unaware of the weight of evidence supporting the benefit of supplementation. Some of the most renowned scientists researching human nutrition felt compelled to counter this widespread anti-supplement myth.[21]

One technical problem leading to this confusion is that *we can't accurately test people for deficiencies of most nutrients.* Tests that accurately identify B12 and folate deficiency are quite new. For some vitamins and minerals, there are still no lab tests that accurately measure whether we're sufficient in these nutrients. The Dietary Reference Intakes are "best guesses," in other words, and sometimes those guesses are way wrong. Even when tests have been developed, they are new enough that too many physicians are as yet unaware of them. Careful dietary analysis by a trained professional can pick up some problems, but others will be missed because individual needs vary and because patients tend to prettify their dietary records.

---

21 "Enough is Enough" Letter to Editor *Ann Int Med,* Jun 2014, http://lpi. oregonstate.edu/news/includes/letter.pdf.

The symptoms of nutrient deficiencies are very important indications. However, while must physicians know that painful muscle spasms occur when a person's calcium level is low, shockingly few physicians tell adults with leg cramps or the parents of children with growing pains that they are probably deficient in calcium. In the face of these realities, making a sound argument against nominal supplementation for everyone is difficult. Far too few health professionals are trained to identify individuals who, for specific health reasons, need more substantive supplementation.

We know many of our patients are deficient. Our tests are inadequate. Our health professionals seldom know how to recognize the clinical manifestations of nutrient deficiencies. In other words, we have a problem.

I understood this malefic nexus of nutritional ignorance. Clinical unfamiliarity, a mountain of scientific unknowns combined with inadequate or unavailable lab testing adds up to a perfect storm of ignorance. However, it was difficult for me to accept that boosting nutrient intake by swallowing vitamins could be advantageous in a land where so many of our major public health problems were and are the result of overconsumption. We have so many choices and eat so much. *How could deficiency of essential nutrients be a common problem?*

One argument is that *poor farming techniques have depleted the soil* and that now our foods are just as drained of nutrients they once contained in abundance. That certainly could be a factor. Soil nutrients vary considerably, markedly influence food quality, and have changed due to farming as well as other human activities.

Another factor could be in the way we live our lives. Our hurried but sedentary lifestyles and exposures to so many new environmental factors, such as the tens of thousands of newly created chemicals and various forms of electromagnetic radiation, might *increase our need* for certain nutrients.

The Rediscovery of Vitamin D

Certainly modern behavior has dramatically *dropped our levels of vitamin D.* As we're rapidly learning, the consequences are far reaching.

When I began medical school, the only concern about vitamin D was bone health. Rickets, a deficiency disease that caused fragile, malformed bones, was the only major disease linked to vitamin D. Rickets was almost entirely a disease black Americans living in the industrial northeast suffered, and it was uncommon. The incidence of rickets, focused so specifically in this population, was the key to unlocking a treasure trove of new understanding, but it was ignored for decades.

The basic human biochemistry of vitamin D is revealed in this medical history. When we're exposed to enough of the right sort of ultraviolet light (UV-B), our bodies convert a form of cholesterol in our skin to vitamin D. Our ancestors spent their lives outside, behavior that led to rapidly aged and damaged skin but high vitamin D levels.

Many now accept that the reason some human beings have lighter skin than others is that the ancestors of those with light skin moved away from the sun-intensive tropics long ago. Their bodies had to adapt to their limited sunlight exposure. None of us are quite pale enough to live our modern, indoor, northern latitude lifestyle. Due to the weak sunlight, even with the lightest skin, it is virtually impossible to make any vitamin D from late fall to early spring if you live anywhere north of Atlanta. It is obvious, then, why people with dark skin, living almost entirely indoors in places with little vitamin D-creating sunlight, suffered from rickets. Women in the sun-drenched Middle East, who carefully cover their bodies for modesty when they are out in public, suffer very high levels of vitamin D deficiency.

Since we recently rediscovered vitamin D, it seems to be related to just about every disease and health problem we investigate. The evidence had been there all along. Those black Americans who suffered from rickets were sixteen times more likely to die from pneumonia. Because of where and how we live, we need to take vitamin D supplements to raise our blood levels into the healthy range.

Nutrient Interactions

Then there is the matter of nutrient interactions. We understand that our intake of one nutrient often influences the need for others. I have had extensive and clinically powerful experience of this issue.

In my residency program, for example, many of our patients were Hmong refugees who had lived under relatively primitive circumstances in the jungles of Southeast Asia. They were often riddled with parasites. Consequently, essentially all of the pregnant Hmong women we cared for suffered from iron-deficiency anemia. Supplementing them with iron treated the anemia but caused many to lose their sense of taste. I recognized their loss of taste as a symptom of zinc deficiency, revealed by iron supplementation, as they interacted and competed with each other. After identifying the cause and explaining it to the other residents, we all prescribed a multiple vitamin containing relatively high levels of zinc to correct this imbalance.

The issue of relative nutrient intake levels isn't just a problem only when there is an overt deficiency, as in those Hmong patients. For example, very high doses of zinc appear to have a powerful impact in preventing blindness in as many as 25 percent of those suffering with a very common form of age-related eye disease (dry macular degeneration). However, long-term zinc supplementation, in the amounts apparently needed for effectiveness, depletes copper. That depletion also has consequences, so it must also be replaced. Too much copper, of course, can create its own problems. Careful and individual attention is required. Obese patients have a much higher incidence of vitamin D deficiency than others, and there is some evidence that obesity is associated with deficiencies of various essential micronutrients, seemingly contributing to the dysfunction of obesity-influencing hormones (insulin, grehlin, and leptin).

Wild Foods—Evidence from Our Primate Cousins

I was wavering but still unconvinced. My resistance to routine vitamin supplement use finally crumbled after reading a very creative bit of animal research. A scientist tracked chimpanzees through the jungle, collecting and analyzing the nutrient content of everything the chimps ate. It turned out that these little ten- to twelve-pound chimps were getting huge amounts of vitamins, including over 600 mg of vitamin C, from the *wild foods* they ate. As humans are over ten times larger than chimps, the eating patterns of our chimp "cousins" suggest that consuming the recommended 75 to 90 mg of vitamin C is probably just a small fraction of our optimal intake. Linus Pauling, the only person awarded two individual Nobel prizes, might have been on to something.

We have learned that the leafy diets of our primate relatives are surprisingly nutrient rich. In addition to the relatively high levels of vitamins and minerals they possess, these leafy primate diets also have surprisingly high levels of protein. With their veggie diets, primates eat more protein for their size than we do. Concentrations of vitamins, minerals, antioxidants, and polyphenols are much higher in the wild precursor plants our ancestors domesticated than in the "healthy" veggies we consume, *sometimes hundreds of times higher.*

Further burdening the unfavorable side of the ledger, our domesticated fruits and vegetables contain much higher sugar levels than their wild counterparts. Long before we reached today's extreme of adding refined sugars, such as high-fructose corn syrup, to our foods, in a more subtle way ancient human farmers started the junk food craze when they began to breed crops more to their liking. Human agricultural practices, altering plants for more pleasing tastes, began squeezing the nutrients out of our diets from the very start.

The evolutionary hints are compelling. If the indications are correct, if we do in fact need much higher levels of nutrients than conventional standards promote, it is extremely difficult or even impossible to achieve those intake levels just by consuming domesticated foods.

Nutritional standards are far from definitive. One problem is that the standards were created in consideration of the effects of *single nutrients* on certain specific diseases. We know that approach is too simplistic to be reliable, because nutrients interact in complex ways. We also recognize that our knowledge is fundamentally limited. We're confident that there are many unknown links between diet and disease. There is a wide gap between treating a disease of nutritional deficiency with immediate effects and creating long-term optimal health through dietary excellence. *We have precious little information using wellbeing as a nutritional target.* When we ignore these unignorable concerns, what do we know about the likelihood of deficiency, as present, narrowly defined standards define it?

Human Deficiency Data

The World Health Organization estimates that over two billion suffer from deficiencies of vitamins and minerals.[22] While the most severe deficiencies exist in the underdeveloped regions of the world, micronutrient deficiencies and health consequences exist in every population everywhere in the world. Even the wealthiest countries have significant groups of impoverished individuals suffering from nutrient deficiencies.

There is still more to the matter. In wealthy countries, the most widespread issue is the phenomenon of overfed but undernourished populations. People consume more calories than they need, but most of those calories come from processed foods. Those foods have had many

---

22 "Guidelines on Food Fortification with Micronutrients" WHO Website, http://www.who.int/nutrition/publications/micronutrients/guide_food_fortification_micronutrients.pdf.

of their vitamins and minerals manufactured right out of them, leaving consumers with deficiencies of important nutrients.

It is well established that large percentages of people in even the wealthiest countries are deficient in a range of vitamins and minerals. With studies showing that 20 to 90 percent of Americans are deficient in any one individual vitamin or mineral, the odds are that every single one of us is deficient in at least two or three of them. Remember that these figures are based on conservative nutritional standards, and consequently they are grossly underestimated.

Food Fortification/Supplementation

If you read food labels (please do), you know that our food supply is already supplemented. If you know the history of our food supply, you also know that food in America has been supplemented for nearly a century.

Iodine deficiency, for example, was common in the United States, leading to epidemic thyroid disease. Thyroid hormones regulate an extensive array of bodily functions. The most obvious physical sign of an underperforming thyroid gland is thyroid enlargement (goiter). Soil, water, and seafood have traditionally been the sources of iodine in human diets. Much of the central part of the USA was called the "goiter belt" even into the 1950s, because there is little iodine in that region, and at that time, there was very little seafood consumption. Adding iodine to table salt markedly reduced goiters and thyroid disease.

Another instance, which few people now recall, was even more dramatic and a *major public health success*. The nutritional disease pellagra, caused by niacin deficiency, was one of the top-ten killers in the southern United States at the beginning of the twentieth century. When manufacturers voluntarily fortified bread with niacin, starting in 1938, the disease nearly disappeared.

Current discussions about vitamin D fortification are nothing new. The American government started adding vitamin D to milk in 1932 to prevent rickets. As so many other impacts of vitamin D come to light, it now appears that an even more aggressive fortification program would have been an even better idea.

In recent years, the United States began supplementing foods with folic acid in a successful campaign to prevent a common neurologic birth defect (neural tube defects). There is evidence to suggest that this program might also have lowered death rates from heart disease. American blood levels of folates are now two and a half times what they were in 1998 before folic acid fortification began in the United States. Low folate levels are strongly linked to cancer risk, complicated by the fact that nearly 20 percent of us don't convert the folic acid typically used in supplements to the methylated form required by our metabolic pathways. There is also the possibility that taking excessive amounts of folate, particularly in the unmethylated folic acid form, might backfire, increasing the growth of small cancers in our bodies.

At this point in time, essentially every American takes vitamins and/or mineral supplements added to their food. They don't usually realize that.

Those who ridicule taking vitamin supplements don't question the wisdom of these nationwide food supplementation programs, probably because they don't realize they are already taking supplements. Critics also appear to have overlooked studies demonstrating the commonality of many vitamin and mineral deficiencies in the United States, and some deficiencies, such as vitamin D and magnesium, afflict the majority of Americans.

Organically certified foods are largely exempt from fortification. Labeling requirements for organics, in fact, preclude fortification. Ironically, while seeking optimal health, organic consumers can find themselves subject to an increased likelihood of certain vitamin and mineral deficiencies. I see this problem most often as iron deficiency among children whose families eat an organic vegetarian diet. B12 and zinc deficiencies also present common, but not insurmountable, nutritional hurdles for those patients.

Nutritional Research Confusion and Controversy

I'm certainly a believer in using clinical research to answer important questions. The big *however* is that nutritional research is notoriously challenging, and there should be no surprise then that different studies yield conflicting outcomes.

Errors of Interpretation

It is expensive but comparatively easy to test a drug by giving it to one group of people, giving a placebo to another group, and then analyzing their responses. Despite the relative ease, there is a sobering high percentage of published drug trials that have turned out to be fatally flawed or massively misinterpreted.

The challenges of assessing the effects of one dietary element out of hundreds of known nutritionally influential substances and interactions among those nutrients on people running around the world, free to eat whatever and whenever they choose, are daunting and actually quite close to overwhelming. Humbly and dismayingly, we should also add the likely confusion caused by presently undiscovered dietary factors. These inherent uncertainties require that we carefully consider the real meaning of research findings. We interpret even apparently clear-cut and compelling data very modestly and skeptically. Eliminating uncertainty is the ultimate goal of research, but even reducing uncertainty can be a tall order in long-term nutritional studies. It is unfortunately easy for nutritional studies to create more confusion than enlightenment. Some examples might be interesting.

The study design makes or breaks any research and is never more important than in a clinical intervention. Although this point is obvious, so too are many of the errors in way too many clinical studies. The frequency of such fundamental mistakes is amazing.

A study of fourteen thousand American physicians who ingested a vitamin C supplement with a vitamin E supplement garnered attention when the authors concluded that the supplements didn't reduce the risk of cancer or heart disease, as some had seen in other studies of these nutrients.[23, 24]

Unfortunately, this very large and seriously flawed study illustrates many of my points of concern. Strangely, although the authors quoted data summarizing the positive effects of a daily dose of 700 mg of vitamin C or more on these outcomes, their study used a dose of 500 mg per day. They didn't control for dietary intake or check blood levels. Many of us believe that the form of vitamin E used in the study was, at best, not very good and potentially harmful. There are also concerns that vitamin C

23   Sesso et al., "Vitamins E and C in the Prevention of Cardiovascular Disease in Men: The Physicians' Health Study II Randomized Controlled Trial," *JAMA* 300 (2008):2123-33. doi:10.1001/jama.2008.600.

24   Gaziano et al., "Vitamins E and C in the Prevention of Prostate and Total Cancer in Men: The Physicians' Health Study II Randomized Controlled Trial," *JAMA* 301 (2009):52-62. doi:10.1001/jama.2008.862.

and E interfere with each other when taken at the same time of day, as in the study protocol.

These details prove that interpreting nutritional data is a challenge. When data from this same trial were published in 2012, this time after fifteen years of study instead of just ten, the *same investigators* reached the opposite conclusion. This time they determined that taking a multivitamin significantly reduced the risk of cancer.[25]

There are other grounds for criticism, most importantly the supplement used. The multiple vitamin used for the study was representative of MVMs (multiple vitamin mineral supplements) in common use. However, based on other scientific findings, their MVMs weren't of the quality I would recommend. Consequently, this MVM was unlikely to be as effective as one would expect a better MVM to be.

Folic Acid Isn't Folate

Vitamin B9 confuses many people. It is often referred to as folic acid or as folate, but the two are not the same.

- Folic acid is synthetic. It is used in food fortification programs and the vast majority of vitamin supplements.
- Folates are a family of chemicals that occur naturally in food.

Trying to avoid untidy confusion, the well-known differences are ignored by most researchers as well as by supplement manufacturers. They refer to "folic acid," instead of using the specific terms folates or folic acid, for the specific, and very different, substances.

Many studies show that folate reduces the risk of a variety of cancers, heart disease, Alzheimer's disease, and birth defects. There are other findings, however, that "folic acid" had no effect. In still others, "folic acid" actually raised the risk of the very same cancers.

Everyone's brain seems to shut off at that point and fall back on his or her biases. Vitamins are bad or vitamins are good. In truth, the response to dietary *folate* is unequivocal. As I discuss under "Nutrients Are Different" on page 128, many of us have a genetic inability to metabolize folic acid, so pre-methylated folate is the best choice as a supplement.

Don't get caught up in this confusion. The ignored "elephant in the room" is that folic acid is not folate. You know better now.

---

25   Gaziano et al., "Multivitamins in the Prevention of Cancer in Men: The Physicians' Health Study II Randomized Controlled Trial," *JAMA*. 308 (2012):1871-80. doi:10.1001/jama.2012.14641

Antioxidants

Many of the key nutritional studies in the past two decades have examined the health effects of antioxidant vitamins. Those that have shown an adverse health effect have gotten a great deal of unwarranted media attention.

For example, a study published in the *Journal of the American Medical Association* in 2007 by Bjelakovic et al. purported to show that supplementing with vitamins A and E and beta-carotene led to a 16 percent increase in the death rate.[26] The study was criticized widely in the scientific community. One formidable weakness was that the conclusions ignored much of the published research. A reanalysis of the very same data found that 36 percent of the studies showed a benefit, 60 percent failed to find a difference, and only 4 percent showed a negative impact. The best studies track patients over time from before an intervention and follow along to observe the consequences. Taking a supplement for just one day during a study interval is obviously not the same thing as daily use for many years. Bjelakovic's design didn't account for this fundamentally fatal flaw.

A 2011 study, designed to address this consideration, followed nearly twenty four thousand healthy people over an eleven-year period.[27] That investigation revealed that taking antioxidant vitamins throughout the time span reduced the death rate from cancer by 48 percent and death from all causes by 42 percent. However, when they analyzed the data from those individuals who had started taking the supplements later in the study, they found that those individuals were more likely to die from cancer or any other cause. The obvious conclusion is that the late users started out sick and that sick people use many means, including vitamins, hoping to get better. Instead of the vitamins making people sick, these people took the vitamins because they were sick to begin with.

Dosage

No matter how good the design, nutritional studies, especially vitamin and mineral studies, are almost invariably based on one or more faulty

---

26   Bjelakovic et al., "Mortality in Randomized Trials of Antioxidant Supplements for Primary and Secondary Prevention Systematic Review and Meta-analysis," *JAMA* 297 (2007):842-57. doi:10.1001/jama.297.8.842.

27   Kuanrong et al., "Vitamin/mineral Supplementation and Cancer, Cardiovascular, and All-Cause Mortality in a German Prospective Cohort," *Eur J Nutr* 51 (2012):407-13. doi: 10.1007/s00394-011-0224-1.

theoretical assumptions. The most common unexamined presumption is that the amount of a nutrient needed to prevent disease is the same as the amount required for well-being. Keeping your wheels from falling off isn't as good as feeling well. Taking enough to survive is not the same as taking enough to thrive. That would seem self-evident, but it isn't.

The adult recommended daily allowance (RDA) for vitamin C is 75 mg for women and 90 mg for men. An intake of that level will prevent obvious disease in 90 percent of us. There is considerable scientific evidence, including data from long-term human studies, that higher intake is even better. For example, an analysis combining data from twenty-nine studies found that a daily intake of 500 mg of vitamin C was more likely to optimize biochemical pathways reliant on vitamin C.

Probably the most serious flaw in the anti-supplement rationale is the fundamental biological truth that we don't know how to determine appropriate nutrient intake levels. Even if we were to measure blood levels in people, there are mountains of evidence that such a simplistic testing strategy doesn't work.

In their published guidelines, the medical organizations that set those nutritional standards routinely include a scientific consideration of the various means of measuring biological adequacy of the specific nutrient under consideration. This scientifically honest discussion is an exercise in hedging their bets, acknowledging their uncertainty about the recommendations later in their text. When we don't even know how to measure meaningful biological levels, how can we confidently recommend specific intakes for disease prevention, let alone optimal well-being?

Testing for Vitamin Deficiencies

Medicine loves tests. Like any other doctor, so do I. Our bodies make symptoms when something is wrong. Clinical experience teaches us how to interpret those clues, what a patient's symptoms might mean, and what to do about them. Laboratory testing and various forms of diagnostic imaging can and should make the process of health care better.

Most patients come in complaining that they are tired. Anything from cancer to a poor diet or stress can announce its presence as fatigue. Asking for more details about the fatigued patient's symptoms can eliminate most possibilities. Clinically sorting out the cause of a

Vitamin References
Further Scientific Reading

Linus Pauling Institute, Oregon State University http://lpi. oregonstate.edu/infocenter/#

Giovannucci et al, "Multivitamin Use, Folate, and Colon Cancer in Women, Nurses' Health Study," *Ann Intern Med* 129 (1998):517–24.

Johnson and Kligman, "Preventive Nutrition: an 'Optimal' Diet for Older Adults," *Geriatrics* 47 (1992):56–60.

Kelly, "Nutritional and Botanical Interventions to Assist with the Adaptation to Stress," *Altern Med Rev* 4 (1999):249–65.

Sebastian et al., "Older Adults Who Use Vitamin/mineral Supplements Differ from Nonusers in Nutrient Intake Adequacy and Dietary Attitudes," *J Am Diet Assoc* 107 (2007):1322–32.

Weisburger, "Approaches for chronic disease prevention based on current understanding of underlying mechanisms," *Am J Clin Nutr* 71 (2000):1710S–1714S.

symptom, such as tiredness, before a patient becomes really sick, is the goal for patients and physicians. Sometimes an excellent clinician will recognize a pattern of symptoms very early in a disease, making a clinical diagnosis before it shows up as an abnormal result on a lab test. Ideally, that early recognition will allow for a proactive, early intervention that can *prevent worse problems* down the road.

Generally, the easier it is for the physician to make the diagnosis, the more difficult life is for the patient. That is because, generally speaking, the specific diagnosis becomes easier to figure out as the patient gets sicker. Laboratory tests can occasionally make earlier diagnoses possible at times when clinical expertise fails. The high tech of laboratory testing complements the low tech of history taking and physical examination. One doesn't supplant the other.

Obtaining reliable information about an individual's vitamin levels would be very helpful for an innumerable number of reasons. Deficiencies of any vitamin cause serious health problems, often over the course of years, which we could prevent by adjusting intake or form of that vitamin. It is well established that individual needs vary widely and that lifestyle, health conditions, and the intake of other nutrient intakes alter those needs. Again, a test to accurately determine an individual's precise need would be invaluable. Dietary cholesterol has an influence on your blood levels, but simply looking at your diet doesn't tell us your level because your metabolism has an equal or greater impact. Similarly, even knowing the exact amounts of vitamins, minerals, and other nutrients you are consuming in your food and supplements isn't enough to be certain that you are getting the right amount for your optimal health.

In the following paragraphs, I will briefly discuss the most useful specific tests presently available. There are other tests, but generally speaking, they are not useful or sufficiently reliable. Laboratory testing to diagnose vitamin deficiencies is far behind where it ought to be. Fortunately, with the increased awareness of nutritional issues, testing for vitamin and mineral levels is rapidly improving. A couple of years ago, there were indications that a reliable panel of a broad assay of vitamin and mineral status might be available soon. Early testing had gone well. While it has yet to appear, I expect our options to continue to improve in this regard, hopefully at an accelerated pace.

Vitamin B12

In medical school I learned not only that B12 deficiency was a significant and relatively widespread health issue but also that blood levels of B12 weren't meaningful. The most reliable test was very complicated, involving injections of radioactively labeled B12. Because of the complexity, essentially no one ordered the test, and B12 deficiency was grossly underdiagnosed. In recent years we have learned that using a panel of tests (methylmalonic acid, homocysteine, 2-methylcitric acid, and cystathionine) is a tremendous help in identifying B12 deficiency and related problems with folic acid and B6. This panel is reliable and a great boon to diagnosing people with B12 and related deficiencies.

Before this panel came along, I had uncovered a very old and neglected part of the physical examination, which helped me find patients who might have a B12 problem. B12 is vital to our ability to sense vibration. The old way of testing for B12 deficiency included applying a tuning fork to the big toe of a patient to see how long he or she could feel it. I use this test every day to determine whether the B12 blood panel is warranted, combining old clinical practice with modern laboratory medicine.

Iron—Ferritin

Iron deficiency is very common. For many years, patients came to me because they had been diagnosed with iron-deficiency anemia and were treated with iron, only to relapse six months to a year later. They were frustrated and sensed that something else should be done. The problem was that their physicians had treated them based on crude laboratory evidence of anemia. After the anemia resolved, the physician told the patient to stop taking iron. Iron is one of the most common minerals in our bodies. Besides carrying oxygen through our blood, making our blood red, we keep more of it stored in our bone marrow, ready to make more of those red blood cells. These patients had been taking enough iron to temporarily restore the circulating red blood cells but not enough to rebuild their supplies to make the red blood cells they would need a few months down the road. Had their physicians known about checking the blood level of the storage form of iron (ferritin) and continuing iron supplementation until their ferritin level was high enough, they wouldn't have become anemic again.

Unfortunately, even if their physicians knew to check ferritin, most labs list the normal range of ferritin far lower than we know it should be. Sports medicine research consistently shows that athletic performance declines when ferritin levels fall below thirty-five and sleep studies show that patients with ferritin levels below fifty are prone to restless-leg syndrome. Some say optimal hair growth requires a ferritin of close to 100. At the same time, many labs indicate that a ferritin as low as ten is normal. In my experience, most patients with ferritin levels below twenty-five or thirty have at least some symptoms, most commonly fatigue, due to their low iron stores. Some hematologists advocate a ferritin level of one hundred or more for optimal health.

Vitamin D

Testing for vitamin D has become extremely popular as awareness grows of the importance of this long-ignored vitamin. Most people can get "close enough" to optimal without testing, but that is the most certain approach. It isn't unreasonable to get tested at least once. There are several forms of vitamin D in our bodies. Testing for the 25-hydroxy form is the most reliable.

You might want to consider getting tested. However, I have found that there are some matters—test quality and uncertainty about optimal blood levels—you should be aware of.

There have been a few controversies about vitamin D testing and not just whether it is worthwhile. One controversy occurred when staff at the largest medical lab in the United States developed their own vitamin D test, which was roundly criticized as inaccurate. That lab eventually withdrew the test (see *New York Times* article[28])

Although the *New York Times* article reported that the lab had notified patients and physicians of the problem and offered to retest for free, none of my patients tested by that lab were offered free testing, nor was I ever notified. Since that incident, other labs and their methods have come under criticism.

Up until March 16, 2006, the lower end of the normal range for vitamin D was 16 ng/ml. Although 16 was sufficient to prevent 99 percent of cases of rickets disease, the only disease clearly linked to D deficiency for decades, new research was beginning to prove that other diseases were linked to D levels above 16. Sixteen was too low. The low end of normal was then doubled to 32. As more research accumulates, linking vitamin D to various diseases, even 32 is turning out to be too low.

What Is a Reasonable Vitamin D Level?

Most of the time I recommend that people try to keep themselves above 50 ng/ml year-round. In some instances, such as for patients with osteoporosis, I recommend trying to maintain a level above 65 or even 70. Our ancestors lived outdoors. Long ago, they all lived in tropical environments. Studies of healthy agricultural workers in Thailand show average levels over 70, and studies of our primate relations show blood levels well over 100. We have learned that our bodies don't begin to store

---

28   Pollack, "Quest Acknowledges Errors in Vitamin D Tests," *New York Times*, January 7, 2009.

vitamin D until blood levels exceed 50 and that optimal bone formation peaks at around 50 to 70 ng/ml.

People with sarcoidosis, hyperparathyroidism, and kidney disease should consult with their physicians about vitamin D. Interestingly, I have seen many patients with mildly elevated levels of parathyroid hormone that normalized after raising vitamin D intake. In their cases the parathyroid hormone elevation was a consequence of low D and then poor calcium metabolism.

When to Test for Vitamin D

Vitamin D rises and falls with seasonal sun exposure. Considering the time of year, your own habits will help you better interpret and time your vitamin D testing. Generally people in the northern hemisphere have the highest levels in mid to late August and the lowest in February or March. A drop of 10 to 20 ng/ml from summer to winter is common, but exactly how far vitamin D falls is profoundly influenced by an individual's habits and skin color. Some people work very hard to protect their skin from the sun for cosmetic reasons, so they tend to have very low levels of vitamin D. They are keeping their skin looking younger and protecting themselves from some skin cancers, but there is also evidence that this habit might make them more likely to develop more serious skin cancers. Others spend much of their time outdoors, and if they live in Hawaii or the most southern parts of the United States, their vitamin D levels can be reasonably good.

Ideally, testing twice a year at the extremes will provide the most concise and usable information. You must remember, though, to consider more than the calendar. If you just returned from a tropical midwinter vacation or spent most of your summer working long days indoors, your vitamin D levels will be altered accordingly. Similarly, I wouldn't recommend relying much on a vitamin D test if you changed your vitamin D supplementation less than a month before.

As toxic levels of D are so far above the normal range, and as you want to stay above the low end of normal year-round, you could decide to test your vitamin D just at the late winter low point. If your D is low and you boost your D supplementation, it is a good idea to retest to see whether your levels have reached a healthy range.

How Much D Should You Take to Raise Your Blood Levels?

It is reasonable to estimate that 100 IU of vitamin D3 will raise your blood to 1 ng/ml. So, if you were at 20 ng/ml and want to be above 50, increasing your daily D3 supplementation by 3,000 IU is a good guess. It is only a guess. If you are bigger or smaller than average, your need might change accordingly. Your own health changes it too. For example, I find that patients with high blood pressure typically need more D than other patients to achieve the same incremental increase in their D levels.

Self-Testing

The populist nature of the Internet has (delightfully in my view) empowered individual health choices. Consequently, you can choose to test yourself without the orders of a physician provided you are willing to pay for that choice. The best example of that may be vitamin D testing available through the Vitamin D Council.[29] There are many other online labs where consumers can order lab testing for themselves.[30]

Telomere Testing

We're just beginning to see tests for telomeres. This isn't a test of vitamins, minerals, supplements, stress level, or physical fitness. For the immediate future, telomere testing might turn out to be the most "bottom-line" test of all. That is because it has become evident that telomere length is, in essence, a marker of biological (as opposed to chronological) age. The longer your telomeres are, the younger and healthier your body is. Quite tidily, each element of a healthy lifestyle appears to influence telomere length. If there can be such a thing as a health "thermometer," a simple single number rating your overall health, telomere length may be it. (See also Chapter 4.)

It might still prove to be a bit more complicated, however. First up is an enzyme, called telomerase. Telomerase is responsible for lengthening telomeres and might be a better measure of the most immediate changes in your telomeres.

---

29 http://www.vitamindcouncil.org
30 http:::://www.directlabs.com, http://www.walkinlab.com

Another consideration is cancer. Cancer cells hurt us because they make more and more of themselves, prolonging their own life. There have been studies showing increased telomere length or increased telomerase activity in association with cancers. There have also been studies demonstrating the opposite. Stay tuned to this one.

My Pragmatic Approach to Vitamins

You need to make the decision, but without spending hours every day studying the nutritional research like I do, how can you? Remembering a few simple principles will help.

Medicine isn't about theory; it is about helping people feel better. Although we're supposed to know more, and hopefully do, every practicing physician is in the same position you are. We have to determine the best course of action with only limited, uncertain knowledge.

Vitamins are, by definition, essential to life. We can't make them ourselves. We have to have them not only to be healthy but also to live and function every day. With the passage of time, we identify more diseases, many of them nonlethal, caused by an insufficient intake of vitamins and a growing list of other nutrients. Ironically, in this land of excess, surveys tell us that nutritional deficiencies are common. As our nutritional knowledge increases, we identify more nutritional issues.

Consequently, when I read a study suggesting that multiple vitamin use might not be good for children, I recall US government survey figures showing that the *majority of children at certain ages are deficient in certain vitamins.* Please note I wrote "majority," not "many." An anti-vitamin study is interesting but almost certainly less important than the massive government survey. So too are conflicting bits of information from all sorts of studies of various vitamins and minerals. We must put each bit of information in context, considering what else we already know. Truthfully, I find the disagreements most informative, as careful thought about the reasons for the disparity usually lead to a much deeper understanding of optimal health or treatment.

Science Is Essential

We cannot simply assume that our individual life experience is universally applicable and that our linkage of apparent cause to apparent effect is truth. Careful scientific investigation generates ideas and can confirm the real-world impact of theoretical principles.

Reality Is Clinical

The test tube isn't the real world. Clinical studies are always flawed, at the very least because *you*, with your precise mix of physiology, genetics, and lifestyle, weren't in the study. Just as I needed many years to accept the connection between the superior health of some of my most elderly patients and their long-term, self-selected vitamin use, we need to cautiously learn from our own experience as well as from the latest academic research. Common sense always has a prominent place at the table.

More Isn't Better

Just because a vitamin is good for you doesn't mean you should take as much as you can. Anything that can help can also harm. Too much can also be a problem. In this case, at least, too much of a good thing isn't.

Everyone Is Different

The science is incontestable. It is absolutely certain that nutritional needs vary from person to person due to genetics, diet, lifestyle, and environmental factors. For example, nearly 20 percent of us lack a certain enzyme, and so those bodies do a poor job of changing folic acid into the form our bodies need. Individuality is basic to the biology of complex biological systems and must be recognized.

Nutrients Are Different

Remember our earlier discussion. Those people lacking that folic acid-converting enzyme are prone to develop heart disease, cancer, and other problems, even when they have a good diet. Most vitamin supplements contain forms of vitamins that are not those our body uses. Some vitamins exist in families (particularly E and the carotenoids). In some cases, research suggests that taking these incorrect forms or incomplete families may be harmful.

The quality of nutrients isn't a trivial matter. It is a vitally important consideration. Independent from manufacturers, the USP 37 certification, for example, guarantees the following:

- The components listed on the label are, in fact, in the bottle.

- Those nutrients break down properly so that your body can absorb them.
- The nutrient levels are not toxic.
- The product was prepared using FDA good manufacturing practices (GMP).

(To learn more about USP testing, also see links in the footnote.[31])

Risk versus Benefit

If, on one hand, you are unlikely to be harmed by taking more of a vitamin or some other nutrient than you really need but, on the other hand, are likely to be harmed if you take too little, taking a supplement of that nutrient is smart. Similarly, if a certain amount is likely to be quite helpful and not very risky but a higher dose is much more likely to be harmful, taking the more modest dose makes sense. There are some dietary components (for example, polyphenols like resveratrol) about which we know only a little but appear to be promising and low risk. Again, taking a moderate dose of those makes sense.

MVM Supplementation—The Bottom Line

Balancing these considerations leads us to simple but well-reasoned multiple vitamin decisions. Look for a multiple vitamin with generally modest levels of specific nutrients (read the label for the "Daily Value Percentage"[32]).

Choose products with higher doses when science shows that customary recommendations are too low (vitamin D) or individual needs vary widely (B vitamins). Specifically, be careful about very high doses of nutrients likely to be toxic (vitamin A) or make you feel nauseated (B vitamins). The nutrients should be present in all their forms. As examples, a supplement should contain mixed carotenoids, not just beta-carotene, fat-soluble vitamin C as well as water soluble C, mixed tocopherols and tocotrienols, not just vitamin E. Certain forms of specific nutrients are better for a variety of reasons, such as vitamin D3 compared to D2 and the methylated forms of B12 (methylcobalamin) and folate (methylfolate).

---

31 http://www.usp.org/usp-verification-services/usp-verified-dietary-supplements
http://www.usp.org/sites/default/files/video/uspvConsumerEducation/index.html
32 "Daily Values," NIH website, http://ods.od.nih.gov/HealthInformation/dailyvalues.aspx.

Chelated nutrients are more readily absorbed. Avoid taking individual nutrients in isolation, as that approach creates relative deficiencies of other nutrients that are linked metabolically. Make certain between your diet, multiple vitamin, and mineral supplements that you cover the *most common deficiencies* (D, magnesium, iron, calcium, and zinc). Don't forget overlooked essentials such as CoQ10 and alpha lipoic acid. Favor products that include components speculated to be important but unlikely to cause harm (polyphenols). Any calcium supplement will need to be separate from the multiple vitamin, partly because calcium blocks absorption of other nutrients and also because we need so much calcium that it simply outweighs everything else. Finally, don't overlook omega-3 supplements, generally emphasizing the EPA component and favoring enteric-coated forms if you are subject to heartburn. Be aware that most enteric coatings currently in use contain phthalates, so ask the retailer or manufacturer to confirm or deny that. *Quality makes a difference!*

Finally, the most important vitamin mineral consideration is for you to remember that *supplements are only a safety net.* I strongly encourage you to view your diet as the all-important foundation of your nutritional program. As Dr. Frankenstein discovered, life is more complex than mixing the right chemicals (or body parts) together. Supplements should be used to overcome dietary deficiency and therapeutically address specific problems. Popping pills of any sort, including vitamins and minerals, isn't a substitute for a healthy diet. Eating a diversity of unprocessed, local, organic food from low on the food chain is the soul of nutritional wisdom. Supplements are useful and can be essential to restoring health and preventing disease, but *they are never as important as eating well.*

What's in a Good Multiple Vitamin-Mineral Supplement?

Moderate to high doses of antioxidants

- 500 mg of vitamin C per day with bioflavonoids and ascorbyl palmitate
- Vitamin E as natural mixed tocopherols, one 400 IU per day (best with tocotrienols)
- Natural mixed carotenoids, 5,000 to 10,000 IU per day (not synthetic beta-carotene)
- Alpha lipoic acid, 150 mg per day
- Selenium 200 mcg per day

Moderate doses of B vitamins (except folic acid and B12)

- B12 as methylcobalamin
- Folic acid as methylfolate

Vitamin K as MK7

Polyphenols (green tea, olive leaf, berries, resveratrol, and so forth)

High doses of vitamin D3 (at least 2,000 IUs in the summer, 1,000 to 2,000 more in the winter)

Iron—maximum 18 mg per day

Zinc—15 mg if you are a semivegetarian

Chelated minerals

Biotin—at least 100 percent Daily Value

Vegetarian capsules

USP 37 Certified

Not one per day—the well-absorbed nutrients on this list are too many to fit into one pill.

Summary

- Too much of a good thing isn't good—excessive nutrient intake can be harmful.
- Everyone is different. Some people need more specific nutrients.
- Nutrients are different. Vitamins often exist in biologically different forms.
- Risk vs. benefit—if taking a supplement has little likelihood of hurting you but might help, give it a try.
- Quality makes a difference.

Chapter 9

Essential Health Habit #5: Avoid the Things That Make You Sick

Over two thousand years ago, in his work titled "On Airs, Waters and Places," Hippocrates told readers that proper knowledge of medicine first required an understanding of the effects of the environment on health. His considerations are subtle and wide ranging. Alterations in our behaviors, environment, and exposures now have influences dwarfing those that caused Hippocrates such great concern.

Taking vitamins and supplements to improve your vitality is pointless if you're not taking care of other fundamentals, including avoiding things that make you sick. If you are being poisoned, you need to figure out that problem and stop it if you can. If you are a smoker, losing the habit is almost certainly the most important thing you can do for your health. Similarly, you are missing the boat if the organic food you eat comes in a can lined with the hormone-mimicking chemical BPA or if your water is poisoned or your house is full of chemicals that harm you and future generations of your family.

I urge you to think more broadly about the health impacts to which you are subject right now and the choices you can make. No one chooses to live next to a toxic waste dump, but too few of us think enough about the kitchen cleaners or toxic waste under our sinks or the chemicals in the cosmetics we use. Prescription drugs are powerful and also potentially toxic, perhaps even in the very low concentrations that leach into the ground water our children drink and wildlife must live in. What about radiation from needless medical testing, the cloud of electromagnetic radiation we have created with our technology, or the uncertain risks of nanoparticles?

How are we exposed? How are we vulnerable? We're part of the world. Our bodies exist in the midst of an environment packed with other living organisms, natural and man-made chemicals, and forms of energy. That is all around us and inside us. We can change some of our exposures, but even living inside a bubble, we would remain a part of the richness of this world and unavoidably subject to its influences. Breathing, drinking, eating, hearing, and touching are wonderful doorways to our environment. Those sensory portals also inevitably open us up to dangers, seen and unseen. Sure, we swim in a soup of sometimes-dangerous chemicals, but it's our soup, and we're the dumplings.

I'm perfectly happy living in the modern world. While I'm scientifically curious about life in the Stone Age, I have absolutely no desire to live there. You can find such conditions without a time machine, in the far corners of our world today, and most of us wouldn't choose to live in such environments. Those of us living in the developed world no longer need to fear infectious diseases in our drinking water, lung damage from a smoky cave, or even the London death fogs of 1879 and 1952.

We do, however, have our own toxic exposures, many of which we can choose to limit. Many people overreact to these threats—in part, I think, because they seem so all pervasive, and simultaneously they are often invisible. It is hard to take it all in without getting overwhelmed and reacting hysterically. As always, it is wise to favor a balanced consideration of the risks while taking useful and positive actions to make things better.

The President's Panel on Cancer released a report in 2010 called *Reducing Environmental Cancer Risk: What We Can Do Now*, which stirred up considerable controversy. For those already aware of the issues, it was confirmatory rather than controversial. The controversy was really just the sound of comfortable delusions shattering. The recommendations were simple and prudent, recommending heightened awareness and avoiding needless exposures to potentially unsafe chemicals until they have been proved safe. Take a look if you want to get a clearer sense of where we stand. (See footnote.[33])

---

33 "Reducing Environmental Cancer Risk: What We Can Do Now," http://
deainfo.nci.nih.gov/advisory/pcp/annualReports/pcp08-09rpt/PCP_
Report_08-09_508.pdf.

In the remainder of this chapter, I discuss

- Environmental chemicals
- Air pollution
- Indoor air pollution
- Antibacterial soaps
- Drinking water
- Getting the best water
- Pesticides, paints, and cleaning products
- Cookware
- Flame retardants
- Electromagnetic radiation
- Medications in your body and in the environment
- Work and play
- Tobacco, alcohol, and addiction
- Summary: how to minimize risk

Environmental Chemicals

The no-brainer strategy to avoid things that make us sick is to just stay away from chemicals. But chemicals are, of course, part of everything. Chemicals make up our foods, our clothing, our homes, our pets, and our bodies. Chemicals aren't good or bad, healthy or unhealthy. You can't stay away from chemicals because you are a big bag of chemicals. Every cell in your body is made of chemicals. The word *chemical* sounds evil because we hear it most often used in some report of the latest discovery that a chemical humans use for *X, Y,* or *Z* has harmful effects.

The news that we have been poisoning ourselves with some previously "safe" chemical has come to be routine. How did we get here? The simple answer is that our efforts to create better lives backfire from time to time. As we move forward, we often stumble backward. The effects of chemicals aren't simple or easily predictable.

Humankind has advanced over the millennia, using our brains to improve our lives by increasing our comforts and efficiency. Most of the time that has worked out pretty well. We have learned what works by trial and error. Learning is easy when the feedback is immediate and dramatic. A very small child has only to stick his or her hand in a fire once to learn that is a bad thing to do. When the bad reaction is delayed, it is much harder to recognize the cause and harder still to make a corrective response. The harmful effects of chemicals are obvious when they make you feel sick right away.

Most environmental chemicals don't walk up and introduce themselves. We can't see, hear, or smell many of them. We can't sense our exposure. We haven't been told we're being exposed. We have no idea what the bad effects might be, because no one knows and those impacts pop up years later. It is a long way from surprising that we're quite ignorant about the hazards of environmental chemicals.

Many of my patients are quite careful, even obsessive about their exposures to unwanted chemicals. They scan the Internet for stories about bad chemicals, learning about their risks and taking whatever action they deem appropriate.

Although learning and taking action accordingly is important, there is a huge knowledge gap. American industrial use of chemicals bloomed in the past half century, and we have been bathed in an increasingly complex environmental chemical soup. The overwhelming majority of these chemicals are new to the human body. With over ten thousand newly synthesized chemicals in our environment to study, it isn't surprising that we know next to nothing about the short- and long-term health effects of nearly all of them. During these same decades, we have observed rising problems with reproduction, genetic abnormalities, immune dysfunction, obesity, brain issues (ADHD, autism, depression, other mood disorders), and cancers in all animals, including us humans.

Federal and state biomonitoring programs have found that everyone tested had significant levels of perchlorates, nearly everyone had significant levels of flame retardants and BPA, and the majority had chemicals used in nonstick cookware and MTBE from gasoline in their bodies.[34]

---

34 "Fourth National Report on Human Exposure to Environmental Chemicals: Updated Tables July 2014," CDC website, http://www.cdc.gov/exposurereport/pdf/ FourthReport_UpdatedTables_Jul2014.pdf

Many states, countries, and the WHO maintain their own biomonitoring and reference programs. [35, 36, 37, 38, 39, 40, 41, 42]

Environmental Health Information Resources

Natural Resources Defense Council: http://www.nrdc.org

Environmental Working Group: http://www.ewg.org

Environmental Working Group: http://www.ewg.org/conG sumer-guides

GoodGuide.com: http://www.goodguide.com

The Case for Concern

The idea of chemicals in our bodies, chemicals we use to kill other species or burn for fuel, is intuitively worrisome. Human health has improved over generations in many ways, but not in others. A very long-term, recurring study of Americans' attitudes toward health show that, decade after decade, we feel less and less healthy. Is there a link between the objective and perceived changes in our health and these new chemicals in our bodies? Causation is very difficult to prove conclusively. Beyond the temporal coincidence, we do have evidence supporting the belief that there is a causative connection.

---

35   CDC: http://www.cdc.gov/biomonitoring/about.html
36   California: http://biomonitoring.ca.gov/other-biomonitoring-programs
37   Minnesota: http://www.health.state.mn.us/divs/hpcd/tracking/
biomonitoring/program.html
38   Colorado: http://www.colorado.gov/cs/Satellite/CDPHE-Lab/
CBON/1251594687726
39   Washington: http://www.doh.wa.gov/DataandStatisticalReports/
EnvironmentalHealth/Biomonitoring.aspx
40   Canada: http://www.hc-sc.gc.ca/ewh-semt/contaminants/human-humaine/
index-eng.php
41   Germany: http://www.allum.de/hbm/HBM_engl.swf
42   WHO: http://www.who.int/ipcs/publications/ehc/ehc_alphabetical/en/

To the human body, many of these chemicals look like its own tightly regulated hormones. Consequently their health impacts are profound and not dose related (in other words, it isn't true that smaller doses have less effects). In fact, the opposite is sometimes true, both of our own hormones as well as of the hormone-mimicking environmental chemicals. In 2009, The Endocrine Society (the world's oldest and largest group of endocrine-hormone researchers and clinicians) published an authoritative and very interesting review of this issue.[43] Among their conclusions was this strong and worrying statement:

> The evidence for adverse reproductive outcomes (infertility, cancers, malformations) from exposure to endocrine disrupting chemicals is strong, and there is mounting evidence for effects on other endocrine systems, including thyroid, neuroendocrine, obesity and metabolism, and insulin and glucose homeostasis.

That organization, one of the scientific leaders on this topic, continues to raise awareness in the academic community, promoting research in the field.[44]

Vulnerability Changes from Time to Time

Variations in the vulnerability of an animal (including human ones) dramatically alter the magnitude of effects of environmental chemicals. Everyone knows it's a bad idea to take alcohol and many prescription medications during pregnancy. The developing baby is just too vulnerable, and the consequences of such exposures can be lifelong or even fatal. Just as pregnancy is a time of unique vulnerability to certain chemicals, all of us are more or less vulnerable to certain environmental chemicals at certain times, or even at specific moments, of our lives. As our bodies go through different daily metabolic processes, the quality of our nutrition and stress levels varies; we're more or less vulnerable to environmental

---

43 "Endocrine-Disrupting Chemicals: An Endocrine Society Scientific Statement," https://www.endocrine.org/sitecore%20modules/web/~/media/ endosociety/Files/Advocacy%20and%20Outreach/Position%20Statements/All/ EndocrineDisruptingChemicalsPositionStatement.pdf#search=%22position%20 statement%20endocrine%20disrupting%20chemicals%22.

44 "Scientists Urge UN to Take Action on Chemicals in Consumer Products and Pesticides," https://www.endocrine.org/news-room/press-release-archives/2013/ scientists-urge-un-to-take-action-on-chemicals-in-consumer-products-and-pesticides.

exposures. Most scientists believe that at any one time, each of us has a small number of cancer cells growing somewhere, which our immune system successfully hunts down and destroys. A poorly timed toxic exposure during a window of vulnerability can create a cancer or hamper the immune system sufficiently to allow one of these preexisting cancers to grow faster than the immune system can eliminate it.

Consequences are Delayed

The effects of these exposures can appear immediately, as in acute poisonings, but more commonly they become evident years later. The delayed effects can turn up as chronic health conditions or cancers. Sometimes the delayed impacts of environmental chemicals are the consequence of damage to an individual's genetic material, his or her cellular blueprint. Such genetic damages will then be passed on to children and grandchildren.

Beyond Genetics

In recent years we have been learning about another means whereby environmental factors can influence our health and that of our offspring for generations to come. These are called "epigenetic effects."

After sequencing the human genome, the next major goal of Human Genome Project (HGP) was to identify the genes causing specific diseases, seeking better treatment and prevention. The HGP has so far taught us a great deal but not what we expected.

We learned that the genetic difference between humans and our primate relatives is much less than we presumed it to be. Disappointingly, we have also learned that the influence of our genes on our health problems is far more complex than nearly anyone imagined. Every genetically linked disease seems to be caused by a number of genes, not just one or two, sometimes in combination. It is rare for any one gene to cause more than a very small percentage of the cases of any genetically linked disease. We can't then reasonably expect that changing any one gene will be a magic bullet against disease.

Most surprising of all is the discovery that factors that turn on or turn off various genes, epigenetic factors, have a greater impact than the simple genetic code. These epigenetic effects can occur immediately. They can be passed down to children. They can even skip over generations. For example, we have learned that enduring starvation makes that person's grandchildren, but not children, more prone to developing diabetes. Environmental chemicals have epigenetic effects.

Atrazine

The herbicide atrazine has been used for over fifty years and is now one of the mostly widely used commercial chemicals in the world. It is the most common herbicide contaminating USA drinking water, detectable in *94 percent* of samples.

Recent evidence has raised concerns that this nearly all-pervasive chemical is creating serious environmental consequences. The greatest concern has to do with its sex hormone-mimicking effects. For over two decades, North American scientists have puzzled over declining populations of aquatic animals, particularly amphibians. Often the animals have become infertile or developed ambiguous genitalia (in other words, is this a male or female?). A study at the University of California, Berkeley, found that atrazine exposure made 75 percent of adult males infertile and turned 10 percent of the males into infertile females.

Another study provides early, inconclusive, but highly disturbing evidence that atrazine might be causing human birth defects. Investigators tracked birth defects and groundwater levels of atrazine in several Midwestern farm states over the same timespan. They found that water levels of atrazine well below the EPA's limit closely *paralleled the rate of birth defects*. Babies conceived in April, May, June, and July were much more likely to suffer birth defects, matching the seasonal fluctuation in atrazine concentrations in the surface water.

Fortunately for us, this nasty chemical is easily removed from our home drinking water by simple and inexpensive carbon filters. There is, however, no such simple solution for all the animals imperiled by atrazine in their aquatic homes.

Roundup (Glyphosate)

The case of Roundup, one of the most widely used herbicides in the world, is very interesting because of the creative thinking of Monsanto chemists. It has been around for decades, but the scientists at Monsanto, the manufacturers of Roundup, had a brilliant new idea to make the chemical even more effective while making more money for the company.

Through genetic modification, crops can be altered to increase their tolerance of Roundup. In this way, Roundup can kill unwanted plants without harming crops, the plants we want, cutting out the competition and thereby increasing production. In many ways Roundup is at the heart of genetic modification in farming, the rationale behind it, and the concerns about it. Some estimate that for over 95 percent of the crops that have been genetically modified, the goal was to make those crops resistant to Roundup. One argument in favor of this approach was that the seeds of such genetically modified organisms (GMOs), resistant to the Roundup herbicide, would allow farmers to lessen their usage of herbicides. In theory, they could use smaller quantities of Roundup in the place of other herbicides. Instead, herbicide use has instead increased.[45]

Monsanto has made a great deal of money working both sides of the street, selling both the herbicide and genetically modified seed crops that are resistant to it. At this point the patents on the chemical have expired, squashing that income stream, but the company continues to earn roughly half of its income from the sales of GMO seeds and Roundup.

Echoing the all-too-familiar pattern, Roundup was first believed to be a safer chemical, but that benignity was probably a naive "first impression." With the slow passage of time, a variety of concerns about Roundup safety have emerged. This includes fetal malformations, endocrine disruption, cancer, neurological damage, autism, and even a possible link to the rising incidence of gluten sensitivity. Most of those correlations are either temporal (increased environmental prevalence of glyphosate at the same time as increased incidence of the disease) or theoretical (biological plausible effects). There is reason to be concerned.

MTBE

Methyl tertiary butyl ether is an ironic example of our scientific ignorance. It was added to gasoline in the United States by government mandate to improve air quality. MTBE helps gasoline burn more efficiently, thereby reducing toxins in the air. Unfortunately, MTBE passes quickly into the groundwater, where it breaks down very slowly, and can then cause other health problems. Because it tastes and smells bad, many of us can sense its presence at extremely low concentrations. MTBE contamination quickly became a problem of such severity that at least twenty-two municipal water systems in the USA, including the city of

---

45   Benbrook,"Impacts of genetically engineered crops on pesticide use in the U.S. -- the first sixteen years" *Environmental Sciences Europe* 22 (2012):24. doi:10.1186/2190-4715-24-24.

Santa Monica, were forced to shut down. MTBE contamination is most common in urban areas, especially for people getting their water from shallow wells. MTBE has been found in concentrations one thousand times greater than the EPA limit, and as mentioned above, national "body burden" testing has shown that the majority of Americans are now carrying MTBE within them. Fortunately MTBE is easily removed from water with simple carbon filters.

Phthalates

Years ago we learned that phthalates, a chemical widely used to make plastics soft and pliable, looked like estrogen to our bodies. As a consequence of mimicking such a strong hormone, phthalates can cause lots of trouble, even in very small doses. We're still learning about the extent of those effects, knowledge that is important because surveys show that the great majority of Americans have significant levels of phthalates in their bodies. Some studies have linked higher blood levels of phthalates with lowered sperm counts. As the average male sperm count is now at a level considered infertile forty to fifty years ago, this finding deserves our attention. Phthalates were voluntarily removed from infant toys but are still common in plastic food wrap, personal care products, medical supplies, and many household items. (See website for product listings.[46])

Perchlorates

Earlier I mentioned the discovery of perchlorate contamination in eighteen of twenty-two samples of organic greens sold in San Francisco Bay Area stores. Unfortunately and ironically, other naturally occurring chemicals (thiocyanates and nitrates) in some greens, including spinach, accentuate the toxic effects of perchlorates. Perchlorates have since been identified in water samples from nearly four hundred sites in thirty-five states, including the Colorado River, which is the source of drinking water for nearly 10 percent of the US population. One 2008 study found perchlorates in nearly three-fourths of various foods tested. Every American tested in recent surveys have had perchlorates in their urine, with the highest levels in children. The *average* level of perchlorates in the breast milk of American women is above the level of exposure considered safe by the National Academy of Sciences. In one study, the CDC found that every sample of powdered infant formula they tested

46 http://www.nrdc.org/living/chemicalindex/phthalates.asp

was contaminated with phthalates. This class of chemicals is used in fireworks, batteries, bleaches, water treatment, rubber manufacturing, and lubricating oils. It also contaminates some commercial fertilizers.

Among their ill effects, perchlorates impair thyroid function, reproductive function, and neurological development. Pregnant women and small children are particularly sensitive to the toxic effects of perchlorates.[47] In a 2006 study, Blount et al. discovered that even very low levels of perchlorates were linked to impaired thyroid function, particularly when iodine levels were less than optimal.[48]

Clinical experience and observation can help us get ideas and determine what is really important to patients. In recent years I have observed that many of my new patients, possibly as many as one-third, have enlarged thyroids. One cause of thyroid enlargement, hypothyroidism, is more common in my practice than it was years ago. That is the reason some of these patients have enlarged thyroids. However, most of these patients with enlarged thyroids are not hypothyroid, and extensive testing of blood work relevant to their thyroid function is normal. For example, they don't have antibodies attacking their thyroids. After a couple of months under my care, whatever the problems were that brought them in to begin with, they feel better, and I feel better because their thyroids have shrunk to normal size.

What is going on? I'm not sure. Maybe it is because thyroid-inhibiting perchlorates are now ubiquitous in American drinking water, and perhaps something in the multiple vitamin supplement I recommend, such as the iodine it contains or something else in it, helps? It also seems that the size of thyroid glands might change more than I was taught, most notably in response to stress.

Although the EPA has acknowledged that perchlorate contamination is a widespread problem, for years it has been simultaneously blocking moves to regulate perchlorate levels in drinking water. The EPA rationale for their inaction is that regulating it won't do any good. Ironically, one of the EPA's own advisory committees (Children's Health Protection) has been pushing for stricter standards and enforcement.[49]

---

47   "Office of Inspector General Scientific Analysis of Perchlorate," EPA website, http://www.epa.gov/oig/reports/2010/20100419-10-P-0101.pdf
48   Blount et al., "Urinary Perchlorate and Thyroid Hormone Levels in Adolescent and Adult Men and Women Living in the United States," *Environ Health Perspect* 114 (2006): 1865–1871. doi: 10.1289/ehp.9466.
49   "Protecting Children's Environmental Health," EPA website, http://www2.epa.

When the EPA proposed a standard of 24.5 parts per billion (ppb), the chair of the EPA's Children's Health Protection Advisory Committee wrote that this standard "is not supported by the underlying science and can result in exposures that pose neurodevelopmental risks in early life," advocating a level that was much lower.[50] California (6 ppb) and Massachusetts (2 ppb) have established their own standards. As in other cases, the EPA may attempt to force the states to loosen standards, bringing them into compliance with national standards—that is, if they actually decide to establish and enforce any.

With levels as high as 100 ppb in the Colorado River, which is the source of drinking water for tens of millions, there have also been discussions about lowering levels to 1 ppb. The EPA continues to wrestle with this issue.[51] In 2011, the EPA announced that it would set a perchlorate standard under the Clean Water Act, but the level at which it would be set was uncertain, and in 2015 the EPA still hasn't done so.

Instead of waiting (and waiting) for the EPA, it is better to take action on your own. If you have perchlorates in your water, reverse osmosis filtration is the best way to remove these chemicals, although some ion-exchange systems might also be effective (see "Getting the Best Water" on page 162).

Dioxins and PCBs

Dioxin and dioxin-like chemicals (such as PCBs) are produced as by-products of burning and manufacturing, including bleaching paper products. These dioxins are fat soluble, so most of the dioxin entering our bodies comes from the fatty foods we eat. Although this problem is certainly outweighed by other benefits, infants receive considerable doses of dioxin in breast milk. Other exposures, such as damaged power transformers or Agent Orange, are less common but more severe. Dioxins then collect in our body fat, which keeps body levels high for years or even decades after exposure. Aging, increased weight, and cigarette smoking are associated with increased body levels of dioxins.

Dioxins cause acne, diabetes, cancer, liver damage, and disruption of many hormones (thyroid, estrogen, and testosterone). Animal research

gov/children.

50 Letter from M. Marty to S Johnson, March 2006, http://www2.epa.gov/sites/production/files/2014-05/documents/30806_3.pdf

51 "Office of Inspector General Scientific Analysis of Perchlorate," EPA Website, http://www.epa.gov/oig/reports/2010/20100419-10-P-0101_glance.pdf.

shows that dioxins are some of the most powerfully carcinogenic chemicals known. Dioxins also increase the carcinogenicity of other chemicals and block the immune system's ability to eliminate cancerous cells. Human studies have shown increased risks of lymphomas, multiple myeloma, breast cancer, lung cancer, rectal cancer, and leukemia.

Every day the average American adult takes in somewhere between thirty and three hundred times the amount of dioxins the EPA considers safe. The average nursing infant takes in three thousand to five thousand times the EPA safe limit every day. We recently discovered that people living in the British Isles a thousand years ago had higher levels of dioxin exposure than any other known society at any point in time. It turns out that burning peat from the bogs to keep warm in the cool, damp climate generated a tremendous amount of atmospheric dioxin. Although environmental levels are declining, because of dioxin's toxicity and persistence, it is a good idea to take action and reduce your exposure. Limiting fat consumption, particularly animal fats, leads to a marked reduction in dioxin exposure. Successful efforts to reduce dioxins include banning open burning and avoiding products that create dioxins like chlorine bleaches.

Bisphenol A (BPA)

BPA was developed in the 1930s as a synthetic estrogen. Then along came diethylstilbestrol (DES). Bisphenol A was temporarily abandoned in favor of DES, because it was found to be more powerful and therefore "better." The "better" chemical, DES, is now infamous because it proved to be a multigenerational hormone toxin prescribed to millions of pregnant American women over the course of 33 years. More applicable to its current usage, scientists later discovered that BPA could be used as a polymer to form certain plastics, especially polycarbonates.

Since it was developed as an artificial estrogen, it is then no surprise that BPA continues to act as an estrogen in the environment, even when we don't want it to. BPA has led to unhealthy prostate growth in older men, accelerated the onset of puberty in girls, increased rates of endometriosis, lowered sperm counts, and damaged chromosomes.

BPA disrupts the normal division of chromosomes so one daughter cell will have increased numbers (as in Down syndrome). However, an increase in the incidence of otherwise-unexplained cases of Down syndrome has not accompanied the widespread use of this chemical. While that report is reassuring, it could be that other chromosomal abnormalities result from bisphenol A exposure or other problems, as noted above.

BPA has the potential to cause liver toxicity, diabetes, and heart disease, but we don't yet know just how powerful an influence BPA is on our health. As with similar information coming to light about another chemical (DORC) used in nonstick cookware and stain-free fabrics, we need to be aware of the risk, but we still know too little to claim definitive understanding of how bad a problem BPA is.

Three million tons of BPA are manufactured each year for use in baby bottles, refrigerator shelving, tooth sealants, fire retardants, pesticides, lined metal food cans, water bottles, kitchen utensils, nail polish, CDs, DVDs, and so forth. Ironically, as we became aware of the risks of phthalates and moved away from soft, phthalate-containing plastic bottles, we moved to stiff BPA-containing polycarbonate water bottles. At this point in time, we think polyethylene and copolyester plastic bottles are safe, but I prefer stainless steel myself and never heat food in plastic containers.

Dealing with another source of BPA is more difficult. BPA is also a significant part of carbonless sales receipts. One study found that half of the sales receipts from purchases at a wide range of stores and banks contained up to 2.8 percent BPA, 41 mg by weight. This is an incredibly high dose and well over a thousand times more than we find in BPA-lined food cans. If an average adult ate just one of the high-concentration BPA receipts, that person would have a blood level over ten times higher than the official safe limits of BPA (which may well be too high anyway). It appears that this source might be our greatest exposure to this hormone-disrupting chemical. In one study only receipts from ATMs were consistently free of BPA. It is also remarkable that these studies were conducted years after the largest manufacturer of these "thermal paper" receipts, supplying 40 percent of the market, had dropped BPA because of their own concern. We have also been surprised recently to learn that BPA is well absorbed through the skin. Don't accept receipts if you don't need them. Wash your hands after handling receipts. The largest manufacturer of these receipts recently began including small, visible red fibers in their paper allowing us to recognize their safer BPA-free receipt paper. Perhaps this is an insidiously unhealthy side effect of consumerism?

Replaying the familiar cycle, bisphenol-S (BPS) is replacing BPA, its chemical cousin. Once again early indications are that the "safer" replacement may be even worse.

Unfortunately, this designation scheme has a problem. If you guessed the problem is with "Other" (#7), go to the head of the class. There are some new vegetable-derived, compostable plastics in the #7 category. They are good. Other #7 plastics aren't.

Plastic Recycling Codes and Safety

Code Number	Name	Safety	Why Not Safe?
#1	PETE or PET	Single use only	carcinogens
#2	HDPE	Yes	
#3	PVC	No	phthalates
#4	LDPE	Yes	
#5	PP	Yes	
#6	PS	No	styrene
#7	Other	No	BPA and so forth

Heavy Metals

The Romans and Greeks knew lead was toxic to humans. It is still a problem two thousand years later. As the perpetrators of this poisoning, we're our own worst enemies. The ancient Mediterranean peoples used lead in their plates and used it to sweeten their wine. Over time, we learned to use lead in ever more creative ways, forgetting the part about its toxicity.

During my residency training, I had many patients with lead poisoning. Some cases were small children who were eating lead-containing chips of paint flaking off the walls of their homes. Also, many of our patients were refugees from Southeast Asia, who used lead in some of their traditional medicines. Some of them were infants too small to crawl around and pick at the paint.

In 2006, a Minneapolis four-year-old died of lead poisoning after swallowing a heart-shaped charm made in China.[52] Millions of toys were

---

52 Lemagie, "Reebok's Deadly Lead Charm Draws $1 Million Federal Fine," *StarTribune*, March 18, 2008.

recalled in the USA alone in 2007 due to lead contamination years after the issue had first come to light and manufacturers' voluntary self-regulatory efforts proved ineffective. Highlighting regulatory problems in the midst of that recall, the acting commissioner of the Consumer Products Safety Commission (CPSC) asked the US Congress not to increase the CPSC budget.

There is less lead contamination in our environment since it was removed from gasoline and paint. Consequently, blood levels in children are also falling. This is very good, as it is now accepted that lead is toxic at levels much lower than we had believed.

In my medical training, we were taught that a level of 50 mcg/dl was the threshold for concern, but maybe even 25 wasn't so good. Later the consensus was that even 25 was too high and that 10 was an appropriate upper level. By 2003, we had clear evidence of reproductive and IQ effects down to a level of 1. Children with lead levels of 1 had IQ scores averaging 7 points higher than those at a blood level of 10. Much of the impetus for the increased awareness of lead's toxicity at very low levels can be credited to the work of Herbert Needleman, MD, who since the 1970s persisted despite conventional disregard and personal attacks.

Given these declining "safe" levels, the reasonable conclusion is very simple: lead is bad for us, and we need to avoid it. Lead is especially harmful to children, and they must be carefully protected. Often children are exposed to lead when a parent working with lead in some industrial setting (metal workers, soldering) brings it home on his or her clothing. Lead poisoning also sickens adults, producing high blood pressure and neurological damage.

If you work around lead or other metals, wash your body and your clothes after work and before hugging your kids. If you live in an old house (built before 1978), be very careful about lead exposure during construction. Almost every home built before 1940 has enough lead to cause serious problems. Lead lingers in the soil. Wipe your shoe, or, better still, take them off and leave them by the door. Minerals interact with each other in our bodies. Deficiency of essential minerals increases our vulnerability to toxic minerals. Most specifically, iron, calcium, and zinc deficiencies are common, and these deficiencies make children more vulnerable to lead exposure.

A new source of lead is the artificial turf fields increasingly used at school and public athletic fields. The materials used in these fields are mostly recycled, including old car tires. That's a fantastic, environmentally conscious idea, but unfortunately these materials are often contaminated with heavy metals, including lead, arsenic, cadmium, and chromium. Showering immediately after playing on one of these fields and washing clothing by carefully turning it inside out during removal so as not to inhale any dust containing these metals will help. Wetting down the turf will reduce the exposure to the players by keeping the metallic dust in the turf, but then again, that step can increase local groundwater contamination from the lead-laden runoff.

The EPA has some information and advice about lowering risks from environmental lead.[53, 54] As small metal toys, ceramic dinnerware, and painted objects from underdeveloped countries often contain significant amounts of lead, testing these items with one of the various home kits on the market is a good idea; this step is even more important if there are small children in your home.

Mercury

During the 1950s, a major outbreak of mercury poisoning in Minamata, Japan, was one of the landmark events in environmental toxicology. The incident created such an impact that Minamata disease became the name used for mercury poisoning.

The first clue that there was a problem was when the cats began behaving bizarrely with strange body movements. The cats of Minamata soon began to die. The movement disorder and deaths were the result of nervous system damage caused by mercury. As years passed and children as well as adults began suffering problems with coordination, trembling, and seizures, it became apparent that some sort of neurological disease was at fault, and it was spreading. People began to die, some in days; others died slowly over years. Some children were born with the disease.

Eventually the mysterious disease was identified as mercury poisoning. A local factory had released the mercury into the environment. The fish and shellfish took up chemical waste discharged into the bay. As they accumulated it in their bodies, mercury concentrations rose higher still in the bodies of animals, including humans, who ate the local seafood. After the cause was identified, the company didn't stop dumping mercury

---

53   "Lead," EPA Website, http://www2.epa.gov/lead.

54   "Evaluating and Eliminating Lead-Based Paint Hazards," EPA Website, http://www2.epa.gov/lead/evaluating-and-eliminating-lead-based-paint-hazards.

for many years. Between five hundred and one thousand people died, while perhaps as many as twenty thousand suffered mercury poisoning.

Mercury poisoning is still a problem. Several years ago a house here in the quiet little city of Santa Rosa was so badly contaminated by mercury that it had to be torn down. There was no other way to detox the property. Public health physicians, while taking care of children from one family, who were suffering from severe mercury poisoning, decided they needed to test the home. Their investigation determined that the family's home was contaminated with extraordinarily high levels of mercury, which was coming from ceremonial candles. The most common source of mercury exposure today comes from seafood as in Minamata, although at drastically lower levels. By avoiding or limiting consumption of certain fish, you can be safe while still enjoying the health benefits of seafood (see "My Guidelines—Fishy Advice" on page 100 in Chapter 7).

Cadmium

The fast-food giant McDonald's gained unwanted publicity when they recalled millions of glasses given away to customers because they were contaminated with cadmium. Even if you weren't a beneficiary of McDonald's generosity, cadmium could be a risk. The 2009 CDC biomonitoring survey found that 5 percent of US adults had levels of cadmium above that known to cause kidney damage, probably most of which came from cigarette smoking. Of less importance, because the exposure levels are much lower, many plants and medicinal herbs are contaminated with cadmium. This is a reminder to use only the best quality herbs, certified for purity (See also "Safety Issues" on page 260 in Chapter 18).

Methyl Iodide (Iodomethane)

This chemical is yet another instance of the seemingly endless cycles of our ignorance about chemicals we use. Methyl iodide first gained consideration attention as the replacement for a similar chemical (methyl bromide, a.k.a. bromomethane) that had appeared safe, at least at first. Methyl bromide had been phased out from 1991 to 2005 because it was depleting the ozone layer in our atmosphere. Methyl bromide also caused severe lung and neurologic damage.

Well, it turns out that the replacement, methyl iodide, is worse, causing those problems plus hormonal effects and cancer as well. Methyl iodide has been used primarily in strawberry farming, one reason to favor organic strawberries. In a proactive move that surprised many, because there was no governmental action involved, in 2012 the manufacturer suspended US sales. A consumer lawsuit and presumably the company's own internal research revealed a level of toxicity sufficient to engender this rapid and prudent withdrawal of the pesticide.

Air Pollution

Polluted air was probably the first and certainly the most convincing evidence that we were soiling our environment and harming ourselves. Air is beautifully invisible. So when soot from burning wood and coal darkened the skies, it was clear to everyone that something was wrong. In the fourteenth century, the English king banned fires for a time when the London air got too bad. As "death fogs" and less dramatic but more widespread problems like asthma became more common with industrialization and population growth, developed countries took steps to cut back on pollution. Appalling images from Chinese cities show frightening images of just how bad things can get. Los Angeles used to look that way in the early 1960s.

We don't always get visual cues that something is wrong with our air. Like other environmental chemical pollution, most of our air pollution problems are invisible. Chemicals like carbon monoxide, carbon dioxide, nitrogen oxide, and ozone are invisible. The small concentration of lead in gasoline, released by combustion and spread widely through the air, became a major environmental pollutant. Very fine particulate matter turns out to be even more deadly than similar quantities of visible soot.

In the 1990s, the US government estimated that invisible particulate air pollution was killing over sixty thousand Americans a year, mostly by causing heart disease and strokes. Deaths from lung cancer, another major consequence of air pollution, weren't included in that sixty thousand.

The good news is that we have made substantive progress in reducing air pollution in this country. In the past twenty years, overall air quality in the United States has improved. This is most notable when compared to increases in population, annual vehicle miles, and energy production, all of which should increase air pollution levels directly or indirectly. Carbon monoxide, nitrogen dioxide, and sulfur dioxide are all much lower than in the past.

There are unfortunately a couple of items of bad news tarnishing the good. Ozone levels and carbon dioxide emissions have risen significantly. In 2008 (the most recent US EPA survey), approximately 120 million Americans were living in counties with ozone levels above targeted air quality standards. Outdoor air pollution still takes the lives of hundreds of thousands of Americans each year.

The atmosphere, our air, doesn't recognize political boundaries. The great lesson of acid rain pollution in the Great Lakes was that air pollution from other states or even some other country can severely damage air, land, and water far away from the source of the pollution. Today the same processes of industrialization and population growth in many developing countries create deadly air pollution afflicting citizens of those countries. Proving that we are "one world," this soiled air floats around the globe, visiting lesser but still significant health-damaging effects upon the rest of us.

Our awareness of environmental pollution led to the positive societal action required to start cleaning up the air. That success has deluded many into the false belief that the job is done. Further action is needed in the United States as well as internationally.

Awareness of air and other forms of environmental pollution has also misled us to think that pollution happens outside, not inside, the safe nest of our homes. In reality our greatest exposures to environmental toxins occur inside our home environments, particularly from indoor air pollution. That is where we're most vulnerable. Don't tear your hair and gnash your teeth over this reminder that more needs to be done. Far from being powerless, you have more control over your home than any other environment. Once you become aware, you can make massive improvements to greatly reduce your exposures.

Indoor Air Pollution

Several years ago English researchers, inspired by new legislation regulating smoking in bars and grumbling from smokers, measured particulate air pollution before and after the ban. They found that prior to the ban, particulate air pollution in the bars was many times worse than the dirtiest city air.

In the early 1980s, I attended one of the first medical conferences on indoor air pollution. A speaker voiced the radical opinion that radon gas might account for as many as ten thousand deaths from lung cancer each year. We now believe this was a gross underestimate. It appears that radon gas, seeping in through basement walls, kills twenty-two thousand annually, with nonsmokers accounting for nearly three thousand. Only cigarette smoking causes more lung cancer deaths.

In 2004, a very interesting study looked at the effects of air pollution inside the cars of highway patrolmen. As expected, it found that particulate air pollution was much lower inside cars, but that levels of hydrocarbon pollutants, carbon monoxide, metals, and nitrogen dioxide were all higher *in* patrol cars than outside them.

This study was also interesting because it applied a new measurement technique, which might give us more immediate information on health impacts rather than on having to wait years to uncover long-term damages. It might also give us insight into other aspects of our physiology, especially neurological or heart function. The interesting measurement is called *heart rate variability* (HRV).

Your heart rate normally varies somewhat from moment to moment. One sign of physiological stress is that our heart rate loses some of that healthy variability. When you monitor it, the little hills and valleys flatten out. Some top-level bicycle racers use that flattening out as a gauge of maximal heart training or fitness level. In medicine, we're learning about HRV as an early and highly sensitive warning of health problems. Investigators studying the highway patrolmen found that their heart rate variability decreased as levels of pollution inside their vehicles increased and recognized that as a warning sign.

Reducing your indoor toxin exposure is generally an easy and very simple process. Because you spend more time in your home environment than anywhere else, the importance of making your home healthy cannot be overstated. Learning where your risks are coming from is the first step. The second is then reducing exposures to yourself and your family by carefully choosing what you allow inside your home. This can be as straightforward as taking your shoes off at the door and as tedious as investigating the relative harm of various types of nonstick cookware. You decide how important it is to you and accordingly how much effort you want to exert. Finally, there are measures you can undertake to remove toxins from your home environment.

Radon

As mentioned earlier, radon gas, produced from the decay of radium, is a serious problem in the United States. It is also easy to test for. It is also relatively easy, inexpensive, and low tech to remove; think fans and plastic bags. So, there are no excuses. Get to it. The one complication is that radon can also get into your home dissolved in your water. Taking a shower can give you significant and ongoing exposures to radon gas. It isn't a bad idea to get your water tested for radon, especially if your water comes from a private well. If your water comes from a shared groundwater source (as opposed to a river), call your supplier and ask for the results of their radon testing. If there is radon in your water, put a carbon filter on your showerhead. (To learn more, see the link in the footnote.)[55]

Furnaces, Fireplaces, and Ovens

Our days of sitting around an open fire burning in some smoky, chimneyless cave are long gone. Today our furnaces, fireplaces, and ovens or stoves keep us from the cold, but they continue to threaten our health. Burned things, including firewood, don't just vanish. They are never simply gone. Even when they are "gone in a puff of smoke," there is still that pesky smoke to deal with. Burning stuff always leaves undesirable residues, especially in the air. Carbon monoxide, nitrogen dioxide, and sulfur dioxide are highly toxic but invisible by-products of fireplaces, gas furnaces, and stoves. Besides being invisible, the deadly gas carbon monoxide is also odorless.

There is much we can do to lower our risks from these appliances so essential to our comfort and our well-being. Electric heating and cooking are much cleaner than gas. Fireplaces are fascinating and attractive but not healthy. Don't even think about heating your house with your gas stove. Use exhaust fans. Charcoal barbecuing is more fun outdoors, and that is the only place it is safe. If you burn wood or use any gas or propane appliances, buy a carbon monoxide alarm and remember to replace it every few years, as needed.

It is shocking how infrequently my patients remember to change the filters on their furnaces. Way too often a patient doesn't even know there is a filter on his or her forced-air furnace. Neglecting the filter turns the

---

55   "A Citizen's Guide to Radon," EPA Website, http://www.epa.gov/radon/pubs/citguide.html.

plus of a nice warm home into a dirty minus. Besides not cleaning the air, filthy filters make your furnace burn less efficiently. That inefficient burning leads to more nasty chemical by-products in your air. Remember that any and all filters need to be replaced or cleaned.

Speaking of forgetting, let me say that my reminder here includes your water filters and humidifier filters as well. Finally, don't forget about HEPA filters, especially in bedrooms. They can greatly improve the quality of the air you breathe throughout the night. (HEPA means a specific grade of filtration – High Efficiency Particulate Arresting).

Fungi

Fungi (a.k.a. molds and yeast) are everywhere, but we usually don't see them. Some are quite harmful, even lethal. In our air or food, most of them are not harmful as long as we keep their numbers down. Some of us are more sensitive to them than others.

Fungi can also be powerful healers. Most people know that many of the antibiotics we use were first identified as chemicals fungi produced to protect themselves. We have learned that some of them not only taste good (think mushrooms); extracts from fungi strengthen the immune system and have anticancer effects. Paul Stamets and others are quickly stretching our knowledge about the potencies of these humble living organisms. They appear to be useful in cleaning up toxic spills, recycling plastics, and maybe even saving bees from Colony collapse disorder.

Moldy food has long been feared as a source of disease. In the Middle Ages, mold growing on grains created what looked like epidemics of insanity. Although we don't usually think of hallucinations and psychosis as epidemic diseases, when food molds create LSD-like toxins, such bizarre incidents can occur. Many believe that a mycotoxin, produced by moldy rye, caused the behaviors culminating in the Salem witch trials, the Great Fear during the French Revolution, and other frightening episodes during the Middle Ages. As recently as 1951, "cursed bread" affected 250 people, putting 50 in insane asylums and killing several.

This toxic effect is horrifying, at least when unexpected. Humans sometimes intentionally seek the hallucinogenic properties of various fungi. For centuries, if not millennia, before Alice's toadstool-powered trip, human beings used fungus-derived psychoactive chemicals to change themselves and experience the world in different ways.

Aflatoxin is a deadly mold that grows on peanuts, corn, rice, and milk. The odds are high that you eat most, or even all, of those foods. That specific mold, then, is a concern in our food.

In the United States, mold exposure is most likely to affect our respiratory tract (lungs, sinuses, and nasal tissues). Even very low levels of mold, invisible to the naked eye, are proving to have a serious impact on asthma rates and hospitalizations. The warm and damp air we create indoors to make our homes comfortable is even more appealing to molds. You can clamp down on mold growth indoors by keeping the humidity low and cleaning up mold when it becomes visible. Eliminating water leaks, using air filters, and dehumidifiers are all worthwhile measures to reduce mold exposure.

Antibacterial Soaps

Triclosan is a chemical often used in antibacterial soaps, many cosmetics, and some antibacterial clothing. As is customary with chemicals that kill some bacteria, the use of triclosan increases bacterial resistance to antibiotics. Only the strongest, nastiest bacteria survive triclosan. Ironically, the popularity of this chemical as an agent to reduce infection has made it one important factor in rising antibiotic resistance. Instead of making us safer, it increases the danger we face from bacteria. Also, like so many recently discovered but widely used chemicals, it is an endocrine disruptor, especially affecting the thyroid. Over 75 percent of Americans have it in their bodies. There is also evidence that triclosan is harming other living creatures because of its hormone-like effects as it spreads through the environment.

Washing your hands *with regular soap* reduces the risk of the most common infectious diseases (diarrhea, colds, pneumonia, skin infections) by around 50 percent. That is big time. There is a great deal of consumer passion for antibacterial this and antibacterial that. However, there is formidable evidence that using antibacterial soap doesn't add to that considerable benefit. It does, however, add needless risk.

Drinking Water

We all know we have to drink enough water to be healthy, but what about the quality of the water? Like the air we breathe, the water we drink permeates our bodies, taking unwanted chemicals along for the ride. Our need for water makes us vulnerable to impurities in the water.

In his or her very first chemistry class, every student learns that water is extremely simple, just two hydrogen atoms and one oxygen atom. Students also learn that we live on "the water planet" because there is so much water. Many chemicals, both good and bad for human beings, dissolve easily in water. Unless it has been distilled, water is never just H_2O. The other, non-H_2O stuff can be quite harmful.

Worldwide, the most commonly harmful water contaminant is bacteria of one sort or another. These microscopic creatures love and need water just as much as we do. Many bacteria don't hurt us, and some are actually very important to our health (recall the probiotic discussion earlier in this book). We want no part of others because they are so very harmful. In fact, the leading cause of death among children in the poorest parts of the world is diarrhea, which they catch by drinking unclean water.

In the developed world, bacterial contamination isn't as much of a problem. Although we have had problems with nonbacterial infectious diseases spread through the water supply (like the 1993 cryptosporidium outbreak in Milwaukee that killed over sixty-nine people and sickened another four hundred thousand),[56] our chief concerns about water come from things we add to the oxygen atom and its two hydrogen pals.

Chlorine

In the mid nineteenth century, Dr. John Snow fought off the London cholera epidemic by convincing the local council to disable the pump local residents used to draw their water from a contaminated well, and he then poured chlorine down the well. Nearly eleven thousand had died, so Dr. Snow's intervention was one of the great landmark successes in the history of public health.

Ever since, public agencies have been adding chlorine to water supplies to prevent the spread of disease through drinking water. Although different means of water purification had been used for nearly two thousand years, chlorine was clearly more effective and easier to use than those other methods. Adding chlorine to public water supplies is now the standard worldwide, and 98 percent of Americans drink chlorinated water.

---

56   Behm, "Milwaukee Marks 20 Years Since Cryptosporidium Outbreak," *Milwaukee Wisconsin Journal Sentinel*, March 2013.

Unfortunately, a chemical like chlorine, which kills bacteria, can also harm humans. Highly toxic chlorine gas has been used as a weapon in wars from World War I to twenty-first-century terrorist attacks. Chlorine is much less toxic when it enters the body through the digestive tract. It is still toxic, though. A 2003 article published in the *Journal of Epidemiology and Community Health* pooled data from six studies and found that drinking chlorinated water increased the risk of bladder cancer—by 40 percent in men and by 20 percent in women.[57]

Chlorine becomes a gas at room temperature. If you have ever smelled chlorine from a swimming pool or in the shower, you know what I mean. When chlorine moves from the water in which you are swimming, bathing, or showering into the air, you breathe it into your lungs, which are exceptionally vulnerable to the ill effects of chlorine. Physicians formerly recommended that children with asthma take up swimming to build up their lungs. In recent years it has become evident that chlorine exposure in youth swimmers actually increases their risk of asthma and other respiratory diseases. We now know that *if you can smell chlorine, the concentration in the air has surpassed the threshold of harm.*

The by-products of chlorine use can also cause problems. As governments try to reduce spending, community water systems often squeeze their purification programs by dropping water filtration, instead relying on higher doses of chlorine to kill whatever microbes are in the water. Unfortunately, this compromise leaves a higher concentration of organic contaminants, like dirt and bits of plants, in the water. Chlorine transforms those organic contaminants into cancer-causing chemicals including trihalomethanes. A 2004 study found that pregnant women were more likely to deliver a dead baby if they drank water containing higher levels of trihalomethanes.

Chlorine is a simple and effective means of water purification, but it is far from ideal. It really isn't good when the water is poorly filtered before it is chlorinated. You shouldn't smell it.

Fluoride

The vast majority of Americans drink fluoridated water. Excepting Britain, fluoridation is uncommon elsewhere in the world. The theory

---

57   Villanueva et al., "Meta-analysis of Studies on Individual Consumption of Chlorinated Drinking Water and Bladder Cancer, " *J Epidemiol Community Health* 57 (2003):166–173. doi: 10.1136/jech.57.3.166.

that fluoride might painlessly rid American children of tooth decay, leaving us all with "Hollywood-white smiles," was a winning argument.

Fifty years ago, as American cities began to fluoridate their water supplies, only a lunatic fringe opposed the process. A character in the film comedy *Dr. Strangelove* exemplified this obsession, ranting about the communist plot to adulterate our pure American water.

The last large city in the United States to accept fluoridation was Brainerd, Minnesota. In 1984, after fighting for thirty years, opponents finally relented only when the state of Minnesota stepped in, forcing the city to fluoridate their water. I knew some of those who had led the Brainerd fight, including a very feisty woman in her eighties. Like my friend, many in that city had a strong, independent character. They were highly skeptical of any sort of government intrusions into their lives, rejecting the rationale for fluoridation and very concerned about uncertain risks. For Brainerdians, the bottom line was that they saw no need to fix a problem that didn't exist by an intrusion that might be harmful.

Ironically, in 1983 the CDC recognized a still-mysterious diarrheal disease following an outbreak afflicting over 120 Brainerd residents. Since then, outbreaks have occurred in several American towns, with those afflicted suffering symptoms for as long as two years. Although no cause has ever been proved, the best guesses are that "Brainerd Diarrhea" is some sort of infection linked to raw milk and untreated water. As fluoride isn't used to kill unwanted microorganisms, there is no known link between water that hasn't been fluoridated and Brainerd Diarrhea.[58]

There are reasons to question the wisdom of mass fluoridation. One might even argue that those Brainerd "crazies" were the smart ones, asking justifiable questions.

For a number of years, the medical convention was to administer fluoride to prevent fractures in patients whose bones were weakened by osteoporosis. Fluoride did make the bones of these patients thicker. However, it also made their bones more brittle and more likely to break, thus terminating the practice. The evidence against fluoride treatment of osteoporosis is compelling.

An English review of fifty years of published human research on the long-term effects of fluoride confirmed the expectation that fluoridated water reduced tooth cavities by about 15 percent. That study also found

---

58 "Brainerd Diarrhea," CDC Website, http://www.cdc.gov/ncidod/dbmd/diseaseinfo/brainerddiarrhea_g.htm.

that nearly half of those drinking fluoridated water had mottled, discolored teeth (dental fluorosis). American studies find a rate of dental fluorosis of just under one-third.

A 2008 study by the National Academy of Sciences (NAS) suggested that the link between fluoridated water, particularly higher exposure associated with dental changes, and lowered IQ was strong enough to warrant more careful investigation. The NAS found that the water in twenty-five of America's largest cities contained more fluoride than was safe for infants. They recommended that fluoride levels in the water should be reduced or eliminated and replaced by fluoridated toothpaste, as that approach would maximize the dental benefit while reducing broader adverse health effects.

Also worrisome is the fact that some studies have linked fluoride to osteosarcoma, a very rare bone cancer.[59] Other studies refute that connection.[60, 61] Conclusively proving a connection to such a rare cancer is statistically extremely difficult. Questions about the influence of fluoridated water on other cancers and bone health are unresolved, but if there is an effect, it seems to be subtle.

While fluoride might not have much of an impact on the rate of cavities when added to drinking water, it does substantially reduce the risk of cavities when applied directly to the teeth. Topical fluoride is clearly more effective, especially when dentists perform the application. Topical fluoride reduces cavities for children who drink fluoridated water but still have many cavities.

The risk-benefit ratio for fluoridated water isn't good. There is a reasonable argument for considering individualized use of fluoride toothpaste to prevent cavities. Adding it to the water supply and exposing everyone just doesn't make sense.

Even if fluoride might be useful, a little bit more thought is necessary. We first learned of fluoride's effects on the teeth from observational studies of areas with naturally high levels of fluoride in the water. One

---

59   Bassin et al., "Age-specific Fluoride Exposure in Drinking Water and Osteosarcoma (United States)," *Cancer Causes Control* 17 (2006):421-8.

60   Levy and Leclerc, "Fluoride in Drinking Water and Osteosarcoma Incidence Rates in the Continental United States Among Children and Adolescents," *Cancer Epidemiol* 36 (2012):e83-8. doi: 10.1016/j.canep.2011.11.008.

61   Blakey et al., "Is Fluoride a Risk Factor for Bone Cancer? Small Area Analysis of Osteosarcoma and Ewing Sarcoma Diagnosed Among 0-49-Year-Olds in Great Britain, 1980-2005," *Int J Epidemiol* 43 (2014):224-34. doi: 10.1093/ije/dyt259.

of the most popular suppliers of bottled water in Northern California was forced to shut down their plant and alter their water processing to reduce unsafe levels of fluoride naturally occurring in their water. Your family might already be drinking naturally fluoridated water. Adding more, then, would be a bad idea. If you are on a well, you should have your water tested for fluoride before assuming that fluoride toothpaste is a good idea for your children.

The most important point in the fluoride debate is that people ignore the importance of more general health measures. Healthy dietary habits, especially avoiding sugars while getting sufficient mineral nutrients, can't be replaced by taking fluoride. Oral probiotics, shifting the bacteria living in the mouth to species more harmonious with our wellbeing, is another emerging and sensible approach.

Arsenic

The Bhopal Disaster of 1984 is infamous as the worst industrial poisoning to date with four thousand to fifteen thousand deaths and another five hundred thousand harmed. Over seventy million people living in that deeply suffering region presently face arsenic poisoning from their food and water. The problem extends further than the industrial accident. This region has high natural levels of arsenic. Still worse, arsenic accumulating from fertilizers used to increase crop production and alleviate ever-recurring famine conditions is exacerbating this environmental nightmare.

Naturally occurring arsenic is present in groundwater throughout the world. Arsenic is extremely toxic, particularly as a carcinogen, so even low levels are problematic. Government water agencies in the United States set allowable limits, but there is strong evidence that *those limits are far too high*. Individual wells, tapping the underground water table, are just as prone to high levels of arsenic. I recommend that you target two parts per billion (ppb) as an absolute maximum, but the lower the better.

Miscellaneous Water Toxins

The list of toxins in our water goes on. Many chemicals used by industry end up in our water. More than just our cities are affected. Water contamination occurs just as frequently, perhaps even more often, in rural America because of the widespread use of herbicides, pesticides, and fertilizers. Radioactive gas wafting out of the soil can be a water-quality issue. Earth is "the water planet," so there is a high likelihood that everything eventually ends up in the water. When the teaching assistant in my undergraduate biology class told us that the water the people in New Orleans drank had been flushed down the toilet seven times before it got to them, the concept was both clear and disturbing. I was thankful to live in Minneapolis, at the other end of the Mississippi River.

Getting the Best Water

The best water is just water. Plain old H_2O is the best, with maybe just a teensy bit of minerals mixed in. We get lots of minerals in our diets, so the minerals in the water are not so important. H_2O, just three very simple atoms combined, is so very simple. As is so often the case, achieving such simplicity is complicated. The first step is to consider the source of your water.

Bottled water has long been symbolic of healthy water, maybe even the supreme icon of health-conscious consumerism. It is ironic, then, how contestable the wisdom of choosing bottled water actually is. Despite the pretty images on the labels and names suggesting a pristine wilderness origin, most often bottled water comes from the same sources as municipal water supplies. Bottled water is usually no more pure than tap water, and it's often less so. Searching out independent chemical analysis of your water, bottled or tap, is wise. You should be concerned about the chemicals in the plastic bottle seeping into the water. When water sits in a container for a long time, often stored in a warm environment, the concentration of chemicals leached from the bottle into the water becomes significant. Lengthy storage times also heighten the problem of bacterial contamination.

Well water might sound like a fantastic idea, but only if you don't know any better. The reality can be seriously disappointing. A well taps into local underground water. This water can be absolutely pristine, or contaminated by the chemicals seeping into the ground from the faraway factory that closed down under court order a generation ago. High levels of naturally occurring minerals or bacterial contamination can also make well water hazardous to your health. Again, the solution is knowledge. Get your well water tested and test it at regular intervals.

Community water supplies have drawbacks, but the convenience outweighs those drawbacks for most of us. Depending on local recommendations, these sources are often subject to required testing at regular intervals.

You can use that publicly available information about your water supply to select a water purification system for your home that will give you water that is truly excellent. For the majority of Americans, a two-stage filtration setup, using a 10-micron carbon filter followed by a 0.5- to 1.0-micron carbon or ceramic block filter, will do an adequate job. These are widely available, just read the labels on the products you buy to be sure you picked out a good one. Don't forget to change the filters regularly to avoid bacterial buildup. To create the best drinking water for yourself, consider the specific characteristics of your water supply. A system that is adequate for someone else's water might not be for you. What is in *your* water? Even the best carbon block filtration won't remove arsenic or fluoride.

Every approach to water purification has its limits. For example, reverse osmosis (RO) systems remove contaminants missed by other approaches, so one might assume that RO is the way to go. Not so fast. The very common and potentially dangerous by-products of chlorination are removed by simple carbon filtration but *not* by the fancier and more expensive reverse osmosis. Reverse osmosis systems also waste a great deal of water. Generally speaking the RO technique is the best and it's usually needed to clean up most water supplies. However, RO should be used in the right way and only when the water needs RO processing.

Some systems use ultraviolet light to kill bacteria or viruses in the water. In theory, this is a good concept. I'm concerned, though. At the end of processing, today's underfiltered community water supplies contain much more residual organic matter than in the past. Sure, the energy from the ultraviolet light ionizes the bacteria and viruses, killing them, but it also ionizes the residual organic matter. It is reasonable to assume that ionized organic matter might be cancer causing. Ionization creates cancer-causing free radicals.

I was not at all reassured when I contacted both the California and US government experts (FDA and EPA) about this. They told me I had raised "an interesting question," one that hadn't been investigated. You probably don't want to be a guinea pig. Thorough point-of-use filtration in the home, removing the organic remnants, might eliminate this possibility. The commercial-filtered water dispensers you see in most

Toxin-Specific Water Filtration

Contaminant	Distillers	Reverse Osmosis[1]	Water Softeners	Carbon Block	Ozone/UV	US Millions with Excess Exposure
Arsenic	+	+				114
Atrazine Alachlor Herbicides	+	+/-		+		28
Benzene				+		5
Chlorine Chloramine Trichalomethanes	+			+		207
Chromium		+	+			75
Cryptosporidium Giardia	+	+		+[2]	+[3]	2-45
Fluoride	+	+				200
Lead	+	+		+		102
MTBE/VOCs				+		150
Nitrates, Nitrites	+	+				4
Radium	+	+	+			92
Radon				+[4]		20-92
Perchlorates	+	+				21

Table Notes

+ = removal, +/- = partial removal

1. Chlorine damages the membranes used in most reverse osmosis systems. Chlorine must be removed first. The exceptions are RO systems with a cellulose-acetate membrane.
2. It must be certified as absolute: one micron/micrometer filter. Granulated carbon is insufficient.
3. Don't use ozone or ultraviolet light unless the water has already been carefully filtered to remove any organic materials (so ceramic or carbon + ozone/UV). Oxidizing unfiltered organic material in the water is unsafe.
4. Carbon removes the radon gas produced from decay of radium, but not radium itself. Carbon must also be changed regularly to avoid increasingly high levels of radioactivity trapped in the carbon.

stores rely on this technology, so I recommend avoiding them, at least for the time being.

To learn more about the contaminants that are likely to be in your water and how to remove them, the Environmental Working Group's website is a practical and useful information reference. As it includes data even from extremely small water suppliers, it helps you find and interpret reports on your water. That site also helps you choose the correct water purification for your needs. Sadly, the site needs updating, but it still gives you a sense of local water concerns, and I've yet to find another with more useful information.[62]

Although less easy to navigate, minimally interactive, and essentially online brochures, the EPA websites are very informative. I highly recommend exploring them.[63, 64]

Pesticides, Paints, and Cleaning Products

Some indoor poisons shout out their toxicity. When fumes from paints and cleaning products burn your nostrils and make your eyes water, there is no doubt that you should be somewhere else. Similarly when an insect curls up and dies moments after you squirt it with a pesticide, little insight is needed to comprehend that the chemicals in that spray aren't good for other living creatures, like you for example.

The reason that these chemicals are so obviously toxic is because they are highly volatile (in other words, they move from liquid into the air rapidly), and once they are in the air, they make the air smell bad. We use the term VOCs (volatile organic compounds) to refer to these chemicals. VOCs are toxic in just about every way imaginable. They irritate our respiratory tracts and cause rashes, digestive symptoms, and neurological damage. They cause cancer.

Staying away from VOCs is clearly an excellent idea and relatively easy to accomplish. Avoid them in the first place by choosing safer products. Use the Internet to learn about options to VOCs. If you feel you must use them, buy products with the lowest levels, such as "low VOC" paints.

62 "EWG National Drinking Water Database," Environmental Working Group website, http://www.ewg.org/tap-water/.

63 "Drinking Water Data & Databases," EPA website, http://water.epa.gov/scitech/datait/databases/drink/.

64 "Local Drinking Water Information," EPA website, http://water.epa.gov/drink/local/index.cfm.

Use them in the smallest amounts you can and in the safest way possible. Don't get them on your skin. Use them in very well-ventilated spaces. Use a respirator. Dispose of them safely. That way no one, including you and your neighbors (humans, animals, insects, and fish) will come to harm.

As so many products have undesirable chemicals in them, a simple "smell test" can be a handy warning. I'm sure you've purchased some item (shoes, electronic equipment, a new mattress, or even a car) that came with an unpleasant chemical smell. When you notice that, do something about it. Park the new running shoes, TV, or whatever out in the garage until it smells less. Sniff the mattress in the store. If it smells weird, think hard about whether you want to inhale those aromatic chemicals eight hours a day for the next several years.

Heat makes these chemicals move into the air more quickly. When I see patients suffering ill effects from the chemicals of new construction (carpeting, curtains, or building materials), I remind them to run air filters and also to use the properties of the chemicals to reduce their exposure.

If you use VOCs, turn up the heat, leave, and before you settle back in, crank up the fans, blowing out the room air. This approach will move the chemicals out of your immediate environment a bit quicker.

Bugs can really be annoying. Describing something as "bugging" you is a natural outgrowth of human experience and universally understood. I'm sure all of you have images of someone you know, often an older man, walking around his home or property with some sort of aerosolized bug spray, hunting down his tormenters. Other options exist, including ultrasonic repellents and chemicals derived from the insect repellents produced by plants. Do him a favor. Hide the bug spray and teach him some safer options.

Cookware

Nonstick cookware is a nice idea to improve the quality of our lives by relieving the drudgery of cleaning while making tasty food for the smiling family. Unfortunately, reality is again harsh. Like the chemicals that make fabrics stain resistant, the chemicals (PTFE) that keep food from sticking to pots and pans tend to be harmful. Year after year, cookware manufacturers promote their "new and advanced" materials as the latest breakthrough. Then those pronouncements are soon followed by new research showing that the materials are not quite so perfect because they

Household Product Safety Information

US Department of Health and Human Services, Household Products Database, http://hpd.nlm.nih.gov/

Environmental Working Group, Guide to Household Cleaners, http://www.ewg.org/guides/cleaners

Healthy Stuff, http://www.healthystuff.org

are associated with health risks. With these continuing cycles of excitement and disappointment, skepticism should be at the top of the menu.

Canaries were used to monitor toxic gasses in mines. The birds were more sensitive to the toxins than the miners were. So if the canary was okay, the miners should also be fine.

Although the nature of the work is different, songbirds, like canaries, can teach us about the safety of our pots and pans. When a company comes out with a new nonstick coating, promising this one is truly safe, one way I investigate its safety is by scouring the Internet for reports from bird owners. To be nontoxic, these chemicals need to be stable. We want them to stay in the pots and not end up inside us. If a nonstick coating is truly stable and nontoxic, it won't vaporize into kitchen air. Bird owners are quick to discover whether they do. Their birds don't develop vague long-term symptoms; they die. I then have no interest in participating in a long-term human toxicology experiment (in other words, cooking with this material).

A close chemical cousin, perfluorooctanoic acid (PFOA), is a by-product of manufacturing nonstick chemicals like Teflon. PFOA is also produced when our bodies try to rid themselves of various nonstick coating chemicals accidentally consumed in our food. PFOA persists in the environment and is yet another endocrine disruptor, affecting the thyroid and reproductive organs as well as being carcinogenic and causing kidney damage. It is also used to line microwave popcorn bags as well as to make carpeting and clothing stain resistant. *About 98 percent of Americans have PFOAs in their blood.*

PFOA also appears to suppress immune function. A Danish study of Faroe Islanders found that children with higher levels of PFOA in their blood don't acquire immune protection from vaccinations as well as other children. Those "higher" levels are still very, very low and lower than that found in the blood of an average American. This also raises a warning flag. Might these chemicals then lead to other immune dysfunctions such as allergies, asthma, or even autoimmune disease?

As nonstick materials aren't really getting safer, there is a lot to be said for old-style cookware. For example, many adolescent females and health-conscious adult women are iron deficient. Cooking in cast-iron pans and eating acidic foods like tomatoes can add a significant contribution to your daily iron intake. A properly seasoned cast-iron pan is effectively nonstick as long as you don't turn the heat up too high and do clean the pan properly. As those are the same restrictions advised for nonstick cookware, the only significant hardship is the weight of the pans. While they don't give you any supplemental iron, I also like enamel-clad cast-iron pots and pans as a less sticky choice.

Flame Retardants

In this book I have gone over a number of unwanted health effects arising from our use of fire. Those are all subtle in contrast to the damage fire causes when it burns our homes or us. It was said that the punishment Prometheus endured for bringing the gift of fire to humanity was to have an eagle pick away his liver each day and then regrow it each night. Prometheus was not the only one to suffer the consequences of his gift.

I worked in a burn center for many years, treating the most severely injured patients. It was very difficult work because the patients, who were fortunate enough to survive, endured extreme pain, long-term rehabilitation, and often a lifetime of disfigurement. Many didn't survive. I am extremely sympathetic to all approaches one might take to prevent such horrors. Unfortunately, chemical flame retardants are badly flawed, harming us in exchange for their protection against fire.

The class of chemicals used most widely as fire retardants are polybrominated diphenyl esters (PBDEs). Used with this intent for over thirty years, these chemicals have spread throughout the environment, with PBDEs now detectable in the blood of nearly all Americans. We learned nearly as long ago that they put us at risk for liver, thyroid, neurological, and hormone-related diseases. Because of high concentrations of PBDEs in household dust, blood levels in children, especially toddlers, are much higher than in adults. Unfortunately children are also more vulnerable to the ill effects of PBDEs. Studies have shown that the average American has blood levels of PBDEs that are ten to seventy-five times higher than levels in Europeans, where they are banned. Californians lead the way with average levels two hundred times higher than those found in Europeans.

Like so many toxic chemicals, PBDEs accumulate in breast milk. The discovery that PBDEs had increased sixtyfold in the breast milk of Swedish women between 1972 and 1997 was the shock that led to a European ban on PBDEs.

A UC Berkeley study linked women's PBDE blood levels with their inability to become pregnant. Every tenfold increase in blood levels of PBDEs was associated with a 30 percent decreased likelihood of achieving pregnancy each month.

The most commonly used high-quality padding used in furniture is flexible polyurethane foam, which can be over one-third PBDE. Two forms of PBDEs, as well as some similar chemicals, have already been banned from American-made products, and eight states currently ban some PBDEs. However, they continue to enter our bodies from imported and American products as well as from some foods (meat and poultry). PBDEs are slow to biodegrade, so they linger in our bodies and in the environment.

Other products, mostly TBBPA (tetrabromobisphenol-A) and HBCD (hexabromocyclododecane) are increasingly used to replace PBDEs. However, they inevitably, it seems, carry their own significant risks. HBCD was recently shown to promote dramatic weight gain (30 percent more than controls) among mice exposed to the chemical. As this is an endocrine-disrupting effect, other hormonal damages should be expected.

Electromagnetic Radiation

If VOCs, with their noxious odors, are at the brightly visible end of the perceptible-harm spectrum, electromagnetic radiation (EMR) is probably at the other end. We spend our lives immersed in energy fields of all sorts, from the magnetic fields created by the earth and sun to those created by human technology. Also, like all other living cells, our bodies use electromagnetic energy for even the most basic functions. Some electromagnetic radiation, such as sunlight, is easy to see (and in fact is essential), but visible light is just a tiny part of the spectrum of electromagnetic radiation. The subtle but all-pervasive nature of electromagnetism in the environment and our tissues makes it extremely difficult to determine short- and long-term effects on our health both positively and negatively.

Marie Curie made many pioneering and enlightening discoveries in the field of electromagnetic radiation, specifically ionizing radiation. Sadly, one of her discoveries was the accidental finding that such radiation is lethal to humans. She died from radiation-induced aplastic anemia, a disease in which bone marrow stops making blood cells. The horrors of Hiroshima and Nagasaki also should have made us frightfully cautious. They didn't. Since we were slow to learn the lessons of radiation toxicity, in the following decades, US soldiers were purposefully marched into atomic tests, and American children had their feet measured using x-rays in shoe stores and their acne and fungal infections treated by "therapeutic" radiation in doctor's offices.

As they say, hindsight is twenty-twenty. That is true only if we learn the lesson in full. Nuclear disasters such as Chernobyl and Fukushima highlight the incredibly high risk our technological incompetence is and the eons before these and other sites that will no longer threaten the health of humans and the environment.

Shouldn't we also approach other forms of electromagnetic radiation with a certain degree of caution, humbled by the mistakes of the past? Thirty-five years ago I remember asking my mentor what he knew about the health effects of microwave ovens. His response was that there was a big experiment in progress. He meant the microwave-using US populace. I chose to sit out the test and waited many years to start using microwaves. Now we know better how to use microwaves: test them periodically for leaks, limit the loss of nutrients by keeping cooking times short, and minimize the water added. Of course, the very best approach is to take time to prepare excellent food instead of using a microwave to "nuke" processed foods.

Our passion for electronic devices increasingly consumes us. One must question whether there might not be adverse health consequences down the road. It is naive to assume there won't be any.

The question of whether cell phones cause cancer is probably *the* technological cancer controversy of recent years. Over two thousand studies have been published in the medical literature related to health effects of cell phones. Many of those studies weren't about distracted drivers. They were investigations of the effects of the radiation exposure cell phones create. Many of them have been studies at the tissue level, showing that such radiation can alter cells. Several human studies suggest a significantly increased risk of brain tumors. More specifically, some of those studies have found an increased risk of tumors of the type, and in the locations, speculated to be most powerfully affected by electromagnetic radiation from cell phones. There are also many other studies showing no increased risks of cancer from cell phone usage. The bottom line is that the matter is unresolved at present.

The next step then is to decide what to do in that state of fretful uncertainty. My opinion is that there is sufficient justification to be cautious and limit your exposure to all forms of electromagnetic radiation. Turning off unused electrical devices is good for the environment and probably also for you. Stay as far away from these things as you can. Check your microwave to make sure it isn't leaking. Electric fans are relatively low tech, but they make big electromagnetic fields.

When buying a new phone, look up the specific absorption rate (SAR) value on those you are considering and favor those with lower SAR values. Use a corded earpiece to keep the phone away from your head and reduce your exposure. One company (Pong Research) accepted the scientific reality that we can't simply erase a phone's electromagnet radiation and has developed a case that redirects the phone's EMR away from the user's head.

For nearly all of us, our most intense electromagnet radiation exposure will occur in a health-care setting, especially x-rays and CT scans. There are even some, at this time minor, questions about the effects of MRI, mostly connected to the heating of cellular tissue created by MRI. Limit the medical imaging you and your family undergo. Ask your doctors, "Is this test necessary? How will the test results change what we do? Is there another diagnostic option?" (Also see "Thoughts on Prevention—A Stitch in Time Saves Nine, or Not" on page 33 in Chapter 3.)

Food Additives

Avoiding things that can harm you has to cover everything you put in your body, including food additives. The first point to remember is that artificial flavors, colors, and preservatives aren't food. Salt, the first food natural additive, has been used to prolong the shelf life of food since way before humans had shelves. Even an essential like salt has become a problem for some, because they eat huge quantities of processed food, containing way more salt than they need. Other additives, especially those with impossible-to-pronounce chemical names, are just plain nasty. They are obvious on the label, and you should follow your gut's inclination to avoid such weird-sounding chemicals.

Why worry about them? Some problems created by some food additives are immediate and clear. Sulfites, added to foods to keep them from turning an unattractive brown, commonly trigger asthma, diarrhea, and allergy symptoms. Most often the effects of food additives are more insidious. Like other environmental chemicals, prolonged exposure, even at low levels, can generate bad health consequences. As food additives are so widely used, prolonged, low-level exposures are common, even the rule. Also, the lack of dramatic and sudden effects makes such long-term exposures extremely difficult to study. Falling rain will wash away a mountain, but we can't usually see this process as it happens. The effects are dramatic but not obvious, particularly when so many choose to look the other way, presuming that ill effects are impossible.

Sweeteners like high-fructose corn syrup, aspartame, acesulfame K, saccharin, and sucralose are all linked to adverse health effects of varying severity. Cancers and damage to the nervous system, liver, and kidneys have all been documented as potential risks. Plain old sugar isn't so great for you, but it is a better than these alternatives. I sometimes quite selectively recommend xylitol a "sugar alcohol" as an alternative for diabetics. Sorbitol is another of those, but it has a undesirable tendency to create gas in those who consume it.

The bottom line is simple. Eating fresh, attractive food is good for you. If it needs preservatives, colorants, or sweeteners to be appealing, you are being deceived and possibly putting yourself in harm's way if you eat it. Don't waste your money or your health that way. (See also Chapter 7).

Cosmetics

We are vulnerable to hazardous chemicals in personal care items, such as cosmetics, partly because we can't just say no. Any anthropologist can testify that human beings have always adorned their bodies. Some in fact claim that this habit is a defining characteristic, separating humans from animals. The desire to look good is instinctual. In their very first session learning how to examine patients, medical students are taught to comment on the patient's hygiene and clothing. That certainly isn't because doctors are fashionistas. Neglecting one's appearance is usually a reliable reflection of ill health, either mentally or physically.

We apply so much of this stuff directly to our skin, the risk of toxic effects is relatively high. We can suffer local reactions akin to poison oak or ivy, such as contact dermatitis, even when the offending substance is completely natural. Systemic absorption of harmful chemicals in cosmetics is an important issue as are concerns about the latest nano-technology widely used in body care products.

Treating patients with contact dermatitis, I learned that US companies are allowed to keep some of the ingredients in their products secret to protect their commercial interests. With so many chemicals in personal care products, it can be quite a challenge to identify whatever it is that is causing the patient's problem and then just as difficult to determine which products contain the offending chemical.

For example, a patient with an underarm rash related to deodorants tested positive for sensitivity to cinnamon and cinnamon-like chemicals. This also accounted for the patient's occasional mouth and lip soreness. Although we think of cinnamon as a widely used flavor, it is also nearly ubiquitous in fragrance mixes. Consequently, this patient and others who are sensitive to cinnamon must avoid all cosmetics using fragrances to avoid contact with cinnamon. Cinnamon is seldom listed when it is present because there is no government requirement to do so, and products labeled as "unscented" are not fragrance free. That fact defies common sense, of course, but the disconnect between common sense and labeling is frustratingly familiar to us all.

Hormone-mimicking chemicals such as phthalates are used in many cosmetics, as phthalates make cosmetics spread smoothly over the skin. They have been frightfully common in lipsticks and are then highly absorbed into the person's body. Lead and chemicals known to cause cancer and liver and nerve damage are found in many of the most popular cosmetics. It is difficult to imagine a more perfect way to maximize our risks than to apply them to our lips and other skin surfaces.

Nanotechnology

This is a good point to discuss nanotechnology because nano-chemicals have very rapidly become ubiquitous throughout the cosmetic industry.

The word *nano* means little, dwarfed, or small. It typically refers to particles, materials, and technology distinguished by their extremely small size. To get a sense of the relative size of nano-products and learn more, visit the US government nanotech website.[65]

Since 1990, when there were only a handful of patents and almost no scientific articles on nanotechnology, the incredibly small has become incredibly big. There are now thousands of each annually. The excitement and the fear generated by nanotechnology, just like previous cutting-edge technologies, border on hysteria. Typically, such extremity of opinion is an outgrowth of current ignorance. As the facts become better known, we approach consensus.

The potential applications of nanotechnology are absolutely revolutionary. In health care alone, nanotechnology could lead to safer and more effective medications and unique materials for diagnosis and imaging. It is possible that we might be even able to *repair* defective genes, reaching even beyond our recent aspirations to replace defective genes.

Nanotechnological products are widely used. The reason sunscreens no longer look like white paste is nanotechnology. Many nutritional supplements are available in highly absorbable nano-forms. The technology is being used to make clothing and automobile paints more resistant to stains and damage. Sporting goods such as golf clubs, tennis rackets, and fly rods use nano-materials. In addition to sunscreens, nano-materials are now used in every category of cosmetic and personal care products.

The key to understanding nano-materials is to understand that size does make a difference, a big one. Describing the size-induced changes in the realm of nanoparticles, Dr. Chad Mirkin, the Director of the In-

---

65 "Size of the Nanoscale," National Nanotechnology Initiative website, http://www.nano.gov/nanotech-101/what/nano-size.

stitute for Nanotechnology at Northwestern University, told the *New York Times* that "everything, regardless of what it is, has new properties."[66]

Materials behave profoundly differently when they are dramatically smaller, including a material as simple as paint. Medieval artisans were unwitting nanotechnologists when they mixed a form of gold with molten glass, producing a red pigment from the gold. Gold was no longer gold. Gold became red.

Once you grasp that even our most basic understanding of the characteristics of a material (color, electric charge, and melting temperature) fly out the window, it is easy to see why so many are anxious about the uncertain effects of widespread nanotechnology. The nano-world is effectively an alternate reality with very different rules, very few of which we have learned so far. These particles are so small that they can slip through the membrane wall of every cell in our bodies, most often in a manner that kills the cells. In the February 2009 issue of *Nanomedicine*, scientists from the University of Minnesota wrote, "Despite the massive research effort in nanotherapeutic materials, there is relatively little information about the toxicity of these materials or the tools needed to assess this toxicity."[67] There is growing concern about the safety of nanomaterials in health care.[68, 69]

The bottom line is that we know enough to be afraid without knowing enough to understand how big or small our fears ought to be. We are placing ourselves at risk of unknown consequences, understanding that our bodies seemingly have no defense against these nanoparticles. Optimistically, they are so small that nanoparticles might be irrelevant to our physiology. That viewpoint is probably wishfully naive. If nano-materials can influence how our bodies work, as more rapidly absorbed nano- supplements have already proven, how can they not also carry the risk of making things go awry in yet unknown ways? Indeed, early

---

66   Chang, "Tiny Is Beautiful: Translating 'Nano' Into Practical," *New York Times*, Feb 22, 2005. http://www.nytimes.com/2005/02/22/science/22nano.html?_r=0

67   Maurer-Jones et al., "Toxicity of therapeutic nanoparticles," *Nanomedicine* 2 (2009):219-41. doi: 10.2217/17435889.4.2.219.

68   Fadeel and Garcia-Bennett, "Better Safe Than Sorry: Understanding the Toxicological Properties of Inorganic Nanoparticles Manufactured for Biomedical Applications," *Adv Drug Deliv Rev* 62 (2010):362-74. doi: 10.1016/j. addr.2009.11.008.

69   El-Ansary et al., "Toxicity of Novel Nanosized Formulations Used in Medicine," *Methods Mol Biol* 1028 (2013):47-74. doi: 10.1007/978-1-62703-475-3_4.

reports from animal research indicate that cancers, genetic damage, and asbestosis-like damage might result from nanoparticle exposures.

The government doesn't require manufacturers to label products created with nanotechnology. This absence prevents consumers from making informed choices to use or avoid nanotechnology. Indicative of the times: yes, there is an app for that. The FindNano app was the first to help those who favor nano-products by finding these products and companies. Hopefully there will soon be an app for those hoping to avoid nano-products as well.

Learn More

How Everyday Products Make People Sick, by Paul Blanc

Exposed, by Mark Shapiro

The Secret History of the War on Cancer, by Devra Davis

Cosmetics

Cosmetics Database: http://www.cosmeticsdatabase.com/

Campaign for Safe Cosmetics: http://www.safecosmetics.org/article.php?id=219

Nanotechnology

Center for Nanotechnology in Society (Arizona State University): http://cns.asu.edu

US Government Nanotechnology: http://www.nano.gov/

Woodrow Wilson Project on Emerging Nanotechnologies: http://www.nanotechproject.org

Medications in Your Body and in the Environment

People are increasingly suspicious of the trade-offs they face using prescription medications. Being careful is smart. These chemicals have adverse effects on the environment as well.

Prescription Medications in You

You might have seen the chiropractic testimonial ads that include a line, something like, "Seven hundred thousand died, but no one built a monument for them." That horrifying number very effectively grabs the reader's attention. It creates outrage over such a loss of life and curiosity about how such a thing could have happened. The ad indicts conventional medicine and prescription medications as mass murderers. This number is highly misleading because it includes four hundred thousand poorly defined deaths from things like bedsores and malnutrition in nursing homes. It also doesn't consider what the death rate would have been if these patients hadn't been treated or how many might have succumbed to the disease for which they received the inadvertently lethal treatment. Those are the caveats.

Although that number is highly inflated, the point is still valid. In addition to roughly two hundred thousand American deaths every year from medication errors, hospital-acquired infections, and procedural errors in hospitals, there is general agreement from the most orthodox sources that approximately *one hundred ten thousand Americans die from adverse reactions to medications every year.* Again, the same medications that were lethal to some might have saved the lives of others. However, we must recognize that powerful prescription medications can't just help or do nothing. They can harm patents and often do. In fact, inherent in the appreciation of the effectiveness of prescription medication should be an equal recognition of the wisdom of avoiding them unless they are truly necessary. While we hope the benefit outweighs the damage, it is foolish and irrational not to try safer measures first.

Adding Drugs Subtracts from Your Health

Patients complain, and my experience confirms, that doctors are overly enthusiastic about lengthening the list of medications they take. No matter how long the list or how long a patient has been taking the medication, medical doctors are not very good at trimming the list. Unless the patient pushes the doctor, forcing reconsideration, the list snowballs. Why is that?

Honestly, adding medication is easier than taking it away. Dropping medication takes time. More careful consideration or reappraisal of a patient's condition is harder than simply renewing prescriptions. Then a new problem comes up, for which we add another prescription, and so on. It shouldn't be this way, but *you* need to step in or put your foot down. To slow or even reverse this ever-rising tide, I strongly urge you to insist that your prescribing physician make a formal reassessment of any prescription medications you are taking at least once a year.

We want to avoid needless medication so we can skip the needless adverse effects. The risks of adverse effects from medications don't add up; they multiply. Each medication has its own long list of ill effects; some are minor and some are life-threatening; some are well known but rare, some are common and others still unknown. When medications are combined, unheard-of adverse effects are more likely to appear, and common ones rear up with greater frequency.

Adverse Effects Are Hard to See If We Don't Look

Some adverse effects are not well known and are consequently over-looked. Many years ago I was treating a patient who had developed a blood clot in his arm while taking a common antidepressant. He had no history of injury, disease, or other medication use that could account for such an uncommon problem, particularly in such an unusual location in an otherwise-healthy male. His psychiatrist told him the clot was unrelated to his antidepressant. However, when I looked up the medication in the standard medical drug reference, way down in the fine print, blood clots were listed as a rare adverse effect of that medication. He stopped the antidepressant at my recommendation and decades later has never had another blood clot. We also resolved his depression without medication.

The last thing any physician wants to do is to hurt a patient. However, in the certainty of our good intentions, we can be guilty of turning a blind eye to evidence that our treatments cause harm.

A new patient told me he had become very ill with some unusual symptoms while taking a common antidepressant. Two different psychiatrists and at least one emergency room physician whom he had seen while looking for help had told him to increase his antidepressant dose.

As he was just getting worse, he finally decided to ignore their advice and stopped the medication. Several days later he was much better. It turns out that he was suffering from serotonin syndrome, a well-documented and potentially life-threatening reaction to the most widely prescribed class of antidepressant medications. His other physicians should have recognized this as the possible cause, one so dangerous that the right thing to do was to take him off the medication immediately to find out for sure. If he hadn't opposed their recommendations and stopped the medications on his own, the consequences could have been fatal. A patient taking prescription medication should never stop his or her medication without professional medical advice. However, a physician shouldn't tell a patient to continue or increase medication that causes serious harm.

Paying Attention Leads to Discomfort

Pick any prescription medication, go online, and read through the list of adverse effects it causes. If you are looking at the package insert that came with the medication, you will probably need a magnifying glass because these inserts are printed in miraculously small type on very thin paper.

Few patients who read the full listing of adverse effects feel comfortable taking the medication. Many simply refuse. The most severe adverse effects are rare but frighten patients, so they don't want to take the prescription. Consequently physicians don't like "burdening" patients with this information. It is hard to explain away the fear many informed patients feel when they are confronted with this information. The combination of these issues, the potential for nasty unwanted effects and the fact that physicians hide the facts from patients, probably explains why those who use alternative medicine are, on average, better educated than those who don't. Users of alternative medicine are less likely to accept a cursory justification of the prescription, research the medication for themselves, and then get upset because of the inadequate communication. That sequence raises suspicions, lowers trust and widens the communication gap between patients and physicians.

Things Might Be Even Worse

Unfortunately even these frightening lists don't fully encompass the problems and complexity of the situation. While some complain that the FDA drug approval process is too demanding and slow, there is a lengthy list of medications that passed through that slow process only to be withdrawn later after severe, often fatal, adverse effects appeared with widespread use of the medications. Long-term adverse effects from prescription medication, the most common use of medication, are effectively unknown. That is because such effects are rarely studied, and it is very difficult to establish that medication was the cause. We have reasons to be concerned.

For example, a very large study (ten thousand women) was conducted by investigating the health-care records of women enrolled in a large HMO in the Seattle area.[70] They compared treatment records on women who had developed breast cancer with women who hadn't. Surprisingly, researchers found that the more antibiotics a woman used, the greater the likelihood that she would either develop breast cancer or die from it. Women who totaled more than twenty-five lifetime antibiotic prescriptions had twice the risk of breast cancer. These findings are in agreement with an earlier Finnish study of two thousand women with urinary tract infections treated with antibiotics, who were subsequently more likely to develop breast cancer.[71]

Some other studies have found a slightly increased risk of breast cancer in association with antibiotic use while others have not. Studies of antidepressant medication and blood pressure medications suggest they might slightly increase the risk of breast cancer. Using small amounts of NSAIDs (the common "anti-inflammatory" drugs like Advil, ibuprofen, and naproxen) might reduce the risk, but high doses increase chances of developing breast cancer. The only comprehensive general review of prescription medication use and breast cancer risk was published in 2008.[72]

Although some research has suggested that using statin drugs might lower the risk of some types of cancer, a study of two million Britons found an unexpected increase in cataract and kidney damage among statin users.[73] A study of over two hundred thousand patients using a

---

70   Velicer et al., "Antibiotic Use in Relation to the Risk of Breast Cancer," *JAMA* 291 (2004):827-35.

71   Knekt et al., "Does Antibacterial Treatment for Urinary Tract Infection Contribute to the Risk of Breast Cancer?," *Br J Cancer* 82 (2000):1107-10.

72   Moysich et al., "Use of Common Medications and Breast Cancer Risk," *Cancer Epidemiol Biomarkers Prev* 17 (2008):1564-95. doi: 10.1158/1055-9965.EPI-07-2828.

73   Hippisley-Cox and Coupland, "Unintended Effects of Statins in Men and Women in England and Wales: Population Based Cohort Study Using the QResearch

certain kind of blood pressure pills (angiotensin-receptor blockers) found that they were significantly more likely to develop cancer, including a 25 percent increase for the risk of lung cancer. Other studies have not found that association or even a protective effect of the same drugs.

Why a Connection Makes Sense

There are physiological reasons why these and other medications could increase or decrease the risk of cancers and other diseases. Chronic or frequent infections create inflammation and various favorable and unfavorable changes in the immune system. Drugs and diseases have direct effects on other metabolic pathways, like as hormonal effects on the growth of certain cancer cells, as well many other biological actions. All of these wide-ranging biologic repercussions make some long-term impacts likely. So our knowledge of human biology suggests that a link is plausible. Clear, incontrovertible proof is lacking. At the present time, and for the foreseeable future, medical disinterest limits the scientific data and maintains our ignorance. The only certainty is continued uncertainty.

What to Do

What is the prudent response? It is pretty obvious that the wise choice is to limit your use of prescription medication for this and every other imaginable reason. It would be foolish to forever forswear all prescription medications. They aren't evil. It would be just as foolish to presume that medications are safe other than the already significant and well-known immediate risks. Even when we don't know the specific reason, caution is warranted. We should hold these medications in reserve for when we really do need them.

The latest drug is also the most unknown drug, and it's too likely to be recalled once its nastiest adverse effects come to light. Doctors are easily seduced by the lure of some new drug (or of the sales rep). You need to help your doctor apply the brakes on his or her enthusiasm. Just say, "Maybe not" to prescription drugs.

Prescription Medications in the Environment

In 2008 the Associated Press published a compilation of records from major US cities, showing that twenty-four of twenty-eight had

---

Database," *BMJ* 340 (2010):c2197. doi: http://dx.doi.org/10.1136/bmj.c2197.

detectable levels of various prescription drugs in their drinking water. The relative levels of specific medications in the water of each city inspired humorous, although apparently at least somewhat justifiable, assessments of the distinctive character of each city's populace (San Francisco, estrogen; Los Angeles, antianxiety medication; New Orleans, cholesterol-lowering medication; Minneapolis, caffeine). This is great fodder for comedians, but it isn't really a laughing matter. These chemicals don't just enter our bodies, do their work, and then vanish. That newspaper piece destroyed such simple assumptions. Most of the medication we swallow passes through our bodies unchanged. It then contaminates the waters around us.

The fate of unused medication is possibly more worrisome. While flushing unused medication down the toilet will keep it out of the hands of small children, again the medication isn't just poof! Gone. Medications have to be biologically active to affect us. The biology of living organisms on this planet varies, but there is a great deal of overlap. Consequently, human medications also have effects on bacteria, plants, and animals. Identifying the long-term hazards of human exposure to various prescription medications is challenging. Complex as it is, that task is simple compared to the work of sorting out their much broader environmental consequences.

Part of the solution to this problem is the safe disposal of unwanted medications. There are a few organizations that can accept unused medications and then redistribute then to people unable to afford them. Much more widespread are programs that governmental organizations

Useful Resources

Consumer Justice Group FDA Recalls Timeline http://www.consumerjusticegroup.com/drugrecall/drugrecalls.html

FDA Archive for Recalls, Market Withdrawals, and Safety Alerts. http://www.fda.gov/Safety/Recalls/ArchiveRecalls/default.htm

Medication Toxicity during Lactation. http://toxnet.nlm.nih.gov/cgi-bin/sis/htmlgen?LACT

and some pharmacies have organized to accept and then safely dispose of unused medication. Please look into it. The FDA maintains a web page that will help you get started (see footnote[74]).

Work and Play

Our vocations and avocations are a big part of who we are. In the best way, these activities are expressions of our passions, our love of the world. Conflicts between what we do and how we feel can be more than merely unpleasant. Such turmoil can create serious health problems. How we spend our time defines us in every way. These activities often include some toxic exposures.

The most mundane images of toxic work exposures are the guys out there with the respirator masks. Sadly, the image most of you just conjured in your mind's eye probably showed the mask dangling around the worker's neck. When a mask isn't actually worn, it (surprise) doesn't work. In my experience, workers being lax about using safety masks and goggles is a problem. Such careless self-disregard is actually lessening as awareness of these risks grows.

Don't make the mistake of thinking it is just construction workers or people who work in chemical factories who are threatened at work. Office workers, ensconced in tall, shiny buildings, can suffer when their building is "sick." Indoor air pollution is harder to remediate in a massive building with windows that don't open than it usually is in your own home.

What about your home? People work mask free with noxious chemicals in closed spaces as they go about their various home maintenance projects. Most don't even own a pair of safety glasses. At home, there is no on-site work supervisor to remind us about job safety.

Just because you're doing something for your own enjoyment or benefit, that doesn't make it inherently safe. Remember to wear masks and goggles. Volatile chemicals are dangerous and thankfully often smell bad. Respect that bad-smell warning.

---

74 "Disposal of Unused Medicines: What You Should Know," FDA website, http://www.fda.gov/drugs/resourcesforyou/consumers/buyingusingmedicinesafely/ensuringsafeuseofmedicine/safedisposalofmedicines/ucm186187.htm.

Tobacco, Alcohol, and Addiction

Much like work safety issues, the toxic effects of these chemicals are plain. However, like other hobbies, the toxicity is easily, or sometimes willfully, overlooked.

After decades of government warnings, that is hardly ever true with tobacco. *If you smoke cigarettes, stopping is probably the single most important step you can take to improve your health.* Yes, exercising, improving your diet, and implementing all the other ideas in this book will help you feel better and live longer. Make stopping tobacco the number one on your "to do" list.

Alcohol, on the other hand, has been touted for health benefits, especially to the heart. Ironically, alcohol is itself toxic to muscles, like to the heart, for example. It also depletes our bodies of many vitamins, probably partially explaining the many cancers alcohol causes.

Addictive behaviors have a myriad of unwanted impacts on individuals and collectively on our society. It is impossible to overemphasize the adverse impact of addiction, including tobacco and alcohol, on our health. If you are suffering from any form of addiction, you usually won't have to look far for help.

Summary—How to Minimize Risk

Avoiding harm can seem overwhelming. Several principles can help guide you in the right direction. There are some specific steps that are both simple and effective.

Pay attention to how you feel. There is much we don't know, but we do know that individuals vary in their sensitivity.

General Approach

- Be aware of risks.
- Be cautious in the face of uncertainty.
- Remember that simple equals safer.
- Limit yourself to moderate exposures.
- Take action.

Summary (continued)

- Change when possible.
- Choose what is least harmful.

Specifics

- Make your home safe, especially your bedroom.
- Is radon a risk for you?
- Choose the best water purification for your circumstances.
- Change your furnace filters and run a HEPA air filter.
- Choose safer plastics (don't heat food in plastics).
- Wash your hands with regular soap and water.
- Choose cosmetics and toiletries free of phthalates and other chemicals.
- Minimize your exposure to electromagnetic radiation.
- Demand that products are labeled for your safety.
- Don't take medications unless you *really* need them.
  - Choose "old faithful" medications since they are safer and often better than new ones.
- Don't force the fish to take your medications; dispose of medications properly.
- Keep safe at work.
- Enjoy your hobbies safely.
  - Be careful about alcohol and recreational drug use.
  - Keep learning.

Chapter 10

Essential Health Habit #6: Get Enough Sleep

Sleep may be the single greatest mystery of human biology. To understand so little about such a primary element of our lives and our physiology is remarkable. Why do we sleep?

In recent decades, research has taught us a lot about what sleep is. We have learned about different sleep phases and their characteristics. We can now categorize a broad range of unhealthy sleep patterns. Discoveries about chronobiology (how the cycles of time influence our bodies) help us understand sleep better, as circadian rhythms are intimately connected to the physiology of sleep. Most of what we know about the health impacts of sleep comes not from healthy models but instead from observing the consequences of disrupted sleep. The present medical understanding of sleep, defining a healthy process by what it isn't, is a great big fly in the ointment.

What *Do* We Know?

When we think about sleep from an evolutionary perspective, it is evident that it must be extremely important. Lying there, oblivious to the environment, we are extremely vulnerable. Our distant relatives, whales and dolphins, have learned to sleep with one half of their brains at a time so they are always at least partially alert. A habit like sleep, which places us in so much danger, just has to be absolutely vital. Otherwise humans, subject to the weakness of sleep, would have died out on this planet long ago. Every one of us comprehends from our lives' experiences at the most primal level how important sleep is. Science is still very much in the dark on this one.

The power of disordered sleep has been evident in experimental studies since 1894, when a study revealed that complete sleep deprivation could be fatal to puppies. Only recently has it been accepted that humans can also die from sleep deprivation.

Between life and death is a wide expanse, running all the way from sickness through good health up to optimal well-being. Sleep impacts every person, whether sick, healthy, or better than well. Chronic sleep deprivation impairs mental alertness, emotional stability, and immune response. Essentially every hormonal system in the body (for example, stress hormones, thyroid, sex hormones, and growth hormone) is affected. Sleep deprivation alters appetite-regulating hormones, leading to increased appetite and greater difficulties maintaining a healthy diet. Studies have found that habitually sleeping less than five hours a night was associated with a threefold increased risk of heart attacks, and sleeping less than five hours even twice a week doubled the risk.

Sleep heals. That fact is obvious to anyone who has or hasn't slept, all of us, in other words. Scientifically, we are just beginning to learn about the healing power of sleep. It appears that sleep is cleanup time for our brains.

The importance of this particular aspect of sleep physiology might be relevant to our epidemic of Alzheimer's disease. A protein called beta-amyloid builds up in the brains of those with Alzheimer's disease. In fact, that buildup is a defining characteristic of the disease. Since 2009, studies have shown that beta-amyloid is flushed from the brains of mice almost exclusively while they are asleep. A new literature review by Scullin, out of Baylor University Medical School, suggests that good sleep in young and middle-aged adults might be associated with better cognitive function later in life.[75]

With increased medical attention to sleep, the health consequences of sleep apnea are becoming more and more evident. Technological advances now allow us to easily conduct in-home sleep apnea testing. This has greatly improved our ability to accurately diagnose and treat these patients. Most patients with significant sleep apnea don't know they have a problem. Maybe that seems odd, but as the patient is sleeping, this shouldn't be too surprising. The patient was, after all, sleeping at the

---

75 Scullin and Bliwise, "Sleep, Cognition, and Normal Aging: Integrating a Half Century of Multidisciplinary Research," *Perspect Psychol Sci* 10 (2015):97-137. doi: 10.1177/1745691614556680.

time. Clues that someone might have sleep apnea include snoring, gasping or choking in sleep, dreams of suffocation, difficulty waking (including mental dullness or headache), and daytime sleepiness (particularly when sitting in a car, reading, attending a movie, or after eating). I have had a number of patients with loud, even very loud snoring, who don't have sleep apnea. Like any condition where the treatment has significant downsides (in this case it is complicated and expensive, and inhaling air pumped through plastic tubing eight hours a day seems undesirable), testing to confirm the existence of the problem is shrewd.

For those who have sleep trouble, it is perhaps dismayingly obvious that everything we do affects the quality of our sleep. Work, relationships, the sleeping environment, daily routines, medications, the timing of vitamin and mineral supplementation, and habits of eating, drinking, and exercising all significantly impact sleep. Don't be overwhelmed by all the ways sleep can go wrong. Instead, think of that list of influences as a list of opportunities to tip the balance in your favor.

Creating Good Sleep

A generation ago the book *The Kin of Ata Are Waiting for You* by Dorothy Bryant achieved cult status. The book was, in part, an indictment of the rushed, inconsiderate, conflict-driven modern lifestyle. In contrast, the author depicted a utopian culture, whose people go about their daily lives focused on creating wonderful sleep. Consequently, everyone, except the outsider telling us the tale, is extremely kind, thoughtful, caring, and placid. Although it is a fantasy, the book is usefully thoughtful, provoking the reader by suggesting a radically altered approach to life based on an uncommon set of priorities.

If your sleep is unsatisfactory, you can certainly improve it. Start from the basics. Your bedroom should be cool, dark, and quiet. It should be a place of relaxation. Remember that sleep is a habit. Learn about good sleep hygiene. If you don't fall asleep within fifteen minutes, leave the bedroom. Remember that the evidence is very strong that sleeping medications, though helpful in the short term, are not helpful in the long term and are often more likely to create problems when used more than once in a while. Just like the self-help elements of sleep hygiene, research shows that a technique called cognitive behavior therapy is more effective than prescription medication. Reflecting the profound impact that our mental and emotional states have on our sleep, a recent study showed that practicing meditation had a powerful effect on sleep, much more even than good sleep hygiene.[76]

Summary: Sleep Hygiene

- Regularity—go to sleep at the same time.
- Do not drink alcohol.
- Do not consume caffeine after noon.
- Avoid spicy and salty food in the evening.
- Make sure the bedroom is cool, dark, and quiet.
- Get bright light in the morning.
- In the hour or two before sleep, avoid lights in the eyes (TV, computer, and so forth).
- Leave bed if you can't fall asleep in fifteen to twenty minutes.
- Then get up until tired again (wait a minimum of fifteen minutes).
- Don't nap more than fifteen to thirty minutes.
- Remember that your day creates your night— daytime stress looms larger in the dark.

---

76 Black et al., "Mindfulness Meditation and Improvement in Sleep Quality and Daytime Impairment Among Older Adults With Sleep Disturbances: A Randomized Clinical Trial," *JAMA Intern Med* (2015):8081. Published online February 16, 2015. doi:10.1001/jamainternmed.2014.8081

Chapter 11

Essential Health Habit #7: Be Involved in Your Community

Human beings are innately social creatures. The most independent soul living "off the grid" out in the forest, learned how to survive from a book, another person, or, at the height of irony maybe, from the Internet. In other words, society helped the hermit get away from society. Just because someone is a recluse, that doesn't mean that he or she isn't watching television or You Tube videos all day long.

Each of us relies on others. From the moment we are born we are dependent, directly or indirectly, on the assistance of others. We don't need to reinvent fire, the wheel, or the iPhone. Unlike our hermit, most of us are deeply connected to many other people, and those interactions powerfully influence us. It isn't at all exceptional for a person to feel that relationships have defined his or her life.

Experts anticipated that increasing use of computer technology would lead to social fragmentation and increasing isolation, but it didn't quite work out that way.

Those "experts" failed to anticipate that our instinctive communal drives would morph what they saw as antihuman, isolating technologies into social media. Instead of destroying connections, our social inclinations inspired people to use these tools to expand their communities. Beyond reconnecting with long-sundered friends and family, our social networks stretch far wider than any other time in human history. Community is simply who we are. We're we as much as we're I.

The proof is everywhere you turn. Listen to the conversations in bars and coffee shops. Anytime you visit a general news or information website, turn on the television, pick up a newspaper or magazine, or visit a bookstore (remember those?), you will encounter stories or information about relationships.

High-minded folks might look down their noses at the popular "trashy" obsession with dysfunctional relationships, involving public personalities or bizarre characters. They feel they are above such tawdry interests. The same high-minded folks might instead focus their attentions on the equally pervasive self-improvement literature that teaches us all how not to be like those fascinating, but often pathetically dysfunctional, souls.

It's really the same obsession. The bottom line is identical. Good or bad, trashy or elevated, entertaining or enlightening, we are intensely aware of and curious about interpersonal relationships.

We Sense How Important Relationships Are

Why is this so? My guess is that it is because we all sense the importance of our relationships. We sense that our relationships reflect and impact our enjoyment of life as well as, ultimately, our well-being. Forming healthy relationships is easier for psychologically healthy people. Healthy relationships provide emotional support and stability. We're all far from perfect. One way to learn about ourselves and about the kinks we might want to iron out is by observing our own relationships with others. What sort of bad relationship habits do we fall into over and over? I firmly believe that the only mistakes we make are the ones we don't learn from. Relationships are complex and challenging. Consequently, they afford innumerable learning opportunities.

In the mid-1960s, when scientists were first working out the nature of stress and its impact on us, they asked people to create lists of various life events, rating their emotional impact. Right away researchers were surprised to learn that positive changes, such as getting married, were every bit as stressful as unpleasant changes. Most impressive to me is the fact that the life changes people rate as the most stressful are nearly all about relationships. Of the fifteen most stressful ones, eleven are entirely about relationships, and the other four (going to jail, suffering personal injury, getting fired from a job, and retirement) some would argue are also predominantly relationship-altering experiences.

Relationships Are Even More Important to Women

There is substantial evidence that relationships are even more important among women than among men and that women do a better job of managing relationships. Generally women report that they have more interpersonal relationships than men do, and they rate these relationships as higher quality ones than men do. It does appear, then, that research data supports stereotypes suggesting that socially inept cave males have survived even to the present day.

Science Supports Social Connections

Bolstering pervasive cultural beliefs, medical research shows that individuals with the most extensive social involvement and connectedness are healthier than others. One study, for example, found that the greater number of friends a person had, the fewer colds he or she suffered.[77]

Clearly, the health benefits of friends are significant. Individuals who have the strongest social connections are more likely to survive a heart attack, experience fewer symptoms of depression, suffer fewer infections, and have an overall lower mortality rate. Nearly every study of patients with chronic disease has shown that social support improves the quality of these patients' lives.

A review of twenty-seven studies of friends supporting friends with heart disease found positive effects on activity levels and self-efficacy, with reduced pain and fewer emergency room visits. A Michigan study of adults suffering chronic disease found that teaching families how to better support their loved one in the development of better coping skills and a stronger sense of control over his or her disease led to better health outcomes for the patient. Reviews of the medical literature show that new mothers who felt they had less social support were more likely to become clinically depressed. Studies of breast cancer patients, as yet inconclusive, suggest that social support increases survival rates.

Community-based exercise programs have been shown to accelerate recovery and maximize cardiovascular fitness, muscle strength, and

---

77   Cohen and Brissette, "Social Integration and Health: The Case of the Common Cold," *Jrnl Soc Struc* 1 (2000). Online only. http://www.cmu.edu/joss/content/articles/volume1/cohen.html.

bone density after stroke in the elderly. These community-based activity programs also improved balance, a very important risk factor for injury and impaired functioning among elderly populations. These programs also lead to wider social involvement for these patients

The phenomenon of altruistic behavior, action based on unselfish concern for the welfare of others, is another proof of the importance we place on relationships. By definition, self-sacrifice requires a decision to favor the well-being of others over one's own. Although altruism is an admirable quality, when carried too far, it can create problems when individuals neglect to take care of themselves, applying themselves too much to assuage the needs of others around them. Sometimes such short-term sacrifices are necessary. However, more often these individuals fail to understand that, in the long term, by taking better care of themselves, they will contribute much more to the betterment of their family, friends, and community. Striking a healthy balance is a task we all must face.

The Downside

Our interconnectedness, on the other hand, can create problems. Relationships can drag us down as well as lift us up. A person working to overcome drug or alcohol addiction usually faces pressure from his or her old group of friends. Many of those people are inevitably addicts themselves. They aren't ready to make a change, and few of them are capable of supporting an old "drinking buddy" in his or her efforts to achieve sobriety. Usually people have to build a new social network in those challenging circumstances.

Building healthy social relationships takes time and effort. You can't develop a healthy social network or keep one going without making relationships a priority. Many of us don't do that. We need to give relationships the attention they deserve.

Younger adults are usually much more adept at the early steps in this process. As they move out into the world, exploration and broadening their social connections are strong impulses. However, establishing relationships is only the start. Improving relationship depth and quality requires time.

Older individuals tend to be more satisfied with their relationships than younger people are. However, aging itself creates relationship problems. Social connections strengthen, but they also become fewer with advancing age, illness, and death. The inevitable disruption and narrowing range of intense relationships can be very disturbing. Sadly, those individuals who have been deeply connected to their community often suffer most intensely when those bonds are broken and they need to relearn the process of developing new relationships.

Regardless of our stage of life, we all need to continue to work on the depth and breadth of our human connections.

Social networks can, and should be, of great help. If your friends and family have good health habits, it is easy and healthy to go with the flow. If you take an active role, you can better your own health as well as that of your friends or family.

I see this most often with exercise. Many times I have seen two or more women create a partnership, training to complete their first running race together. Some people join walking groups or tennis clubs, or they join an athletic team because integrating a regular exercise habit into a social network makes them happier and more likely to get the exercise they know they need. There are social websites where people challenge friends to be active by posing specific activity challenges for themselves. What better gift could there be for someone you care about than to join force in this way to feel better?

Summary

- Value relationships.
- Build relationships.
- Use relationships to support your own health.
  - Set goals together.
  - Work together to achieve those goals.
- Volunteer—helping others helps you.

Value your relationships. Build the relationships you already have and be on the lookout to make some new friends. Use relationships to support your health. When you see that someone you know has a quality you admire or does something you would like to be able to do, ask how he or she accomplished it. Set goals together. Make a pact to change a behavior. The connection with a sponsor or mentor is one of the reasons a program like AA is so successful and life-enhancing. Volunteer your time to support some cause or to help strangers. Remember that *helping others is good for you as well as for them*. Look around for someone who needs your help. I bet you won't have to look very far.

Chapter 12

Essential Health Habit #8: Create a Healthy Sex Life

Sexuality is one of the most fundamental parts of being human. Actually, sex is much more basic and essential than that. Sex is more fundamental than being human. Even bacteria have sex. Along the evolutionary highway, sex appeared before breathing. It is no wonder (a no-brainer, even) how much attention humans pay to sex and how important sex is to who we are individually, culturally and as a species.

Such an essential part of biology shouldn't be ignored. We couldn't ignore it no matter how much we wanted to. The power of sexuality is undeniable and a necessary consideration in any comprehensive discussion of health. Nevertheless, some of us still try to avoid the topic. Looking away or puritanically pretending sex is somehow beneath human dignity is just foolish. Oddly, we seem to be pretty good at both obsessing about it and hiding it away at the same time.

Sex Is Natural, So What Could Go Wrong?

It is every bit as naive to assume that because sex is so instinctual, nothing could go wrong. Studies show that only a small fraction of adults at any age don't care about sex (bet that isn't a surprise to you), and the great majority of them believe it is an essential part of a good relationship.

Some religious traditions deride sex. Sex is an unhappily base animal quality, required for procreation but shameful, and it should be transcended. Other religious traditions profess sexual union as the nearest approach to divinity human beings can achieve. Interestingly, these opposing viewpoints are often encompassed within the same religion.

Simply suppressing sexuality, trying to make it go away by ignoring it, is like trying to cap an erupting fire hydrant with a dinner plate. It just doesn't work, and too often those denied but irrepressible sexual urges erupt with destructive force. Some individuals are able to lead a celibate life, successfully redirecting or sublimating this powerful energy, but they are truly exceptional. All of us, though, have the ability to channel our sexual energy in life-enhancing ways.

Why Sex Is Biologically So Cool

What is sex, and how did it come to be so important? Obviously, sex is how we make more of us. Other forms of reproduction existed before sexual reproduction appeared on Earth. But those other means of making more simple forms of life kept them simple. They couldn't adapt and change as rapidly or as profoundly as sexually reproducing life forms can. That's how humans and other sexual species "won."

The biological superiority of sexual reproduction, particularly the *adaptability* it engenders, made it possible for more complex living organisms like us to appear. Sexual activity is *the* biological requirement for continuation and adaptation of the species. Accordingly, the sexual urge is imprinted in the very deepest parts of our biology. Although sexual reproduction requires a sometimes-complicated interaction with an opposite-gender human being, the biology is simple.

The relationship part of sex is where things get complex. As a physician, I'm well versed in the numerous biological problems likely to interfere with sexual functioning and reproduction. However, the range of those problems is much more limited and straightforward than the innumerable permutations of failure that can arise in relationships. Things can go wrong in so many ways and collapsing relationships usually destroy the sexual element of the relationship.

The complexity of relationship dysfunctions, impairing sexual functioning, is a striking parallel to the biologically complex potentials of sexual reproduction itself. When sex is involved, biologically or socially, the options, benefits, and problems multiply geometrically.

What Is Healthy Sex?

Healthy sexual functioning is easier to explain than to define. Healthy sexual functioning depends on everything working well. All of our "parts"—physical, emotional, social, and possibly even spiritual—influence our sexual performance and well-being.

During my medical training I was taught that the biggest sex organ in the body is the brain. It most assuredly isn't the only one. When we consider it in a different way, maybe the entire body is the biggest sex organ in the body.

If you are sick, tired, stressed, or upset with your partner, you are unlikely to be interested in sex. If you are worried about how you look or how well you might perform, it probably won't go well. Although circulatory problems and high blood pressure are notorious for compromising sexual function in males, medications to treat these problems are even more likely to impair performance or desire.

As we age and our relationships evolve, so too does our sexuality. Ironically, as we become more sexually experienced with age, the changes in our aging bodies usually require learning still more about some of the mechanics (especially lubrication and erectile issues). Life offers us many challenges, including those of a sexual nature. These challenges can be opportunities for greater understanding and a means of enriching your intimate relationship(s).

What is healthy sexual functioning? *Sex is healthy when it is satisfying, enlightening, and absorbing; and when it makes your life better.* It can help you relax. It can bring you closer to the person you have already been sharing your life with. Sex can help a couple move past conflicts over mundane worldly matters. Like a meditation or spiritual experience, sex can take you someplace transformative. Some individuals have little interest in sex and are content just getting by. Others are eager to transform themselves, their relationships, and the quality of their lives. Sex is satisfying to those at either extreme.

If you want to improve your sexual life, you need to make an effort—any effort will help. It is easy to find suggestions online or in books or magazines to suit whatever your needs and desires may be. To say that humans are obsessed with sex is a gross understatement. Sex is, after all, what made us who we are.

Chapter 13

Essential Health Habit #9: Remember That Attitude Is Important

Someday, hopefully in the very near future, the present era will be recognized as a dark age in our understanding of the human brain. Why is it so hard to realize that our habits of thought are just one facet of our health? I really don't understand why this is apparently so hard for some to grasp.

Ignore the wisdom of common sense (but only for a moment). Scientific proof of the connection between our thoughts and diseases stretches back two generations or more. The landmark work of Meyer Friedman and R.H. Rosenman established that specific personality characteristics put people at risk for death from heart disease. Their work identifying and investigating "Type A" personalities was the cornerstone, establishing the wide importance of psychosomatic medicine.

Patients often say they come to see me because I understand that the brain and body affect each other. My response tends to surprise them at first.

The Unity of Thought and Health

My response is to tell them that I don't believe our thoughts and emotions affect the way our bodies work. I don't believe this, since the brain is part of the body, right there inside the skull; they are not separate. Thinking is a biological process. The chemicals, hormones, and electrical signals generated by biological processes in the brain or any other area spread throughout the body. For example, just as the chemicals produced when we're happy affect chemical processes outside the brain, the various biological responses to infection anywhere in the body also change the way we think and experience our moods. While some might have the view that recognizing a connection between our physical health and our state of mind is an enlightening step forward, that concept is still too fragmented. They are one and the same. How could the healthy functioning of our brains, expressed by our emotions and thoughts, not be just another facet of physical health?

My view isn't new or unique. Your grandmother could tell you that habits of thought can make life better or worse for you. The wisdom of common sense is too often forgotten.

After I graduated from medical school, I invited some friends over to celebrate. One of my friends, a member of an Irish dance performance group, slipped on a rug while dancing and broke a bone in her foot. It took her many months longer to heal than the orthopedic doctor expected. He told my friend he was confused, asking himself why a healthy young woman could be taking so long to heal. My friend asked whether the fact that her mother was dying of cancer might be the reason. Since there was no evidence at that time that depression would or wouldn't delay healing of foot fractures, the doctor told her this couldn't account for it. Well, in advance of future scientific discoveries, your grandmother could have told you otherwise. There is often tremendous wisdom in common sense.

Habits of Thought Change Brain Anatomy

I am not saying that we are victims of our physiology. On the contrary, we have the ability and responsibility to make changes in our habits of thought every bit as much as in our more obviously physical behaviors.

For nearly twenty years, we have been accumulating evidence that counseling changes brain chemistry and even brain structure. Life experiences, particularly the activities we pursue on a daily basis, change our bodies, our brains included. When a person uses his or her muscles in physical labor, his or her body adapts, building skeletal muscle and restructuring bones, tendons, and blood vessels. With the same remarkable ability, research shows that the brain changes in all kinds of ways, in response to a person's activities. For example, a study of London taxi drivers found that the longer an individual drove a cab, the larger was the portion of the driver's brain that manages spatial relationships. That is common sense, right?

An interesting 2004 study found that depressed patients treated with either medication or cognitive behavioral therapy experienced physical changes in their brains as they improved with treatment. The precise nature of the changes differed depending on the treatment. This study suggests that each approach has its own merits. It might be that one treatment will prove to be superior in the long term or at least superior for some individuals. It might be that some people with certain brain structure could benefit more from a certain therapy.

These findings make sense to me, as they confirm my clinical experience and lessons I learned from yoga and meditation training when I was young. If you are always looking for problems or finding things to worry about, you will be prepared for bad things to happen. You are also going to be more prone to anxiety, depression, and many unwanted health consequences. We need to find a balance, moving away from the darkness and taking care to cultivate more positive thoughts and experiences.

Optimism Is Healthy

Proving the connection between a specific attitude and the consequences, specific health problems or even simply general health status, is fraught with scientific land mines. However, generations of research are quite convincing despite the unavoidable flaws. The weight of evidence is overwhelming. Reviews of the medical studies performed pertaining to stroke, spinal cord injury, and general health consistently find that optimism is healthy.[78, 79, 80]

Another way to consider this influence is to look at it from the opposite side, the dark side rather than the sunny side. Do you know people who always expect the worst? Might that be you? Most of us find it wearing to be around others who are always complaining and finding faults.

78   van Mierlo et al., "The Influence of Psychological Factors on Health-Related Quality of Life After Stroke: A Systematic Review," *Int J Stroke* 9 (2014):341-8. doi: 10.1111/ijs.12149.

79   van Leeuwen et al., "Associations Between Psychological Factors and Quality of Life Ratings in Persons with Spinal Cord Injury: A Systematic Review," *Spinal Cord* 50 (2012):174-87. doi: 10.1038/sc.2011.120.

80   Rasmussen et al., "Self-Regulation Processes and Health: The Importance of Optimism and Goal Adjustment," *J Pers* 74 (2006):1721-47.

Again, the research shows that this habit is consistently associated with feeling poorly.

Maybe it is my own pessimistic streak, but I would be uncomfortable if I didn't mention that naive optimism isn't healthy either. People sometimes make the craziest decisions because they refuse to consider the possibility of a bad outcome. I have seen that too often, especially around risk-taking teenagers. Be optimistic but season your optimism with a little dash of realism.

Coping with Life's Challenges

Nearly every study of patients with chronic disease has shown that patients with better coping strategies enjoy a better quality of life. Their coping skills influence their attitudes and moods, their illnesses and healing. This is true whatever the trouble. It is as true for chronic schizophrenics as it is for patients with spinal cord injuries, cancer, diabetes, or heart disease. Even young athletes recover from injures more rapidly if they possess better coping skills. Regardless of the nature of a health problem, it is less disabling when we respond in certain ways.

Sometimes the events of life are so horrendous that they overwhelm nearly everyone. In those extreme cases, we still have to do our best with the skills we have at hand, and hopefully the people around us can rise together, helping each other. Our response is usually the most important factor in determining the impact of the event. In other words, most of the time *our response* to an experience determines the nature and extent of our suffering.

One of the greatest gifts of being a physician is learning from patients. I have seen patients emotionally crippled by seemingly minor emotional distresses, while other individuals, on whom fate inflicted horrendous trauma, astoundingly emerged changed for the better, sometimes remarkably transformed into truly amazing and inspiring individuals. Events with the same outward characteristics can have entirely different meanings to those involved, impacting them differently and leading to entirely different reactions.

Thankfully, most of us aren't forced to confront such horrors. This world is, however, filled with woe. Life tests each of us, so we must learn how to do our best when the challenges come our way. How can we do that?

Positive Coping Skills—Recipes for Lemonade

Some people do better than others at making the best of a difficult situation. We know that children who grow up in abusive and unstable households have a much tougher time managing stresses throughout their lives. The same is true of adults who have endured extreme psychological trauma.

Thankfully this isn't a one-way street. Psychological hardiness, mental and emotional strength, can be learned. Much of what we can do to get through the short-term crisis helps us in the long-term as well. That's because those immediately positive steps improve our long-term resilience. In other words, healing is both possible and even inevitable as you cultivate healthy habits. Furthermore, many of the habits that build psychological stability and improve one's ability to deflect stressors are the *same principles I have been discussing throughout this book.* One "side effect" of taking action to improve your physical health is that your psychological health will likely improve as well. That isn't surprising given what we know about the reality of our integrated nature. If you are healthy, you are healthy. Resistance to stress, physical or emotional, is both an expression and a consequence of overall well-being.

It All Adds Up

Although a chain is only as strong as the weakest link, human beings are thankfully stronger and more flexible. You don't have to be perfect, but all of your efforts do add up, making you stronger in ways that are not so obvious.

My experience has been that patients who have mastered several health behaviors are less vulnerable to their deficiencies in other areas. Too often, though, people who are dedicated and passionate about one health behavior neglect other important health habits. I have seen many patients who meditate for hours every day but rarely exercise, and others who run ten miles a day but eat poorly or even smoke cigarettes. These individuals need to develop a more balanced approach to health. The reason there are so many cultural traditions and metaphors for such awareness of how to live properly (Buddhist moderation, Navajo walking in beauty, or living in the Tao) is because this underlying attitude or sense of perspective is important for each of us.

Where Are You Now?

Every good health habit makes you stronger and better able to cope; none of it is wasted effort. However, a thorough self-examination is the place to start. Where do you stand? What are your vulnerabilities and strengths? What risks run through your family? A good self-examination will help you better direct your efforts, leading to the optimal outcome for you. Running through a checklist of each of the essential habits I have discussed to identify what you are missing is the first step.

Next, consider your own experience. What helps *you* feel better? Some people notice that eating a food they are sensitive to does more than just give them abdominal symptoms. They feel anxious, irritable, or otherwise unstable. Research by the British government showed that many children became distracted and restless after eating certain foods.[81] Well in advance of the authorities, many parents have long known that even minimal quantities of dietary sugar, artificial colors, or preservatives make their children emotionally unstable. Exercise helps many people stay calm through their most difficult days, whereas they get restless and irritable when they aren't physically active.

Anticipate

Think about the situations that particularly disturb you. After you identify your own vulnerabilities, be proactive. Don't slack off on your positive health habits when you know a big stress is looming over the horizon. That is the worst thing you can do. It will make the challenge more formidable. Consider specific steps you can take to better ride out the "storm" next time it comes and then put your plans into action *before* the storm hits.

Expecting to run a marathon the first time you put on a pair of running shoes is crazy. Similarly, sometimes a situation is simply just too much of a challenge at the moment. A wise approach, then, is to avoid it. I hate to admit that we do have limits, but the reality is that sometimes we do. Learn yours.

---

81 Pelsser et al., "Effects of a Restricted Elimination Diet on the Behavior of Children with ADHD," *Lancet* 377 (2011):494-503. doi: 10.1016/S0140-6736(10)62227-1

The Challenges of Work

The work environment is a major source of stress for nearly every one. That's why someone pays us to do it. Most often the challenges are temporary or surmountable but not always.

Some of my patients have found themselves struggling in jobs that demand personal characteristics they don't possess. Often their work success has led to a new administrative position with responsibilities that are entirely different from the responsibilities of the job they had previously performed so well. Just as I have had to put patients on disability following physical injuries, psychological stresses at work can be every bit as disabling. Several studies have found that work stress can even be fatal, leading to heart attacks, for example.[82, 83] While life is about testing ourselves, stretching our limits, and adapting to opportunities, it isn't healthy to be in a position where your livelihood is dependent on filling a role completely at odds with your temperament. Nor is it wise to place yourself in other situations that are just too much for you to cope with at that time.

A Specific Set of Skills

Beyond the essential health habits, there are coping skills that are specifically helpful. Some of them are habits of thought. Others are more overtly external. One skill, often called "flexible coping," reflects the reality that using a variety of coping strategies is so important that the variety itself should be considered an important skill on its own merit. Flexibility itself is a powerful coping skill.

The give and take of social interaction helps us deal with problems in other ways. Having a sympathetic ear to share your troubles with or someone to hug can make a surprisingly powerful difference for some people. Social interactions teach us about life and about how other people responded to their challenges effectively or disastrously. We can learn from the experiences of others without having to repeat them all

---

82   Kivimaki et al., "Job Strain as a Risk Factor for Coronary Heart Disease: A Collaborative Meta-Analysis of Individual Participant Data," *Lancet* 380 (2012): 1491–1497. doi: 10.1016/S0140-6736(12)60994-5.

83   Virtanen et al., "Perceived Job Insecurity as a Risk Factor for Incident Coronary Heart Disease: Systematic Review and Meta-Analysis," *BMJ* 347 (2013):f4746. doi: 10.1136/bmj.f4746.

over again ourselves. I have found that the process of supporting others is also healing to the individual giving the support. Somehow it seems that providing the kind of support to another person that we might have needed for ourselves at one time, can heal our own wounds.

The internal aspects of positive coping are connected to a *sense of empowerment.* When we feel we cannot control our circumstances, feelings of depression, futility, and anger often arise. Accepting our responsibility to act in whatever manner possible and then figuring out what can be accomplished and how to go about it is empowering even beyond the actual impact on the situation. "Planful problem solving," as this approach has been called, helps us to gain control (over our internal landscape, at least) and move forward.

The term "stress management" encompasses many techniques that help us to cope better and enjoy life more fully. The production of stress management items, including music, videos, and all sorts of devices, has become an industry unto itself. As so many of us feel so stressed, it makes sense that we would support such a concerted and commercial effort.

However, the best stress management doesn't require specially labeled purchases. The best stress-management tools come from you. Anyone who has ever lain on a sunny beach, listening to the water; walked through the forest; or enjoyed the smells knows well that the natural environment has power to wash away our worries. I once knew a highly respected photographer, who titled one of his books of nature scenes *Meet My Psychiatrist.*[84] Whatever method you choose to manage your stress is far less important than the act of doing something, anything at all, to help you seek and reclaim your emotional center.

When life is difficult, it is easy to feel like a victim, as if the misfortune has been specifically directed at us and we're powerless to do anything to help ourselves. There are always limits. However, we know from inspiring tales of people incarcerated, subjected to practically unimaginable torment, that there are always windows and doors open to freedom inside of us. Those remarkable individuals teach us how they determined to take control of the only thing they could—their reactions to situations. Their endurance gives us hope.

Thankfully, the trials most of us endure are not so extreme, and it is then easier to triumph over them. It is tremendously helpful to psychologically shift from feeling like a powerless victim of some situation to

---

84   Les Blacklock, *Meet My Psychiatrist* (Minnesota: Voyageur Press, 1990).

recognizing the possibility of exerting some control. Then the next step, finding or creating a path of action appropriate for you, *transforms* the stress into a life-enhancing experience from which you can learn and derive benefit. The power we gain from meeting such challenges can change our lives. Transformation is seldom a painless process.

The ability to find something positive, the silver lining in the dark clouds, is a powerful coping skill. It is often labeled "positive reappraisal." I like this term a lot. *Reappraisal* of course means that the first impression wasn't so good, it wasn't so much fun. But then the individual chose to go back and look at events differently. Even deciding to rethink a situation is an empowering activity that leaves passivity back in the dust.

I'd like to say a bit more about flexible coping. It isn't terribly surprising that the ability to use multiple coping strategies is more effective than using any single tactic. Psychological flexibility, like a tree bending in the wind, allows us to endure by adapting, by bending without breaking. Any individual coping style has pluses and minuses, and a healthy response at one time will be unhealthy at another time. As with any physician, a number of my patients were abused as children. Whatever their emotional response was at the time of the abuse was appropriate and necessary. However, continuing to respond to the world in the same way, when there is no longer the need for the same self-protective strategy, can be a problem. The ability to change tools in response to different conditions increases the likelihood of successfully passing through the crisis or avoiding it in the first place.

Forgiveness

Alexander Pope was a remarkable person. His body ravaged by tuberculosis, he was a "hunchback" in the terminology of his day, growing to just four and a half feet, and he was subject to a litany of illnesses. He was a Catholic during a time when Catholics were severely oppressed in England. Among the persecutions Catholics endured was segregation (they could live only in certain parts of the country), and they were denied education, either public or private. Pope achieved great respect, overcoming the formidable challenges he faced. He teaches us about forgiveness: "to err is human; to forgive, divine."

Whether accidental or fully intentional, whether personal, political, or systematic, we all suffer wrongs. Sometimes each of has been the party at fault.

On a daily basis, I see patients who suffer because of injustice. Usually they are distressed. Often they suffer health consequences. The damage to their health is seldom directly due to the injustice. They aren't, for example, disabled by badly healed broken bones. The damages are instead self-inflicted in a way. The injustice has so disturbed the patients that there are health consequences from the reaction.

These patients are right, and they are often righteously angry. I don't disagree with them because they *are* in the right. I am sympathetic and empathetic. Their response is entirely understandable. However, their response hasn't gotten them anywhere except sicker than they could be. I have to convince them that they need to set aside their grievances. They need to forgive to move forward.

Sometimes, as in the case of the woman embittered by the murder of her daughter, injustice was horrendous. But, as she saw, the damage to her was ongoing, and accepting that nothing would reverse the tragic event, she had to forgive to move forward.

Other times the injustice is trifling but still hard to drop. Sometimes the person we need to forgive lives in the mirror.

Those of us who have endured emotional or physical traumas early in life are especially disposed to all kinds of ugly feelings about ourselves. Poor self-esteem is the nice way to describe what might often be described as self-loathing, self-hatred, and self-abuse. It's hard to be happy and healthy if that is how you feel. It isn't impossible, but it takes a sustained effort at creating new habits of thought and feeling.

There are many good and healing books on forgiveness. My favorites are *Forgive for Good* by Frederic Luskin and *The Forgiving Lifestyle: How to Forgive Everyone (Including Yourself)* by Marina Michaels.

Recreation Beyond Stress Management

I want to go a bit to move in a slightly different direction. Stress management is a vital skill, which too many of us neglect. In a subtle way though, it is inadequate. It can be too much like taking out the garbage, doing something you *should* do, when it ought be delightful; filled with delight.

Each of us has our own special qualities. That includes aptitudes, interests and passions. Spending some time in activities that have special meaning for us enlivens, transforms, and recreates us. We don't have any scientific explanations for this joy. To me, that lack of understanding just proves how important it is not to neglect these soul-enhancing experiences.

I see many patients who absolutely love to paint, play music, go hiking, or pursue any of a long list of activities. The problem is that they don't pursue the activity. Their rationale is that they are "just too busy." When I ask them to tell me what they really love to do, their faces brighten momentarily and then they slump back to their dimmed, responsible, no-time-for-that, explanation.

You don't have time not to do the things you love. You can't wait for some future idyllic time because you can't count on ever making it there. If you don't live your life in harmony with your own nature, you can't possibly live as long or as well. Don't wait.

Attitude Isn't Everything

It disturbs me greatly that many people who perceive that attitudes affect our well-being fall into the blame-game trap. They blame themselves or others for getting sick. This is as every bit as foolish as it is insensitive and unkind. It is also a pointless waste of time, sort of like sitting by the side of the road and feeling bad because your car tire went flat. Whatever. Just get on with it. Identify the problem and fix it.

At no time since the Middle Ages have humanity's various spiritual traditions, the human cultural elements most devoted to perfecting one's attitude, blamed the sick for their disease. Most traditions teach that death and decay are inevitable. In fact, they use this reality as an incentive (or looming threat), declaring the primal importance of getting your "spiritual house" in order. They say that the material world is transitory; therefore, a spiritual perspective is a smarter bet.

Sadly, we don't need a scientific study to prove that we all die, saint and sinner alike. Nor is it brilliant conjecture to extrapolate that most of us will get sick before we die. No matter how saintly your attitudes, disease and death are the inevitable fate of physical bodies.

Even for atheists, without an outside force to blame or praise for one's health or illness, attitude isn't everything. Your thoughts *are* an important component of your health. However, people get sick, injured, and die regardless of their thoughts and emotions. Your response to circumstances will have a huge impact on the quality of your life and maybe the quantity as well. That impact will be favorable or unfavorable. You get to choose. You can't choose everything that happens in your life. It is what you do that matters. The response is your choice.

Summary

- Develop new coping skills.
- Forgive imperfections in others and in yourself.
- Remember what is really important.
- Do your best and then let go.

Keep it simple.

Chapter 14

Essential Health Habit #10: Develop a Purpose or Spirituality in Your Life

Discussing our most deeply felt beliefs and impulses is a touchy topic, even explosive, like purposefully walking out into a minefield. At one extreme, some feel that any sort of spiritual belief is naive at best, possibly even dangerous. Many of us have strongly held beliefs. Sometimes those beliefs don't allow for other, even slightly different, points of view, religious or otherwise. In my experience religious opinions, including opinions about religion, are the most intransigent ones. Some feel their religious belief is the only correct one and that other people, including those devoted to a different branch of the same religion, are less than human, justifying murder in the name of God. Thankfully, far more of us take more moderate positions, recognizing commonality or at least our own uncertainty.

My opinion, based on my clinical and personal experience, is that dedication to *some* ideals is essential. Some sort of idealism vitally underlies healthy attitudes toward life and the world.

Those who are particularly religious might disagree with me because I insist on stretching the boundaries here. To me dedication to humanistic ideals, without spiritual belief, serves just as well.

Intellectual honesty demands that I admit that I might be a little biased. There is a scant amount of research supporting my opinion or any other opinion on this subject. That's certainly partly due because so many are hypersensitive about this topic. Furthermore, the world's headlines shout the harmful consequences of religious fundamentalism on a daily basis. There is ample cautionary evidence that the good has to be very good to overcome the harm, dare I say evil, inflicted on our world by moral certainty and self-righteousness.

Spirituality and Psychosis

Many psychotic patients have religious or spiritual delusions; including speaking to or believing they themselves are God or some other angelic or demonic force. That doesn't mean all "spiritual experiences" are psychotic. The scientific evidence is otherwise. Studies of such experiences, published in the psychiatric literature, have generally concluded that spiritual experiences themselves are not psychotic.

A Purposeful Life Is a Healthy Life

Religious or nonreligious, spiritual or atheistic, a purposeful life is a healthier life. For example, in 2014, the results of a study following over six thousand adult Americans over a fourteen-year period were published.[84] The self-described "purposeful" individuals defined themselves as planning for the future, feeling there were more things they could still do in their lives, and stating that they lived with clear aims, in contrast to other, more aimless people. After controlling other known risk factors, self-described purposeful individuals lived significantly longer.

Prayer for Everybody, Including Atheists

One of my mentors in medical school sometimes gave a lecture titled "Prayer for Atheists." As an excellent speaker (and an atheist himself), his talk was filled with stories exemplifying the psychological benefits of focused intention. It is well documented that individuals who feel they can influence the circumstances of their lives are happier than those who believe themselves to be powerless. Prayer is one way to seek influence. In some forms it is also a means of setting worries aside. "Let go and let God," "*Deo volente*" (God willing), and "*Insha'Allah*" (If God wills it) are some of the prayer-like aphorisms repeated in various cultures as reminders of the wisdom of being at peace no matter what occurs.

---

84   Hill and Turiano, "Purpose in Life as a Predictor of Mortality Across Adulthood," *Psychol Sci* 25 (2014):1482-6. doi: 10.1177/0956797614531799.

Although my grandfather died forty years ago, I still remember a conversation we had one day about religion and spirituality. He spoke of how he felt he could experience God more readily in the sunlight reflected off the surface of a lake, or in the breeze moving through the trees of the forest, than he could in the perpetually squabbling church he sometimes unenthusiastically attended. For some, spirituality means sensing beauty or harmony in the world. The texts, buildings, or even people comprising formalized religion aren't prerequisites.

Many studies teach us that terminally ill patients have a great need to bring spiritual considerations into their daily lives. Some studies show that many patients, facing serious illness, express a desire for some sort of spiritual interaction with their physicians. For physicians this could be as simple as just acknowledging the patient's beliefs. That isn't much to ask. However, as a profession, physicians are not generally very comfortable with that.

The presence of spirituality or leading a purposeful life seem to me to be mostly about striving to be better or at least doing one's part to help make the world better. Going through life aimlessly and passively is as unhealthy as it is boring. Whatever your beliefs or inclinations, living life with some direction, some intent, or some purpose is more fulfilling and good for all of us. Consider it.

Chapter 15

Achieving Essential Changes

Forget the high-minded goals if you don't have a plan. You might make it from New York to San Francisco just by pointing your feet westward and heading out. Probably not. If you figure out the obstacles ahead, you can equip yourself with the tools needed to conquer them.

Of course, don't forget that a journey has a beginning as well as an end and, well, a journey. Where are you now? You need to know where you are on the map to find the best path to where you want to be.

Self-Assessment

I can't overemphasize how important an honest and thorough self-assessment is when you are trying to make changes. Your self-assessment must be as objective and honest as you can make it. An inaccurate assessment is infected with the seeds of failure. If you think you're in better shape than you really are, the training for that April marathon *will* injure you. You might assume that you aren't eating well enough, but really the bigger issue is your lack of exercise or poor stress management.

Each of us tends to see some problems clearly but not others. We think certain problems are bigger than they really are, and others are completely invisible to us. Trying to sort things out by yourself can be an awful lot like painting a self-portrait without a mirror, or maybe having only a distorted fun house mirror in which to see your reflection.

These distortions and plain ignorance are the reasons so many people find the help of a professional useful. A professional can identify problems and solutions you might not recognize or know about. A professional should have learned from the experience of helping others (as well as himself or herself) and can use that accumulated wisdom to guide you. Seeking the advice of family and friends can also be helpful at times.

Reflection is an inward, ideally a meditative, process. In keeping with that inwardness, we should *start* from the inside, meditating on who we are and who we want to become. My recommendation—why I wrote this book, in fact—is to use the essential health habits as your framework for both assessment and change.

Essential Health Habits

1. Drink enough water.
2. Exercise almost every day.
3. Eat well.
4. Take your supplements.
5. Avoid the things that make you sick.
6. Get enough sleep.
7. Be involved in your community.
8. Create a healthy sex life.
9. Remember that attitude is important.
10. Develop a purpose or spirituality in your life.

Step 1—Set Achievable Goals

After you sort out where you are, you can create an image of where or who you want to be and construct a map to make the transition from here to there. Deciding that you want to be younger isn't going to work any more than deciding you want to be taller or win the lottery. Make your goals *achievable*! That is the first step in goal setting.

In a more subtle way, just deciding that you want to be stronger or thinner or calmer won't work either. There is an art to creating goals that will help you achieve success.

Step 2—Create Specific Goals

If you set a goal but don't have a path to follow toward that goal or don't know when you have reached it, the journey won't go well. For example, maybe you decide that you want to lose weight. You then must sort out how you are going to do that and how you are going to measure it along the way. That way you can correct your course along the way and avoid getting lost or wasting your time.

Let's say you determined that for you the keys to improving your health are to increase your activity and change your diet. Specifically you target eating more vegetables and cutting out soda and alcohol.

As far as the physical activity changes, you could begin by tracking your activity level for a week by wearing a pedometer or using your smartphone and apps. Then decide how much more active you should be. As you set about implementing your new physical training regimen, you have clear feedback and an incentive by simply reading the numbers.

The same applies to your diet. You could decide that you will eat some vegetables at every meal, including two servings at lunch and dinner with a leafy green salad every night. You also determine to limit yourself to no more than one alcoholic drink and one soda a week. All you have to do is look at your plate and into your drinking glass to learn whether you are reaching your goals.

I have a couple of comments about weight loss as a goal. First, it isn't a particularly health-oriented goal, so I don't like it much. As long as you are sort of close to "normal," other factors (especially physical fitness) are much more important than the reading on the scale. There is some evidence that, as long as you are physically fit (in other words, with good aerobic capacity and strength), obesity might not be a risk factor for death, disease, or feeling poorly. The scale doesn't tell you what you are made of—your body composition. Most people who do a lot of strength training are overweight on the charts but have low body fat. Increased levels of body fat are more risky than similar increases in body weight. Many people find that improving their diet and exercise pattern doesn't change their weight as much as it changes how they feel, their physical capacity, and how their clothes fit. Muscle is denser than fat, so patients usually tell me their clothes fit more loosely, even when their weight hasn't changed significantly.

Step 3—Achieve Early Success

To maintain and build on a change, we need positive feedback. If you try to do too much, feel horrible while doing it, and feel worse the next day, how likely are you to try it again? Fine-tune your goals to create and then build success.

Say that you learn you are averaging three thousand steps a day. You should be over ten thousand, but going straight from three thousand to ten thousand is unrealistic. So, an achievable target would be to bump up your daily step count by three to five hundred steps each week (for example, 3,000 a day, then 3,300 a day, then 3,800 a day, and so on).

If you are trying to be calmer when you drive the freeway, make this goal specific and achievable. When you enter the freeway, remind yourself that your goal is to get to your destination calmly. If that is too much to ask, make the goal easier; maybe your goal is getting there without screaming at the stupid drivers.

Creating those specific, achievable goals helps you set in motion a positive feedback cycle. You met your goal. What you did made you feel better. You felt good because you met your goal. You then want to keep it going. Letting yourself feel good about your accomplishment is vital. *Celebrate your successes!*

Step 4—Pay Attention to the Process

Implementing your strategy requires determination, but it also demands gentleness. Living with a drill sergeant isn't going to work, especially if *you* are the drill sergeant. Instead of going AWOL, leaving your grand plans for better health behind you, kick out the drill sergeant. For some patients, I need to be a cheerleader, doing everything I can to convince them of the need for change and applauding their positive steps. For many others, particularly those who are less healthy than they used to be because of age, illness, or just letting themselves go, I have to work extra hard to help them reign in their overenthusiasm.

Particularly with exercise, it is very easy to do too much too fast. The consequence is often an injury, and the time then needed for recovery often sets the patient further back than he or she was to begin with. You will make the fastest progress by going slow. When it comes to increasing physical activity, I tell all but the youngest, strongest patients to increase either intensity or duration by 10 percent a week.

Sometimes changing several problem areas in your life at the same time can be very good and a highly successful approach. Diet changes, in particular, are often most successful when they are dramatic. You feel better quickly, and that experience helps you do more. As you feel the benefit, your commitment will be stronger, and you will have more energy to do more to feel better still. Breaking old habits and creating better new ones sometimes works best when you dive into it as a real transformation.

The greatest wisdom is in simply paying attention to how you feel and adjusting accordingly.

Step 5—Build on Your Short-term Successes

Tied closely to the concept of early success is the distinction between short- and long-term goals. If you're going to be satisfied only when you have fully transformed from couch potato to triathlete, you are going to be unhappy, or injured, for a long time and are probably never going to become a triathlete.

Short-term goals are the steps on your path. Long-term goals are the destinations to where the path leads you. If you think only about the beach, you are going to get lost on the path through the jungle.

Failure

The road of excess leads to the palace of wisdom.
—William Blake

Failure is good. It is good because we have to make mistakes to learn. The only mistakes you make are the ones you don't learn from.

When I see a patient who hasn't implemented my recommendations, I always want to know why. I *must* understand why he or she failed. That's how I can help him or her go further. I don't want him or her to feel bad. I don't want to punish the patient and I don't want the patient to punish him or herself. To be successful we need to figure out the problem and solve it. Failure, mistakes, and then problem solving are each part of doing anything new. If I recommend swimming for a patient with back trouble as the best exercise for his or her condition, but he or she can't swim, what is the point? I missed the boat. If a patient hasn't been using the breathing exercise I recommended because he or she didn't understand how to do it, my job is to make that exercise clearer and easier. If someone is forgetting to take a supplement or medication he or she needs, we have to come up with a plan that works for him or her. You have to find your own ways, the specific steps, on your path toward better health.

Summary

- Conduct a self-assessment.
- Set goals.
  - Make them specific.
  - Make them achievable.
  - Celebrate your success.
  - Channel your inner cheerleader.
- Create long-term goals built on the short-term ones.
- Use failure to achieve success.

Part 3
Consider the Alternatives

Chapter 16

Consider the Alternatives

The old trope "There is more than one way to skin a cat" is one way to frame this discussion of "other" approaches to health. As long as you aren't a cat, it is a useful perspective.

Conventional medical orthodoxy has been pushing toward "practice guidelines" to develop "standards of care," seeking to improve the treatments provided to patients. Clinicians are more than decidedly ambivalent about these efforts because the guidelines too often trash whatever wisdom we have gained from taking care of our patients. (Yes, being under someone's thumb bruises our professional egos.) *Standard* is a dirty word, not just because it means average.

"Standardization" can lead to a rationally considered optimization of medical services. It can also become a creepily "big brother" intrusion between a patient and a provider. After all, that provider knows that individual patient better than anyone else, certainly far better than a board of researchers gathered in some far-removed conference room. Who wants to be standard or average? Do you? Don't you want the best health care possible? *Your* situation is unique, and optimal care for *you* is absolutely at least somewhat different from what your neighbor needs.

When we expand beyond the limited confines encompassed by conventional medicine, the questions become boundless. I'm absolutely certain that the most important things that can give you better health, including habits and treatment interventions, lie outside the boundaries of conventional medicine. Our job is to stretch those boundaries of convention so they become porous. Leaky boundaries are best, because some "unconventional" practices *are* better. We just don't realize that at the moment. We are still learning. Some practices, including many conventional ones, are ineffective or unsafe, and as has happened uncountable times before, they *will* someday be pushed aside. A good health practice is just that—good. Who cares whether it is orthodox or common? Certainly a suffering patient or caring physician doesn't.

In this chapter, I discuss the following:
- What is complementary and alternative medicine?
- Americans and CAM
- Who uses CAM in America?
- Why do people use CAM?
- A third path—you can all take a hike
- American CAM usages—patients and physicians
- Categories of CAM

What Is Complementary and Alternative Medicine?

Though it is easy to ask, this simple and straightforward question just can't be answered simply. In this case the name we choose tells us more about medicine or our own judgments than it does about the variety of healing choices in our world.

The difficultly is evident in the terminology. *Complementary* and *alternative* are words that have to lean on something else for their meaning. In this definition by difference, the "something else" that defines them is conventional Western medicine.

Unconventional was briefly the favored term. That word segregated the conventional therapies used in American hospitals and taught in American medical schools from everything else used either by professionals or the average person, to achieve healing. *Unconventional* sounded dangerous or disparaging. Very simply, it has also been wrong for as long as we know. The other healing approaches are actually not at all unconventional.

In 1995, I led the first survey of alternative medical education in US medical schools and learned that one-third of the schools were already teaching their students about these other forms of therapy.[86] That figure surprised pretty much every one, but it was rapidly eclipsed. By 1998, 80 percent of US medical schools were teaching students about these other therapies.[87]

Alternative essentially means "instead of." "Alternative medicine" is also then an inaccurate descriptor. Most people use these other therapies *in addition to, not instead of,* conventional medicine. It was not so very

86   Carlston et al., "Alternative Medicine Instruction in Medical Schools and Family Practice Residency programs," *Fam Med* 29 (1997):559-62.
87   Wetzel et al., "Courses Involving Complementary and Alternative Medicine at US Medical Schools," *JAMA* 280 (1998):784-7.

long ago when all of humanity used what are now called "alternative" therapies as their only health care. Even today the therapies defined as "alternative medicine" encompass what 80 percent of the world uses for health care. How can something most people do be labeled "alternative"? Is the use of this term motivated solely by antagonism, or does the term have meaning?

Over the years a variety of other terms have been used, including *holistic, integrative,* and *complementary*. Words can cut both ways. The term *holistic* (or *wholistic*) is a good example.

My mentor in medical school, who was unusually open minded toward alternatives, challenged my preference then for the term *holistic*, correctly pointing out that no doctor proudly claimed to practice "halfistic" medicine. He was a wise man. I have seen "alternative" practitioners ignore the complexity of complicated patients. Many times I have seen medical doctors, whose only therapeutic tools were entirely conventional, deeply involved in addressing the broad range of their patients' problems—emotional and even social services issues, not merely the medical diagnosis. Again, labels and words can impair understanding instead of leading to enlightenment.

The issue isn't about science either. The great majority of treatments every conventional medical doctor uses in the United States are not supported by solid research evidence proving they are effective. Does that mean they are ineffective? Does that mean some other understudied approach is ineffective? No and no.

While homeopathic physicians in the early 1800s prescribed the same medicines today's homeopathic physicians use, patients of those "conventional" physicians in the 1800s were treated with bloodletting and toxic doses of mercury and arsenic. It strikes me that homeopathic treatment in the nineteenth and early twentieth centuries looked much more like today's conventional medicine than did the "conventional" medicine of that time. The range of accepted methods of treating patients, the precise boundary between alternative and conventional medicine, is constantly evolving. For many, the term *alternative* emphasizes "otherness" nearly as much as *unconventional* did. Both labels are more political than enlightening.

"Integrative medicine" is probably the most popular label today. As a practitioner who integrates a variety of therapies in my work with patients, I'm comfortable with it. However, from the view of the independent patient, who treats himself or herself with only herbs or homeopathic remedies, *integrative medicine* doesn't fit quite so perfectly.

In many ways the term *complementary* is the most suitable single term. The great majority of Americans and people throughout the world choose a treatment based on its availability, effectiveness, and harmony with their own view of the world. There are circumstances when individuals refuse a particular therapy for any number of reasons (toxicity, expense, discomfort with the therapy, and so forth). They choose unconventional medical approaches when they want something different, something *complementary* to customary Western medical treatment. They might use the treatment instead of, or in addition to, conventional treatment. Consequently, "complementary and alternative medicine" (CAM) is the label I prefer and will use here.

Cutting to the heart of the matter, the editors of the *New England Journal of Medicine* (*NEJM*) wrote that there is no alternative and conventional medicine. There is just good and bad medicine. I agree wholeheartedly. As scientists, we must investigate with open minds, remembering that the patient's well-being is all that matters.

Ironically and perhaps uncomfortably, the opinion of the *NEJM* editors was perfectly harmonious with that of the founder of homeopathy, Samuel Hahnemann. He admonished physicians for constructing theoretical systems and clinging to them instead of focusing on healing patients. He began the book that established homeopathy with the following: "The physician's highest calling, his only calling, is to make sick people healthy–to heal as it is termed."[88] Less elegantly, I say that definitions don't matter. Healing people is what matters. There is a listing of CAM therapies at the end of this chapter.

Americans and CAM

One obvious reason the term *alternative* is misleading is that nationwide surveys over the past two decades have found that Americans visited practitioners of these therapies more often than they saw medical doctors. In 1993, one out of every three Americans sought treatment from a practitioner of "alternative" medicine, spending over $13 billion, which grew to $34 billion by 2007. Insurers and the health care industry

---

88   Samuel Hahnemann, *Organon of Medicine*, 6th ed. trans. Jost Kunzli, Alain Naude and Peter Pendleton. Los Angeles: Tarcher, 1982.

got very excited when they learned that Americans were so enthusiastic about CAM treatment that they spent more than $10 billion of their own money for these services. Americans have been voting for CAM with our bodies and our wallets. Although some felt that the newfound interest of insurers and medical institutions was a cynical cash grab, the outcomes have been positive. Awareness has led to more research delineating when CAM therapies are likely to be useful and to more open communication between patients and physicians.

Complementary and "alternative" approaches have become so common as to now be conventional. In any given year, nearly one-half of all Americans now use some form of CAM. Surveys confirm impressions that CAM popularity continues to rise. CAM is now both firmly established and widespread as an integral component of American health care.

Who Uses CAM in America?

While I have already established that CAM use is the norm in the United States, considering some of the patterns of use in the United States can help us understand CAM better.

The iconic American CAM user is a female between forty and seventy years of age. She has a graduate or professional degree, lives in the western part of the country, and earns an above-average income. Of course, this simple statistical summary is misleading. For example, Native Americans are the most impoverished ethnic group in the United States, but they have the highest rate of CAM use in the United States. Also, many US residents use CAM because they are uninsured and CAM costs them less than conventional medicine.

We should also recognize that CAM is used worldwide throughout developed and underdeveloped regions. The style and prevalence of specific CAM therapy usage vary broadly from country to country and by social class. CAM therapies are far from a uniquely American phenomenon. On the contrary, in many countries CAM therapies are even more highly regarded and accepted than in the USA. For example, Germany has officially recognized CAM practitioners since the 1930s, and in France, the study of homeopathy has been required of medical students for two decades.

Why Do People Use CAM?

So very many of us use CAM that it isn't surprising that there are lots of reasons why we do so. Those rationales influence the nature of therapies we choose as well as how and when we rely on them.

Cultural traditions have the greatest influence on CAM usage. A healing modality that is familiar is comfortable. Cultural institutions, attitudes, and history often maintain it. From the viewpoint of many cultures, conventional medicine is truly the alternative and unorthodox choice. Herbal medicines are the most common indigenous form of health care worldwide and, predictably, the most commonly practiced alternative healing modality used by ethnic minorities in the United States. Acupuncture is far more common among Asians than among other segments of the population. Shamanic healing is exceptionally rare among highly educated Caucasian Americans, but it is common among many other ethnic groups.

Limited access to conventional medicine only excludes conventional medicine. Limited conventional access doesn't mean people lack any care for their ills. Instead people turn to other resources or develop their own. Homeopathic medicine spread across the frontier of nineteenth-century America as mothers treated their families using Constantine Hering's *Domestic Physician*, as there were few medical doctors available. That book was, in fact, the highest-selling homeopathic book in America for well over a century. As the greatest local expertise was often Native American, settlers on the frontier were eager to learn how to use native plants. Those contacts between Native American healers and the Europeans moving out across North America led to the rise of the Eclectic and Thomsonian traditions of American herbal medicine. The process of integrating new information is, after all, what human culture is all about. There is nothing new in that.

Lack of access to health care is often a consequence of economic conditions. The bottom line is that self-treatment costs less than paying a professional. With the access to prescription medications legally controlled, self-treatment has often had to be some form of CAM. New immigrants pack their traditional medicines in the luggage they carry from their old homes to the new ones. They use those medicines guided by need and generations of experience. We can all learn from these unfamiliar therapies, but they sometimes include toxic elements (including hundreds of cases of pediatric lead poisoning).

Toxic and dangerous self-care is also an issue in a developing American cultural tradition. As the Internet has opened a Pandora's box of access to otherwise prescription-only medication, self-treatment with prescription drugs is a rising and risky form of self-care.

Highly educated Americans often choose CAM therapies, hoping to avoid the risk of toxic reactions they believe prescription medications will cause. Some Americans use CAM, not because they are sick, but because they believe they can use CAM for wellness, to become even healthier. Some choose CAM based on a philosophical connection they have to a CAM therapy. Some turn away from conventional practitioners, feeling that CAM practitioners are more supportive and give them more hope.

The number one reason Americans turn to CAM therapies is as simple as can be. They don't feel well, and conventional medicine hasn't helped. The bottom line is getting better. In one review, for example, the majority of patients with back trouble who sought CAM treatment did so because they found conventional treatment to be ineffective. Approximately 60 percent of these conventional-treatment-failing patients then discovered that CAM *was* effective for them. In this review, the most effective CAM therapies for back trouble were chiropractic, massage, yoga, qigong, tai chi, and acupuncture.

A Third Path—You Can All Take a Hike

There is a nearly invisible "elephant in the room" that is important to this discussion of self-care and treatment choices. An experience I had one day years ago shined a light on the "elephant."

It occurred during a talk I gave about homeopathy at a local seniors' center. The group was gathered in a small circle. I sat down in one of the chairs before we began. As the host introduced me, the woman next to me started to gather her things into a shopping bag, clearly preparing to leave. I whispered to her, asking why she was leaving. Her response was as meaningful as it was succinct: "You are a medical doctor." I convinced her to hear me out, and she later became one of my patients.

However, she never set aside her determination to make her own choices, starting at her first visit when I discovered she had what is aptly called "malignant" hypertension. Her blood pressure was 250/130! After

I told her she needed to go into the hospital, probably into the intensive care unit, she countered my plans, saying, "Doc, I'm leaving for vacation in Hawaii tomorrow." She survived her vacation, and we shared many such "interesting" but nerve-racking experiences over the subsequent years.

Her independence exemplifies some findings in David Eisenberg's groundbreaking 1993 US survey of CAM use that were generally overlooked. When patients who had identified themselves as having a "significant health problem" were asked who they saw for health care, 58 percent reported seeing only a conventional physician, 3 percent saw only a CAM professional, and 7 percent saw both. But a stunning 33 percent saw neither. In other words, *one-third of those who felt they had a significant health problem took care of things themselves without any professional help.* This is humbling evidence that the choices American's make in their health care decisions extend far beyond the territory we professionals claim as our own, and people are probably suffering as a consequence of our off-putting arrogance. Sometimes people make this choice because their finances or access to care are limited for some other reason. However, people aren't dissatisfied only with conventional medicines; they are dissatisfied, or at least skeptical, of CAM and physicians or health-care professionals of all allegiances.

Physicians sense this dissatisfaction while experiencing some of it themselves. Increasingly, conventional physicians express an interest in learning about CAM practices, and institutions of medical education are responding to that perceived need. One of the preeminent conventional physicians of the twentieth century, Bernard Lown, authored a book *The Lost Art of Healing*, in which he wrote, "Medicine has lost its way if not its soul. An unwritten covenant between doctor and patient, hallowed over several millennia, is being broken."[89] Later in the book, Dr. Lown expressed, correctly I believe, that part of the impetus toward CAM is the sense we have that in CAM we might regain the connection between patient and physician that we lost with our increasing reliance on medical technology.

---

89   Bernard Lown, *The Lost Art of Healing* (Boston: Houghton Mifflin, 1996).

American CAM Usage—Patients and Physicians

In 1993, the most heavily used forms of CAM in the United States were relaxation and chiropractic medicine, with alternative systems such as acupuncture and homeopathy being much less common. Since that time the alternative systems have become increasingly prevalent. With the glaring exception of herbal medicine, they are still much less widespread than other approaches.

The use of herbal medicines has risen most dramatically (over 500 percent). This is a crucial fact for numerous reasons. Because herbal medicine was already relatively more common than other CAM therapies, its use is now extremely common. Estimates by the American Botanical Council and others indicate that we spend close to $6 billion annually on herbal supplements. One study found that nearly one-half of Americans had, at some point, taken the herb echinacea. The rising popularity of herbal medicines has led to significant issues involving quality, proper identification, adulteration, and contamination.

Chiropractic is one of the most widespread and firmly established CAM therapies. Although survey data don't show any increase in American visits to chiropractors, 10 percent of us visit a chiropractor in any given year. Most conventional physicians aren't happy about that, but frankly, patients don't care.

In comparison, acupuncture and homeopathy are much less common. As fully developed systems of medicine with their own uniquely cohesive theoretical world view and approach to treatment, they are fundamentally different from conventional medicine. Their alternative metaphors for disease and healing make understanding and accepting them more challenging for conventionally trained physicians and patients accustomed to the prevailing Western biomedical model. At times they directly conflict with the assumptions of conventional medicine. Many of us find these challenges to be refreshing because of the fundamental questions they pose. Despite these differences, American acceptance of acupuncture and homeopathy is also rising rapidly, with a three-fold increase in users of each over a recent ten-year period.

As conventional physicians have become more aware of CAM, they have become increasingly anxious about toxic effects of CAM therapies, particularly interactions between herbal products and conventional

233

medicines. It appears that somewhere between 20 and 50 percent of patients taking prescription medication are also taking herbs or high doses of vitamins, while only a minority of those patients (28 to 62 percent) inform their medical doctors about that concurrent usage. From 35 to 45 percent of Americans suffering from anxiety, depression, back problems, or chronic pain conditions seek both conventional and CAM treatment.

Cancer patients often choose to add CAM to their treatments. A Boston University study of patients with thyroid cancer found that over 80 percent used CAM treatments. European studies of lung, colorectal, and gynecologic cancer patients found that 25, 32, and 40 percent, respectively, used CAM, with herbal medicine most popular, followed by homeopathy, massage, spiritual healing, and vitamin supplements. Many US estimates are that 25 to 50 percent of patients with cancer use some form of CAM. Other well-done US and European surveys show that the majority of American and European cancer patients use at least one CAM therapy either on their own or with the assistance of a health-care professional.

By a slim majority, Americans using CAM tend to do so on their own, without the advice of a physician or any practitioner otherwise trained in the use of CAM. This use varies considerably by therapy. Just a small portion of American homeopathy involves the participation of professional practitioners (10 to 20 percent), in stark contrast with acupuncture or chiropractic therapy, which almost invariably does so.

Given the discomfort many conventional physicians feel about CAM, it is ironic then that in a way we are all CAM practitioners. Between 30 and 40 percent of conventional medicines are derived from plants; very few can by synthesized less expensively, and some can't be synthesized at all. Medical doctors are unwitting, part-time herbalists.

Although communication is improving, the patterns of CAM use are still concerning. This isn't true only for physicians with a skeptical or antagonistic attitude toward CAM. As a long-time advocate of CAM, I'm also concerned. My concern is that too many patients with serious diseases are taking powerful prescription drugs, but still not informing their physicians of their use of CAM. There is a very real potential for dangerous, unanticipated interactions. As patients often turn to CAM when conventional medicine has failed them, I'm concerned about the cases where the conventional practitioner has missed the conventional diagnosis. That is a common experience in my practice. While CAM approaches are often superior, informed decisions are essential and dependent on accurate diagnoses.

Unfortunately, the reluctance of patients to discuss their CAM usage with physicians is too often justified. Conventional doctors are still too dismissive or even reactionary. Too many of us maintain that CAM practices don't do anything—that is, except for the times when we rail against them because they are harmful. It is difficult to understand how an ineffective treatment can be harmful, the exception being when a patient neglects an effective conventional treatment. Patients do have the right to refuse effective conventional treatment. Patients are also free to reject treatment more likely to harm than to help, as can sometimes be the case with conventional treatments. Underlying all this, though, is the need to make good decisions, and the crucial importance of physician-patient communication as a true dialog, in both directions, to provide the patient with the accurate information required. Poor communication leads to mistrust and bad decisions, preventing us from learning what works, what doesn't, and when harm might result.

Categories of CAM

A bit later I will go over some more specifics, but with such an immense range of possibilities, it is helpful to consider the widely diverse range of CAM therapies in an organized way. One schema is to group them into five categories.

- There are full-fledged systems of complementary medicine with their own world view and specific theories (for example, acupuncture, Ayurveda, and homeopathy).
- Mind-body medicine includes therapies that work specifically to develop mental or emotional control over symptoms (e.g., biofeedback, dance therapy, prayer, and psychotherapy).
- Biological therapies act through their biochemical effects on human physiology (e.g., dietary supplements, herbal therapies, and vitamins).
- Manipulation or body work involves physical manipulation and movement (e.g., chiropractic, massage, osteopathy, and Rolfing).
- Energetic healing uses subtle energies to promote health (e.g., Jin Shin, magnets, qigong, Reiki, and therapeutic touch).

Conventional Western medicine more comfortably adopts some of these therapies. That is true because they are more palatable to those with a conventional perspective either because they are stylistically familiar in application (herbs and vitamins) or the theories behind them are not so disturbing (massage and biofeedback).

The systems (acupuncture, homeopathy, and Ayurveda) generally developed independently of conventional medicine and have their own comprehensive theory and philosophy. They tend to be firmly established within a regional culture, sometimes for millennia. Consequently, these systems of medicine are more likely to be used as alternatives to conventional medicine than the other forms of CAM. Their "otherness" makes them lightning rods for conventional antagonism. The presumption is that these approaches are so different, how could they possibly be worthy of attention? Homeopathy approaches patients holistically and views symptoms as a functional attempt of the organism to heal itself. Acupuncture and Ayurveda view the patient's disease as an imbalance of the body's various energies and use assorted means to recover that balance. Those concepts are very different from the pure biomechanics of today's conventional medicine.

The list I have constructed herein may be exhausting, but it isn't exhaustive. That is, this list is incomplete and inevitably arbitrary (especially in the categorizations). Exponents of homeopathy, acupuncture, and qigong, for example, often attribute the efficacy of their methods to their impact on energies of the body, so they could be categorized differently, favoring that "energy" emphasis. Even the seeming familiarity of herbal medicine, simply replacing a prescription drug with an herb, is an oversimplification. That limited view is grossly at odds with some "energetic" schools of herbal thought. Anyone who has ever looked for a book on the best diet or considered the variable use of plants for healing across the wide expanse of our planet recognizes the error in such assumptions of standardization. Human beings have developed a variety of methods to relieve their own suffering, and they are as diverse as the earth itself. You could spend many lifetimes studying these approaches without learning all there is to know about any of them.

Mind-Body Interventions

- Art therapy
- Biofeedback
- Breathing techniques
- Dance therapy
- Hypnosis
- Imagery
- Meditation or relaxation
- Music therapy
- Prayer and mental Healing
- Psychotherapy
- Tai chi
- Yoga

Bioelectromagnetic Applications in Medicine

- Biofield therapeutics
- Electrostimulation
- Light therapy
- Magnetic and electromagnetic therapy
- Reiki

Alternative Systems of Medical Practice

- African traditional medicine
- Anthroposophical medicine
- Ayurvedic medicine
- Curanderismo
- Environmental medicine
- Herbal medicine
- Homeopathic medicine
- Native American Indian health-care practices
- Naturopathic
- Santeria
- Shamanism

Alternative Systems of Medical Practice (continued)

- Traditional Oriental medicine
  - Acupuncture
  - Cupping
  - Qigong (asthma, back pain)
  - Moxibustion

Manual Healing Methods

- Alexander technique
- Applied kinesiology
- Craniosacral therapy
- Chiropractic medicine
- Counterstrain
- Feldenkrais
- Healing touch
- Massage therapy
- Network chiropractic spinal analysis
- Osteopathic medicine
- Pilates
- Polarity therapy
- Pressure point therapies
- Postural reeducation therapies
- Rolfing
- Trager

Pharmacological and Biological Treatments

- Apitherapy (bee venom)
- Cartilage
- Chelation
- Diet and nutritional therapy
- Essiac
- Hoxsey method
- Hyperbaric oxygen
- Iscador/mistletoe
- Marijuana and psychedelics

Chapter 17

How and When to Use CAM

There are many adherents of either conventional medicine or CAM therapies that believe patients should avoid "the other side" like the plague. They feel their favored therapy is the only safe or effective means to heal and that the other approaches are ineffective at best. Sadly, it isn't rare (typical?) for a health-care provider to feel that "the other side" is unethical, corrupt, or malign.

We currently hold only fragments of the objective data ultimately required to settle all such disputes. There is basic sciences research supporting the theoretical potential of many CAM treatments. Most importantly, we have clinical studies that establish solid footing for certain CAM treatments for certain conditions (for example, acupuncture for back pain; relaxation, biofeedback, and meditation for lowering blood pressure; red yeast rice to reduce cholesterol; and probiotics for GI infections). We also have studies showing that homeopathic treatment of chronic health conditions is more cost effective than conventional medical treatment. There is new research finding that combining psychedelics with psychotherapy dramatically improves quality of life for terminal patients. The wealth of studies demonstrating the ineffectiveness of conventional therapies for common problems (anti-vertigo medications, antibiotics for ear infections, and treatment of the common cold) proves that looking elsewhere is entirely reasonable. At the same time, we lack the unbiased information that would enable us to make well-informed decisions as to the perfect therapy for every circumstance. As I have written repeatedly, ad nauseam perhaps, this is the reality of medicine, and we must then choose in semi-ignorance.

Over the decades it has become transparently clear to me that no one approach is complete, so we health-care providers should actively

encourage patients to seek out other healers and therapies as warranted. As a conventionally trained medical doctor, experienced in CAM
therapies, my approach has developed as follows:

- Establish the medical diagnosis.
- Understand conventional treatment options.
- Evaluate CAM providers.
- What about self-care?
- With choice comes responsibility.
- Steps to manage your health care responsibly.
- When is which therapy a good option?
- For physicians.

Establish the Medical Diagnosis

People suffer from any number of a long list of symptoms for a variety
of reasons. Fatigue may be the most common symptom any of us experience. It can be caused by cancer, depression, poor diet, heart disease,
food sensitivities, sleep disturbances, influenza, or literally a thousand
other possibilities. Neglecting any of the essential health habits can lead
to fatigue, but so too can nearly any medical problem. Pretty much the
same can be said of all the common symptoms human beings experience,
including headaches, body pains, and sleep and digestive disturbances
among them. *Understanding the cause for your symptoms* is a vital prereq-
uisite to selecting a treatment. If your symptoms are due to a bad health
habit, taking a prescription drug won't fix it, and the adverse effects will
probably make you feel worse.

Patients don't turn to CAM just because of an idealistic impulse;
they do so because they hope for a treatment that is gentler but at least as
effective as conventional medicine. In line with survey findings, patients
usually come to me for CAM treatment because conventional medicine
didn't help them. In many of those cases, the previous physician missed
his or her diagnosis. In some cases, a safe and effective conventional
medical treatment, one perhaps acceptable to the patient, was available
if the disorder had been recognized. The medical diagnosis can be one (a
vitamin or mineral deficiency, for example) where the treatment must
replace the missing nutrient. At other times, when the missed diagnosis
is a life-threatening condition, like some cancer, for example, it is vital
for the patient to understand what the options are.

In truth, I share some concerns with the most CAM-phobic physicians. There is a significant risk when we presume that symptoms are benign and aren't caused by a serious medical condition. Establishing the diagnosis is more than merely prudent. It also allows patients to understand their options and the consequences of their treatment choices.

No matter what I, some other physician, or anyone else believes, some patients will make opposing decisions, some that seem unwise. I have had entirely rational patients make health care decisions that would seem bizarre to others (sometimes including me). We are free to make our own decisions, but no one should do so without understanding where he or she stands—what *is* going on. If a patient elects to try a CAM therapy without seeing a medical doctor, it is important for the patient or CAM provider (if there is one) to be wary. Remember that persistence of even a minor symptom could indicate that a more serious problem is brewing. In any event, sticking with an unproductive treatment, conventional or CAM, isn't a good idea.

Ironically, of course, my experience counters at least part of my own argument. If patients are seeking CAM after their conventional MD missed the diagnosis in the first place, what is the point of sending them back to a conventional doctor? My conventional training, coupled with the disproportionate number of patients seeking treatment for missed, often unusual, medical conditions, has sharpened my diagnostic abilities. Despite the advantages of my experiences, I'm as imperfect as any other health-care provider. We all make mistakes. Maybe the greatest wisdom is *caveat emptor*. In other words, the patient should look out for himself or herself and avoid placing too much faith in *any* healer. He or she should look for some other option if the treatment isn't progressing as expected.

Understand Conventional Treatment Options

After the medical diagnosis is established, making choices is far easier. If you know where you stand (diagnosis), it is possible to make a pretty good guess where you are headed (prognosis). With that map, recognizing the consequences of your choices, you can make better decisions, the ones that are best for you.

Generally speaking, conventional medicine's greatest strength is treating serious injuries and immediately stopping life-threatening disease. If you are in such a circumstance, conventional medical treatment is absolutely warranted. Applying a risk-benefit decision strategy is best. If the conventional treatment is unlikely to be helpful and likely to make you feel worse, you're less likely to want to charge down that path. If conventional medical treatment is likely to help with only a minimal risk of bad effects, those less severe than the disease, it becomes more appealing.

The same is true of CAM therapies. Sadly, the volume of relevant medical data is almost invariably much, much smaller. That lack of information alters the decision-making process significantly. The data on treatment efficacy is usually far too sparse to lead to easy decisions. Most often the consideration boils down to balancing the unclear possibility of the CAM therapy helping versus what is better known about the therapy's adverse effects and cost in comparison to conventional treatment.

Evaluate CAM Practitioners

In the face of uncertainty regarding the method, seeking expert opinions is an excellent idea. In this case, that means asking those who use CAM. Clinical experience and clinical research are both limited and potentially misleading. They do, however, complement each other. Ideally, clinical research helps us objectify the experiential truths of clinical practice. Clinical research of conventional and CAM treatments is limited by complexity; it is simply too difficult and expensive to conduct adequate clinical trials capable of testing every situation that arises in even the most routine clinical practice.

The clinical knowledge of highly experienced clinicians stretches far beyond the reach of clinical research. We have all treated patients with a broader range of problems than clinical research can ever encompass. Clinicians must continually make decisions based on their best judgment with or without the support of research. Sick patients cannot and shouldn't wait. Experienced clinicians will know what *appears* to work.

How about objectivity? As health-care providers almost certainly believe in what they are doing and make a living in that work, why (and when) should a patient trust the judgment of any clinician?

The best clinicians learn the most from their patient care experiences. Even a mediocre clinician has to be circumspect. To provide the *best* care, a good clinician will critique his or her experience. Any clinician who is honest with himself or herself will form opinions about what works for what and when, as well as what doesn't work for what and when. Starting from the foundation of medical training and reading medical literature, he or she learns what truly works in the real world by the experience of treating patients. The wisdom gained from open-eyed experience is invaluable. Based on such experience, a good practitioner, CAM or conventional, can give you a reasonably good idea whether he or she is going to be able to help you.

The best clinicians are confident but, at the same time, sufficiently humble that they recognize their limitations. Acknowledging our deficiencies is essential for learning. Otherwise, why bother? Recognition of our limits leads us to seek out other clinicians, hoping they might know something more. That something more, something beyond the individual physician's current experience, might be the missing ingredient to help patients unrelieved by the best care we know. This desire to learn more, to help patients we have been unable to help so far, takes us beyond our present boundaries. That is where the best clinicians, conventional or CAM, meet each other and learn what the other might be able to accomplish.

As the best clinicians, conventional and otherwise, learn about each other, we can guide our patients toward the best care available. When I moved to California, I asked a local doctor, whose judgment I valued, to give me a list of conventional medical specialists she thought were the best locally. That gave me a very good start, helping me make certain that my patients received good medical care. Over the years, the feedback I got from patients who shared the experiences they had with other providers added tremendously to my fund of referral information. Patients and the local health food stores also accelerated my learning by telling me who the best CAM practitioners were. It is an ongoing process and one of my most important responsibilities to my patients.

Professional reputations are established over time and represent the opinion of the community. Communal wisdom is often phenomenally accurate. It would be foolish to ignore it.

From the other side, the practitioner side, I still recall one day when I asked a new patient how he or she came to see me. He told me that someone at his work had recommended me. After that another friend, who didn't know his work friend, had recommended that he see me. He finally decided to make an appointment to see me on the day a guy was delivering water to his house, heard him sneezing from allergies, and told him he should see me.

The following outline will help you identify and sort through prospective CAM providers:

Evaluating CAM Practitioners

Find them.

- Ask your friends, family, and coworkers.
- Visit health food stores.
- Consult professional organizations.
- Look online.

Talk to them.

- Find information about the practitioner.
  - How did you get your training, and how long did it take?
  - How much experience have you had?
  - How much experience have you had with patients like me?
  - How do you feel about my using conventional medicine?
- What is going to happen?
- What do you do during the visits?
- How many times will you need to see me?
- How long should it be before I feel better?
- What sort of adverse effects might I experience?
- Are there supplements, medications, or other items I will have to buy?
- How much will all this cost me?
- Can you suggest something for me to read?

What about Self-Care?

Much of CAM use in this country is in the form of self-treatment. That idea, of course, makes health professionals very nervous. We all have horror stories of tragic cases where a person ignored a serious health problem. The reality is that *you* are in charge of your health. Furthermore, no matter what any health professional thinks, me included, you provide nearly all of your own health care. You bandage your own cuts, you choose what to eat, and when things get bad enough, you decide whether to get help from a professional like me.

Recognizing that reality, I urge you to be the best self-doctor you can be. We learn from each other. In the past people learned how to take care of themselves mostly from parents, family, and friends with occasional help from a local, semi educated healer. Such cultural healing traditions have been increasingly fragmented and degraded as our cultures scramble and reconnect. Asking others is always a good idea. Books partially replaced the neighborhood gossip circle, and now, more dramatically, the Internet has done so.

Unlike some other doctors, I love how patients use the Internet. Typical of the profession's stodgy conservatism, the prevalent tone of commentary about the Internet within medicine has been a whine or loud moaning that the Internet is a Pandora's box that overwhelms patients with misinformation. I disagree. To me, it is actually a marked improvement. In the past people would uncover just a little bit amount of information from a limited number of sources, including neighbors and books. Much of that information was good, and some of it was bad. Today there is a lot more bad information available, but in the information avalanche that is the Internet, much more of it is genuinely excellent. You can learn just about all you want with a computer and an Internet connection. In a way, the volume of conflicting information a person confronts on the Internet teaches her or him to think critically.

As a professional, in an instant I can find information that even ten years ago would have required the resources of a large medical library, the assistance of a medical librarian, and days of work. To be honest, it is better than that. Even all that time and effort wouldn't have led me to the mother lode of shared experience, research, and wisdom that is the Internet.

The strength and weakness of the Internet is its sheer size. The best resources can become echo chambers for bad or misinterpreted information, establishing falsity as truth. Bear in mind that many sites merely recycle the content of other sites. When you see the same exact phrases, that content came from the same source. Electronic plagiarism isn't higher truth. Don't get fooled into thinking that another independent expert reached the same inevitable conclusion. With even a cursory attempt at digging just a bit, comparing sources, and thinking critically, you will be able to uncover a range of opinions on any topic. Then the Internet will become the greatest source of useful, accurate, and practically free information you have known since your parents taught you to walk and speak.

Again, when a problem is persistent or severe, please consider seeing a conventional physician to get a medical diagnosis. That is why over-the-counter medications always carry a warning about not using them for more than a few days without seeing a doctor.

With Choice Comes Responsibility

When you make the decision to treat yourself or to try something different, you have to accept responsibility for those decisions. This is a good thing. Far too many patients simply turn all the decision making over to their conventional medical doctor. No matter how good the physician is, not only do you know more about you, but the outcome of treatment is more important to you than anyone else. Why then wouldn't you want to take as active a role as possible?

Medical doctors in the USA moan about patient compliance. They can't get patients to exercise or change their diets, so they've given up trying to convince them. Many patients never get their prescriptions filled, and most stop taking their medications, even when their MD still wants them to take the pills. Studies show that patients seeking homeopathic treatment in the United States are far more likely to follow the homeopath's recommendations. In fact, homeopathic patients are more likely to do what the homeopathic recommends than they are to feel better from the homeopathic treatment.[90]

---

90   Goldstein and Glik, "Use of and Satisfaction with Homeopathy in a Patient Population," *Altern Ther Health Med* 4 (1998):60-5.

What are the reasons for these differences? Maybe the most important is that the normal mode of patient-physician interaction in conventional medicine assumes or at least encourages submission and dependence. "Fix me, Doc" is the patient attitude. The doctor becomes a Medical Deity, and the patient becomes a passive recipient of our good works. Inevitably, this passive role is reflected in poor compliance. When health care is done to you, why would you do anything? While that is a good model for the care you receive in surgery, the rest of the time passivity is the arch enemy of well-being and good health care. It's your body. You are in charge. No one expects those in charge to stand idly by in a time of crisis. Why would you when your health is threatened?

Steps to Manage Your Health Care Responsibly

I encourage you to take formal steps to make better decisions. It's such a good idea that you really should put some work into it and do it right. The process of assessing your present condition and sorting out your goals and expectations about the path toward achieving those health goals will keep you on track and minimize the odds of making mistakes along the way. This awareness will also help you get back on course more quickly if you do go astray.

Evaluating Treatment

Initial visit—how are you at the beginning?

- Keep daily symptom diary, rating symptoms one to ten.
- Make a record of treatment goals.

Return visits—how are you now?

- Review your symptom diary.

Discuss with provider perceived benefits and adverse reactions.

Consider other treatment options, if needed.

Where are you now? What is the main problem? What are your other concerns? Make a list rating the intensity and frequency of your symptoms. You can use that for later comparison. What are your expectations? How long before you expect to get better? What would better look like? What are you going to have to do? What is it going to cost you? At what point are you going to consider other treatment options? Periodically reevaluate your condition and review your symptom diary, reactions to treatment standing relative to your desired outcomes. Then consider whether now might be the time to change treatment strategies.

You can apply this approach all across your health care. You can use it as a means to keep on track with self-care. You can also apply it when someone else is treating you. You can use it to better manage treatment by a conventional physician or a CAM provider.

When Is Which Therapy a Good Option?

You need to make choices about what you should do. My job here is to help you. First, remember that a practitioner's ability and availability are paramount. Acupuncture might be great for your problem, but if there isn't an acupuncturist nearby, you need to pick another option. Second, my recommendations are a combination of science and experience.

Although we all complain about the lack of research on CAM treatments, there is a lot of research. Scientific proof is a nearly insatiable hunger. Our methods are too uncertain to lead to definitive conclusions without massive accumulations of data, data, and still more data. Additionally, the scope of these methods dwarfs conventional medicine, multiplying the number of studies required to reach similar levels of certainty about their effects. You can dig through some of the most useful careful scientific reviews by going to pertinent pages on the websites of the National Center for Complementary and Integrative Health and the Cochrane Library (search "complementary and alternative medicine"[91], [92]). Research evidence partly supports the list that follows. That isn't enough, though.

---

91   National Center for Complementary and Integrative Health
https://nccih.nih.gov/health/providers/litreviews.htm
92   Cochrane Collaboration (complementary and alternative medicine)
http://www.thecochranelibrary.com/view/0/index.html#http://www.
thecochranelibrary.com/view/0/browse.html

Clinical experience, despite its subjectivity, extends further than research and warrants respect. My clinical experience has influenced

Mind-Body Interventions

Art therapy—depression, Alzheimer's dementia, stress management

Biofeedback—pain management, anxiety, stress, blood pressure regulation, migraines, bladder control, peripheral circulation (for example, Raynaud's)

Breathing techniques—anxiety, asthma, high blood pressure, stress reduction

Dance therapy—psychological and physical outcomes in cancer patients, ADHD, PTSD

Hypnosis—bed wetting, smoking, drug addiction, labor and delivery, migraines, pain management

Imagery—anxiety, immune augmentation with cancer, sports performance, pain management

Meditation/relaxation—hot flashes, pain, back pain, anxiety, insomnia, pain management

Music therapy—autism, cancer quality of life, pain, anxiety with medical procedures, depression

Prayer and mental healing—anxiety, stress reduction

Psychotherapy—anxiety, depression

Tai chi—Alzheimer's disease, back pain, fall prevention, anxiety

Yoga—back pain, anxiety, insomnia, arthritis, fall prevention my list. Even though I have four decades of experience along this path, that is not enough to know everything, not even close.

For a time I consulted with a company whose business was to, in turn, advise health insurers and large provider organizations about the integration of alternative medicine into their coverage. It was very interesting work. It was so interesting because the company collected a panel of experts in various fields of alternative medicine, me among them. We then sat together and determined which therapies might be best suited for various medical conditions. The experts were all quite circumspect in their perceptions of their own field. These honest assessments by the most highly regarded experts in these therapies were invaluable. Those collective opinions have also influenced the following list.

Despite all this input, I still ask for your forbearance. Please forgive me as the possibilities are endless. Although I'm confident about the content of this listing, I'm supremely confident that my listing is woefully incomplete.

Please view this list through the lens of your experience and that of people you trust. What have you and they found helpful? Just because there is no research evidence that you will feel better by setting aside the worries of your day and going out dancing with your friends certainly doesn't mean dancing is worthless.

Patients often tell me they got better from something I don't know very well or something I've consistently not found helpful for others.

Bioelectromagnetic Applications in Medicine

Biofield therapeutics

Electrostimulation—pain, depression

Jin Shin—pain, anxiety

Light therapy—depression, insomnia

Magnetic and electromagnetic therapy

Reiki—pain management

Alternative Systems of Medical Practice

African Traditional Medicine—prevention of sickle cell crises, anxiety

Anthroposophical Medicine

Ayurvedic Medicine—general well-being, digestive complaints

Curanderismo

Environmental Medicine—allergies, any symptoms influenced by location and season

Herbal Medicine—too many to count

Homeopathic Medicine—adverse effects of radiation and chemotherapy, anxiety, insomnia, digestive disorders, croup, otitis media

Native American Indian health-care practices—depression, stress management

Naturopathic Medicine (practice encompasses many of these therapies, so broadly useful)

Santeria—anxiety, depression

Shamanism—depression, stress management

Traditional Oriental Medicine

- Acupuncture—chemotherapy's adverse effects, smoking cessation, insomnia, back pain
- Herbs—chemotherapy's adverse effects, cancer survival, ulcerative colitis, small bowel obstruction
- Qigong—asthma, back pain
- Moxibustion—Cephalic version (repositioning breech babies)

Manual Healing Methods

Alexander technique—pain

Applied kinesiology

Craniosacral therapy—headaches, colic, post-concussion syndromes, head trauma, pain management

Chiropractic medicine—back pain

Counterstrain—back pain

Feldenkrais healing touch—pain management

Healing touch—pain management

Massage therapy—anxiety, back pain

Osteopathic medicine—pain, headaches

Pilates—musculoskeletal pain, fall prevention

Pressure point therapies—pain

Postural reeducation therapies—back pain, stress

Rolfing—pain, headaches

That doesn't mean it didn't happen. I don't know it all. Maybe it's just that the people who were helped didn't need to see me because they were already relieved from that other treatment. I only saw those who didn't get better. Even if it was a placebo experience, that patient *did* get better. *That* is the bottom line. When patients report such outliers, such atypical experiences, I don't immediately change my opinion. Instead, I note those experiences, hoping to learn more from those patients, and move forward with a healthy uncertainty. That is my job.

It is imperative that you think carefully about the risks of your choices. Remember my patient with the malignant hypertension? Ignoring that problem wasn't a good choice. She also harmed herself in other ways.

Pharmacological and Biological Treatments

Apitherapy (bee venom)—arthritis

Cartilage—arthritis

Chelation—diabetics with heart disease, kidney disease

Diet and nutritional therapy—gastrointestinal cancers, cancer survival, chemotherapy's adverse effects, autism, death from infectious disease, insomnia

Hyperbaric oxygen—cancer survival, musculoskeletal injury, skin ulcers, skin infection

Iscador (mistletoe)—breast cancer quality of life

Marijuana and psychedelics—chemotherapy nausea, end of life anxiety

Once, for example, she applied an electrical current (not a little trickle of voltage—I mean from an electrical outlet) through her body, hoping to burn a skin cancer off her nose and avoid surgery. Yes, she *did* end up in the hospital that time, with heart failure.

For Physicians

My patients often tell me they have found one of these CAM therapies helpful, frequently in a life-changing way. I am thankful they have shared their experiences with me so I can learn from them and help others. I'm just as grateful that patients have felt comfortable relating their experiences to me. Physicians are supposed to be health experts in the broadest sense. We need to gather knowledge and experience to help our patients find healing. Patients chose CAM treatments. Doctors must learn to help patients find the best therapies and the professionals with the skills to provide the care the patients need.

My bottom-line advice to physicians is to try to remember that medical doctors don't know it all, and no one else does either. You work for your patients, not the other way around. Support them and keep them realistically informed about dangers. Remember to grit your teeth and swallow your pride. These steps will make you a wiser and more effective physician. Also, your patients are more likely to listen to your criticisms if you scrupulously critique conventional medicine at the same time that you consider the potentials of these other approaches to healing. Yes, we are members of the Western medical fraternity, but we are also part of a much larger healing tradition, one that includes other healing professionals.

Physician Evaluation of CAM Practitioner Referrals

Find them.

- Ask your patients.
- Visit health food stores.
- Consult professional organizations.

Talk to them and ask questions:

- How do you feel about your patients using conventional medicine?
- What problems do you think you can best help?
- What problems do you think you are unlikely or unable to help?
- What are appropriate referrals?
- How did you get your training, and how long did it take?
- What do you do with patients?
- How much experience have you had?
- What much will your help cost patients?
- What can I read to learn about your approach (include research)?
- How can I help make your treatment successful?

Physician Evaluation of
CAM Practitioner Referrals (continued)

Evaluate referrals.

Establish a baseline before the initial CAM visit.

- How is the patient now?
- Keep daily symptom diary, rating one to ten.
- Make a record of treatment goals.

Reassess at return visits.

- How is the patient now?
- Review the symptom diary.
- Discuss perceived benefits and adverse reactions.

Consider other treatment options, if needed.

Summary

- There is good reason to consider CAM.
- Responsible use relies on clarity.
  - Known diagnosis
  - Specific goals
  - Fair evaluation
- Tap into community resources and knowledge.

Chapter 18

Herbal Supplements

Herbal medicine is common, widespread, and ancient. Some estimate that herbal medicine constitutes the health care of as much as 80 percent of the world's population. Human beings have been using plants to treat illness as far back in time as we can determine. It is probably the oldest method of healing. The use of plants for healing is so extensive and archaic that humans cannot even claim exclusive rights to the discovery. There is evidence that monkeys and other animals will seek out specific medicinal plants when they are ill. Not only is there consistency in the plants these animals select, but also scientific testing has found that these plants often have biologic effects (for example, antibacterial) that one would expect to help that sick animal. If you want to learn more, search the Internet for the term *zoopharmacognosy*.

Most Americans who use herbal medicine do so without the direction of a medical doctor. Many use herbs without the guidance of *any* health professional. The most widespread use of herbs in the United States has been among the elderly. Ginkgo had long been the most popular single herb in the United States, until echinacea recently outpaced it. Ginkgo is most commonly used to improve memory. Ginseng and garlic are used primarily for aging-related concerns, and they are nearly as popular as ginkgo.

The coincidence of the greatest usage by the portion of the population most likely to also use prescription medication highlights and justifies concerns about interactions between prescription medication and herbs. This evidence makes medical doctors anxious, afraid that patients to whom they prescribe medications are highly likely to use herbs at the same time. Medical fears of drug-herb interactions are heightened because we're still early in the process of learning about the extent and nature of herb-drug interactions.

- Traditional use
- Scientific investigation

- Conventional medicine and herbs
- Safety issues
  - Proper identification
  - What part of the plant?
  - Contamination
  - Processing
  - Extracts?
  - Adulteration
  - Herb-drug interactions
- Herbal safety—solutions
  - Noble cultivars
  - Certification
  - Avoid proprietary blends
  - Herbs plus prescription drugs
  - Herbs from China
  - Summary—herbal safety issues and solutions
- How to read a label
- Long-term concerns
- Summary
- Further information

Traditional Use

> What is a weed? A plant whose virtues have never been discovered.
>
> —Ralph Waldo Emerson

If we adapt Emerson's comment to today's world, it might be more accurate to say that a weed is a plant *we* don't know how to use. In keeping with the regional variation of plants, many generations of human beings learned to use their local plants to address their health problems. As Western medicine became more closely married to chemical refinement and synthesis, we have neglected and forgotten knowledge our ancestors acquired from experience over millennia.

The similarities and differences in regional usage of herbs are very interesting. For example, ginseng and rhodiola are quite different botanically and chemically and in their geographic distribution. However, populations living in the areas where these herbs are native use each herb for similar purposes. On the other hand, there are many instances where native populations, separated by just one hundred miles, use a certain specific herb, or a very similar sister plant, for different purposes.

Finding the "right stuff," the right plant for the purpose, has always been the task. Just as animals know where to go to find what they need, modern humans have convenient access to herbs at health food stores, pharmacies, and online sources. However, lacking connections to the original source of the herb, we have to rely on herb suppliers to provide the herbs we want and label them properly. Unfortunately, this modern convenience isn't so reliable.

The wisdom of traditional use is indispensable. The specifics regarding the plant—where it is gathered and when; which part of the plant is used; how it is processed; and when, how, and to whom it is given—are an immense fund of knowledge. We would be worse than foolish to disregard such an invaluable wealth of experience. We have a great debt to those who came before us. We owe it to ourselves and our ancestors to preserve this knowledge.

Scientific Investigation

From the very outset of scientific study of herbal medicine, research has confirmed the efficacy experienced herbalists claimed. There are now many thousands of conventional medical studies, published in the most demanding medical journals, which document the effectiveness of many herbs. In many cases the evidence of efficacy for these herbs is every bit as strong as the evidence of efficacy for the prescription medications used for the same conditions. In numerous direct comparisons of prescription medications and herbal preparations, the herbs proved superior in effect and in their adverse-effect profile.

Scientific study can be used to build on and optimize traditional uses of herbs. The traditional lore about plant collecting, processing, dosing, and so forth is the foundation. Just like a house, we want more than a foundation for our medicinal use of herbs. Comparing traditional usage patterns from one population to another can suggest the herbs that most consistently offer beneficial qualities. Scientific study can also teach us how to use the herbal components in even more powerful, but potentially more risky, ways.

That potential for increasing the power of an herbal component and attendant risks may well be *the* defining characteristic of the confluence of pharmaceutical science and herbal medicine. Traditionally, herbs are used after only a small amount of processing in the form of a tea or poultice. Every plant contains dozens of chemicals, and those chemicals always interact in some way. Usually those interactions are highly complex and entirely uninvestigated. When we try to discover the "active" chemical components of an herb, with the goal of isolating that compound and so heightening its biological impact, we also heighten the risk of this imbalanced, now pharmaceutical, agent.

Conventional Medicine and Herbs

As conventional and alternative medicine come together, evolving into what is simply better medicine for us all, it is important to recognize that conventional physicians have always been herbalists, although unwittingly. The roots of all medicine are firmly planted in the soil of herbal medicine. We just forgot that fact. Between 30 and 40 percent of currently used prescription medications contain active components made from processed plants. Very few of these chemicals can be synthesized less expensively. Some just can't be produced synthetically.

Scientific investigation followed by clinical application is leading to new uses for old herbs. Butterbur, for example, was traditionally used for treating colic and asthma. It has now been found to be very effective for the treatment of allergies and migraine headaches. St. John's wort was traditionally used for emotional disorders and pain. We now have evidence that it seems to have potent effects on regulating blood sugar and insulin sensitivity.

Safety Issues

One of the most powerful and common factors motivating people to use herbal medicine is their fear of toxicity from prescription medication. Ironically, herbal medicines also have their own toxicity issues, but this doesn't have to be the case.

Proper identification

As any nervous parent knows, it isn't safe for children or anyone for that matter to go out and randomly start eating plants, whether the person is in the woods or in his or her own garden. Pretty flowers and the wrong kinds of mushroom can be deadly. Similarly, proper identification of herbs is the first step toward the safe usage of plants.

In 1993, a number of patients at a weight-loss clinic in Belgium died of kidney failure after they took an herbal mixture containing Aristolochia instead of a similar herb Stephania.[93] Due to the potential confusion between these herbs, one high-profile herbal manufacturer decided to stop selling Stephania. Although those in charge of that prominent company were confident about their own ability to identify the herb, they feared that by selling Stephania, they would be encouraging its use and consequently increasing the likelihood of someone accidentally purchasing the misidentified toxic Aristolochia from other manufacturers.[94]

When St John's wort first surged into the American consciousness, the *LA Times* purchased seven bottles of St. John's wort from various stores and then had the herbs chemically analyzed.[95] Three of the seven bottles didn't contain any measurable quantity of St John's wort. They didn't determine what herbs *were* contained in those bottles.

In 2003, the *Archives of Internal Medicine* published an investigation of the herb echinacea.[96] It was not a clinical or scientific trial of the effects of the herb, but it was important for fundamental reasons. There are different forms of echinacea—the most common are *Echinacea purpurea*, *Echinacea angustafolia*, and *Echinacea pallida*. Each of these herbs has somewhat differing biological effects. In this study, *none* of the fifty-nine samples purchased from local stores contained what the labels said they contained. Half of the time, the wrong species of echinacea was identified. Six samples contained *no* echinacea at all. The quantities contained were also often substantially above or below what was listed on the labels. This is seriously bad and the rule rather than the exception.

---

93   Vanherweghem et al., "Rapidly Progressive Interstitial Renal Fibrosis in Young Women Associated with Slimming Regimen including Chinese Herbs," *Lancet* 34 (1993):387-391.

94   Kerry Bone, personal communication to the author, October 15, 1998.

95   Monmaney, "Labels' Potency Claims Often Inaccurate, Analysis Finds Spot Check of Products Finds Widely Varying Levels of Key Ingredient," *Los Angeles Times*, August 31, 1998.

96   Gilroy et al., "Echinacea and Truth in Labeling," Arch Intern Med 163 (2003):699-704. doi:10.1001/archinte.163.6.699.

What Part of the Plant?

The proper part of the medicinal plant must be used. Different chemicals are present in different parts. Sometimes the plant must be collected at a specific season or time of day. Then the herb must be processed in the correct way. For example, the hairs of ginseng are traditionally thrown away, as they are believed to be ineffective or even harmful. However, many ginseng products widely sold today are produced exclusively from these hairs (clue: they are surprisingly inexpensive).

Contamination

Another recent survey found that samples of echinacea contained significant lead contamination. A colleague who runs an herbal supplier told me once that he and his staff had to reject over one-third of the herbs his company purchased from China and India, because they were either misidentified or contaminated.[97] Heavy metals are the most common contaminant, especially lead. Studies of Chinese herbs distributed in Asia, Europe, and the United States have found that 3 to 10 percent of samples were contaminated with lead. Many other heavy metals have been discovered in herbs (arsenic, mercury, cadmium, thallium, and copper), sometimes at quite dangerous levels. Contamination with herbicides or pesticides is commonplace as well.

Processing

We typically have little, if any, idea which of the hundreds of chemicals in any one herb creates the herb's beneficial effects. The optimal effect may depend on some combination of those chemicals. Consequently, traditional herbal wisdom is the best starting point.

Dried herbs usually have the best balance of chemical components. This form is then usually the best source material for the processed herbs you buy at the store.

Companies have been working to identify what are called "marker compounds," which we can test for and possibly reflect the herb's biological activity. After discovering whether these marker compounds are present, we can then *semiconfidently* determine which herbs are reliable. We can attain semiconfidence only as we lack certainty about the importance of the marker compounds. Individually and collectively, they are our best scientific guesses at this point. For many herbs, there is more

---

97   Kerry Bone, personal communication, January, 2005.

than one marker compound. For example, we look for anthocyanosides in bilberry, echinacoside in echinacea, escin for horse chestnut, kava lactones in kava, ginsenosides in *Panax ginseng*, eleutherosides in Siberian ginseng, hypericin and hyperforin in St John's wort). The presence of established levels of marker compounds in the final product can also reassure us that the processing didn't remove the chemicals most likely to be helpful.

Extracts?

The question mark above represents our considerable uncertainties about extracts. When we process herbs and use their extracts, we are medicalizing them. We hope to extract their powerful essence and thereby maximize the beneficial impact. The formidable problem is that we seldom know which chemicals are vital, so our ignorance easily leads to miscues. Also, this extractive process usually creates an imbalance of the normally present compounds in the herb. That imbalance can make us more vulnerable to toxic effects that are less likely using the entire herb.

I'm comfortable with most extracts, as they are still very much like the whole herb. These extracts are in essence simply "condensed" for easier usage. However, I am concerned about the safety of extracts that have been heavily processed, with the specific intent of dramatically raising levels of certain chemicals thought to be therapeutic. Consequently, I use such preparations rarely and only with great care. (See "Extract Ratios" on page 269 to learn more about the meaning of the numbers used to describe extracts.)

Adulteration

Adulteration of herbs is a serious problem, especially in herbs coming from Asia. A study of over 2,600 samples of traditional Chinese herbal medicines in Taiwan found that 24 percent had at least one conventional prescription medication in the mixture.[98] A similar study in California found that 7 percent of the 251 samples analyzed contained prescription medication that wasn't listed among the ingredients.[99] Among the pharmaceuticals commonly found in these herbs are steroids, diuretics,

---

98   Huang et al., "Adulteration by Synthetic Therapeutic Substances of Traditional Chinese Medicines in Taiwan," *J Clin Pharmacol* 37 (1997):344-50.

99   Ko, "Adulterants in Asian Patent Medicines," *N Engl J Med* 339 (1998):339:847. doi: 10.1056/NEJM199809173391214.

pain medications, and drugs used to control seizures. The worst of the worst are tableted herbs from China.

One of the most notorious episodes of adulterated herbs occurred with the product PC-SPES, which was used to treat prostate cancer. Initial scientific studies and clinical reports looked very promising, and researchers at the University of California, San Francisco (UCSF) started a clinical trial. The trial itself generated a great deal of excitement for a couple of reasons. First, it was the first serious investigation using herbs for cancer treatment at a major medical institution. Second, this combination of herbs appeared to have effects that none of the individual herbs had alone. Demonstrating synergistic effects of combined herbs would have been a great leap forward in scientific investigation of herbal medicine.

The study was a comparison of conventional antihormonal treatment of prostate cancer using DES (diethylstibesterol) with the PC-SPES herbal combination. As the study was underway, early results showed that men using the PC-SPES were doing much better than the conventional treatment group, with twice as many patients showing a 50 percent drop in their prostate specific antigen (PSA) levels. *However,* following up on a recent report of adulterated lots of PC-SPES, the investigators analyzed the PC-SPES they were using for their study. They discovered that their PC-SPES contained DES. They immediately stopped the study, and the manufacturers of PC-SPES went out of business.

Sadly, there is still uncertainty about whether PC-SPES might actually have been helpful, either alone or in conjunction with DES. The early data indicated that there was a benefit. In previous studies different batches of PC-SPES seemed to have been more or less effective. After the evidence of DES adulteration was revealed, investigators in the other studies examined their PC-SPES, some finding evidence of DES contamination of PC-SPES, while others didn't. The men in the UCSF study who had received the DES-contaminated PC-SPES received only a few percent of the dosage of DES the men in the DES group received. Given the suspicions and bad feelings engendered in this incident, it is impossible to see any study clarifying potential benefits of PC-SPES in the foreseeable future.

Herb-Drug Interactions

Several years ago, you may have heard about the controversy surrounding kava. There were reports of liver damage coming out of Europe. Despite hundreds of years of widespread use of kava across the South Pacific, this problem was previously unknown. Swiss researchers eventually linked the kava liver toxicity to the process of extraction used in Germany and Switzerland. The highly toxic chemical acetone was used to extract what they determined were the active components of the kava. It is still controversial whether every one of the patients who experienced this life-threatening problem was also taking prescription medication. Most of them were taking prescription sedatives notorious for adverse effects on the liver.

Prescription medications are often highly toxic. Herbs can be so, but rarely. The combination, however, can be dangerous, because the herbs can alter the metabolism of the medication. Ironically, this potential has falsely led many physicians to become highly critical of herbal medicine when in actuality it is our prescription medication that is primarily to blame.

We need to step beyond the presumption that herbs and prescription drugs must interact in a detrimental way. As scientists started investigating drug-herb interactions, they have also found many beneficial interactions. This shouldn't be at all surprising. The very first serious drug-herb interaction observed was the tendency of St. John's wort to lead to the rejection of donated organs. This rejection was a consequence of St. John's wort making the liver work more efficiently, so that the liver more quickly metabolized the immunosuppressive medication that was meant to block organ rejection. That consequence wasn't good for those rare patients, but improving liver function is likely to help many other patients.

Herbal Safety—Solutions

Although trying to use herbs safely and effectively is a challenge, it is not an insurmountable one. There are several prudent steps we can take in this regard. Some of them are long-standing traditions, others are especially suited to modern circumstances.

Noble Cultivars

Herbal quality and safety aren't new issues. How did our ancestors solve these problems?

As humans recognized the utility of plants, they also recognized the limitations, variable effects, and toxicity. Over time communities learned to optimize their usage. They learned to collect the plant at a certain time from a certain location and process it in a certain way. They also discovered that certain plants of the very same species were slightly different. Some were more effective or less likely to cause unwanted symptoms than others. People would then selectively breed these plants to further improve their efficacy and safety. Those specific plant lineages were handed down through generations.

We call them "noble cultivars"; in essence, they are plant royalty. Noble cultivar may sound strange, but you are already probably familiar with the concept of noble plant cultivars in the world of fine wines. The six historical noble grape cultivars were Cabernet Sauvignon, Chardonnay, Merlot,Pinot noir, Reisling, and Sauvignon blanc.

Similarly, each island in the South Pacific has its own noble cultivar of kava. After some European kava extracts were found to lead to liver toxicity, the Australian government eventually recognized that it was a processing issue and lifted their ban of kava, *provided the kava was a noble cultivar.* This was an excellent, well-considered application of centuries of knowledge.

Certification

Independent confirmation of the safety and quality of herbal products, as with dietary supplements, is a good idea. Manufacturers have been developing voluntary good manufacturing practice (GMP) guidelines, and the FDA is proposing mandatory GMPs. While this will create major financial problems from small herbal suppliers, overall it could be a good step forward.

The United States Pharmacopeia certifying process (USP) is very useful for chemically simple products like vitamins, minerals, and many dietary supplements. USP certification of herbs, which are more complex products, is considerably more challenging and hasn't yet been achieved. USP has assembled an expert committee to achieve this goal. There might be a "middle ground" option whereby USP could certify levels of established marker compounds in herbs and an absence of contaminants.

That has long been the approach of the best companies supplying herbs to the world market—using chromatography and other scientific methods to precisely identify herbs. They also analyze the herbs for contaminants.

You can also learn about the contents of some products through an organization such as ConsumerLab.com, which independently analyzes herbs and supplements. The number of products and the sources of those products they analyze is rather limited, but the information still quite useful.

Avoid Proprietary Blends

In the interest of maximizing profits, herbal manufacturers in the United States are allowed to sell blends of herbs without telling the consumer how much of each herb is included. To me this is as bizarre and irresponsible as it would be for me to tell a patient to just go to a certain drugstore to buy that store's "special blend" of antibiotics to treat his or her pneumonia. Would you go buy Super Bob's Antibiotic Blend because it had an attractive label, unconcerned about whether it had the right amount of the right antibiotic to treat your infection? Fortunately for them, citizens of other countries are better protected.

Herbs plus Prescription Drugs

Simply put, the bottom line is that for your own safety as well as the education of your physician, you really must tell him or her whether you are using any herbs while you are also taking prescription medication. Tell the pharmacist as well because he or she is most likely to have the latest updated information about interactions between drugs as well as between herbs and drugs. Although *generally* herbs, with their complex mix of chemicals and long history of use, are less prone to serious adverse effects than prescription medication, the combination can create serious problems.

Herbs from China

If you insist on using herbs imported from China, select loose herbs instead of tableted ones. Try to find GMP-certified herbs. If the herbs were recommended by a professional, ask whether she or he can vouch for the quality and safety of this specific source of herbs.

Summary—Herbal Safety Issues and Solutions

These issues of quality control severely impact your health. If you take an herb contaminated with pollutants or prescription medication, it is likely to hurt you. If you take the wrong herb, it won't work. If you take the correct herb but it is relatively inactive because it was processed incorrectly or because the wrong part of the plant was used, it won't work. If poor-quality herbs were used or good-quality herbs were used incorrectly, studies conducted to learn how well an herb works will reach the wrong conclusion.

Guidelines for Safe Use of Herbs

Remember that herbs are powerful and deserve respect.

- Don't take them without a specific need.
- Take care to use them properly.
- Choose high-quality herbal products (remember, noble cultivars).

Read the labels.

- Is the herb identified fully (name and plant part)?
- Is the production process specified?
- If it is an extract (as usual), is the ratio specified? (see Extract Ratios below)
- Is it made from dried herb or fresh? (Dried is usually better due to chemical balance.)
- How much is in a dose? ("Proprietary blend" means they won't tell you.)
- Was the extract cold?
- Was the extract made using ethanol, glycerol, or aqueous solution?
- Are marker compounds identified?

Buy from the best possible sources.

Avoid tableted herbs from China.

How to Read a Label

The best "medical" herbs (in other words, ones that have been carefully processed for use by professionals treating diseased patients) will have detailed and reliable information on the label about the herbal preparation inside the bottle. They are usually sold as extracts, listing the nature of that extract and identifying the quantity of any "marker compounds."

As I mentioned earlier, marker compounds are thought to be the active substances in the herbs, the chemicals that create the desired clinical effects. So, good manufacturers will analyze the extract to ensure that sufficient levels of these marker compounds are present in the final extract. In addition, they will include this information on the label, generally specifying a minimal concentration of those compounds.

You are wise to avoid proprietary blends of herbs. If the label says "proprietary," try to find another product that fully discloses the contents. This will make the label easy to read, as there is no information. Walk on by; don't buy it.

Extract Ratios

Remember that the numbers by "extract" tell you a great deal about the strength of the product in your hand. A 100:1 extract means that the product has been concentrated to a strength 100 times that of the source material. So, 1 mg of a product labeled as a 100:1 extract came from 100 mg of herb. Conversely, when the ratio is the other way around, for example 1:4, it means that each 200 mg tablet contains 50 mg of the herb.

Turning this into a math problem should make it easier to understand.

Extract Ratio = Weight of original dried herb/weight (or volume) of finished product

Weight of original dried herb = A
Weight (or volume) of finished product = B
Extract ratio = A:B

Now, let's turn the math around:

Example 1: If A:B = 1:2, the one part of the herb you started with ended up contained in a volume twice as large.

MORE SPECIFICALLY: One kilogram of herb was extracted into two liters of water. One liter of water weighs one kilogram. So, that one kilogram of herb is now spread through two liters (two kilograms) of water. This is a 1:2 extract. The herb is one-half as concentrated as it was before processing.

Example 2: How many mg is that?

There are one thousand milliliters (ml) in every liter and one thousand grams in every kilogram. So, one ml of a 1:2 extract contains one-half of one gram of the herb. In medicine we usually measure medication doses in milligrams (mg). So, one-half of a gram is the same as 500 mg. That means that one ml of a 1:2 extract contains 500 mg of the original dried herb.

Example 3: In this case a 4:1 extract. So, A:B = 4:1.

Here 4 kg of dried herb is processed into 1 kg soft extract or spray-dried powder.

A 250-mg capsule, filled with this 4:1 extract, then contains 1 g of that dried herb.

There is one g of dried herb in:

2 ml of 1:2 liquid

or

1 ml of 1:1 liquid

or

250 mg of 4:1 soft extract

or

200 mg of 5:1 spray-dried powder

Long-Term Concerns

The good news is that we're investigating the medicinal uses of herbs at a pace never seen before. That is great, but unfortunately, there is bad news as well. Resources are vanishing even faster than the pace of our learning.

Economic factors, including the limited financial gain possible for those who might fund research, are slowing down clinical investigation of herbs. Recently, poor worldwide economic conditions have not favored costly medical research. It is impressive how much we have learned despite these obstructions.

We are losing medically important plant species every day. Climate change and expanding development into wilderness areas, especially the rain forests that hold the huge preponderance of the world's biologic diversity, are burning down our botanical "warehouses."

It isn't only plants that are lost when the environment changes. The repository of traditional wisdom about the effective usage of medicinal plants has been the memory of elders living alongside those herbs. As encroaching development gobbles up these regions of botanical diversity, the human experts are vanishing just like the plants. The old ones are dying without heirs to receive and build on their wisdom. The successes of conventional medicine and the allure of civilization markedly reduced the number of individuals willing to apprentice with these healers to learn the knowledge of generations they carried forward. This loss might be even more devastating than the loss of the plant habitat. Many plants, once identified, can be cultivated. However, the loss of millennia of human knowledge cannot be regained. Because the knowledge isn't written down, it is as if human libraries are burning down.

Summary

- Herbs are the most widespread method of healing.
- Herbal medicine is the most ancient method of healing.
- Conventional medicine is founded on herbal medicine.
- Herbal medicine has risks.
- Respect the power of herbs.
  - Be selective about sources.
  - Consult with experts if you are seriously ill.
  - If you are also using medications,
    - consult with experts.
    - tell your doctor.

Further Information

The American Botanical Council is an independent organization dedicated to providing unbiased educational information on herbs to the public, professionals, and the media. I strongly recommend them to you.

Chapter 19

Homeopathy

Aude sapere (Dare to taste and understand).
—Hahnemann's motto for homeopathy

Homeopathy is growing in popularity in the United States. That is largely because the approach is so different from conventional medicine. A good deal of the difference is the focused, individual attention the homeopathic physician gives to the patient. That is refreshing for patients and physicians who feel that conventional medicine has grown cold, corporate, and impersonal. Also, it is easy for anyone to learn enough about homeopathy for his or her own personal use, treating colds, injuries, and other minor health conditions.

For the benefit of laymen, back in the nineteenth century, homeopathic pharmacies learned to make homeopathic remedies even easier to use. They made homeopathy so simple that, in my experience, most people who use homeopathic remedies know close to nothing about the principles behind homeopathy. Most users simply see homeopathy as a safer, more natural alternative to prescription drugs. They aren't the only ones. Physicians as well as laypeople are typically confused about what homeopathy really is.

- Confusion about homeopathic principles
- Definitions
- Hahnemann's story
- Homeopathic principles
- Homeopathic view of health and disease
- Homeopathic survival
- What is homeopathy good for?
- Optimal use of homeopathy for self-care

Confusion about Homeopathic Principles

Although many tenets of homeopathic philosophy are debatable, antagonism toward homeopathy is surprisingly uninformed. It is ironic that conventional medicine's summary judgment against homeopathy is based on a misunderstanding of homeopathic principles. Thoughtful consideration of a system of healing requires an understanding of the method, including its principles and clinical practice. The system of homeopathy is so complex and different from conventional medicine that it requires careful thought to either intelligently accept or reject its principles.

The most frequent misconception has been that "homeopathic medicine" is synonymous with "natural medicine." That pleasant-sounding assumption is entirely wrong. But even if it were true, what would that mean? What exactly is "natural medicine"? Naturopaths, the most established group of health professionals specializing in "natural medicine," study homeopathy as only one of many therapies during their training. It is true that homeopathic medicines, or "remedies" as they are often called, are frequently manufactured from naturally occurring materials, but "natural" isn't a requirement of the homeopathic pharmacopoeia. There are homeopathic remedies made from antibiotics and other prescription drugs. Homeopathic theory advocates using remedies to heal the patient by stimulating his or her own healing powers. Based on this theory, homeopathic treatment would affect a "natural healing," but what would that mean compared to other forms of "natural medicine"? This confusing imprecision makes the "homeopathy is natural" definition more misleading than helpful.

For many generations, the first exposure an American medical student had to homeopathy was when she heard the phrase "homeopathic dosage" used to castigate a physician who prescribed a subtherapeutic dosage of a conventional medicine. She learned that homeopathy has something to do with using inadequate quantities of medicine. If the student investigated a bit further on her own, she was likely to learn that homeopathic manufacturing involves a process of serial dilution of the medicinal agent, sometimes to an improbable extreme. It was extraordinarily unlikely for her to investigate further, given the certainty that this pharmacologic nihilism must be a therapeutic blind alley.

In truth, the controversial process of dilution doesn't define homeopathy. Herein lies the irony—conventional medicine's rejection of homeopathy has been based on the issue of ephemeral dosages, although such dilutions are actually not essential to homeopathy. If homeopathy cannot be defined simply as the use of fantastical dilutions, then what is it?

Definitions

Despite the confusion, defining *homeopathy* is really quite simple. The word does it for us. *Homeopathy* means "similar to disease" or "similar to suffering." It is the clinical application of this principle that defines homeopathic medicine.

Use of this essential homeopathic principle extends well beyond the "confines" of the two-centuries-old, multicontinental homeopathic medical tradition. The approach, applying "likes" to the treatment of "likes," was one aspect of ancient Greek medicine and the Ayurveda system of India. Hahnemann sometimes referred to the concept of likes to cure likes as the *similia* principle.

As a unified and distinct system of medicine, homeopathy originated in Germany with the experiments of Samuel Hahnemann. Reviewing Hahnemann's life story is a good place to start.

Hahnemann's Story

Hahnemann was a conventionally trained physician practicing the medicine of his time. These methods included a variety of practices that had changed only a little over centuries. Patients were bled to reduce lung congestion, whether that was caused by pneumonia or heart failure. Various noxious agents were applied to the skin to create blisters, believing that they would purify the body by making it secrete toxins. Chemicals such as mercury and arsenic were given to patients in poisonous doses. History records the deaths of many people, including heads of state, whose deaths were hastened, if not directly caused, by the medical care they received during this time in the history of conventional medicine.

As Hahnemann observed the clinical response of his patients to these treatments, he was understandably disturbed. Frequently, the only apparent effects of these treatments were adverse ones. Pressed by the economic necessity of providing for his young and growing family, he was caught in a moral dilemma. His practice of medicine was no different from that of the rest of his medical community, but he perceived that this standard care was harmful to his patients. If he acted in accordance with his beliefs and the Hippocratic dictum of "First do no harm," he would have had to eliminate much of his medical practice. On the other hand, he needed to support his family. Why should he suffer economically while his colleagues harmed their patients, made a living, and won praise for their injurious methods?

Hahnemann wrote of his decision,

> To become in this way a murderer, or aggravator of the sufferings of my brethren of mankind, was to me a fearful thought,—so fearful and distressing was it, that shortly after my marriage I completely abandoned practice and scarcely treated anyone for fear of doing him harm, and—as you know—occupied myself solely with chemistry and literary labors.[100]

Hahnemann possessed an easy facility with languages. He put this gift to use when he decided to abandon his clinical practice and earn his livelihood translating medical texts into German from French, Latin, Italian, and English. His work as a translator provided his family with adequate means for their survival and simultaneously allowed him to remain true to his convictions.

Hahnemann gained more than economic subsistence from this work. The translations brought him into close contact with the ideas of the most prominent physicians of his time as well as the masters of antiquity. These ideas influenced his subsequent medical practice. As his clinical practice changed, Hahnemann acquired a reputation for unorthodoxy.

Hahnemann vigorously espoused unpopular opinions criticizing conventional medicine. His forceful declarations understandably antagonized the medical community. When he lectured in the University of Leipzig, he was described as a "raging hurricane." Hahnemann's fury and his apparently foolish ideas made him a lightning rod for ridicule. It is interesting that much of that ridicule was for ideas we now accept as conventional medical advice.

One of his unorthodox opinions was his conviction that peoples' environment and behaviors could profoundly impact their health. Con-

---

100 Dudgeon, ed. and trans., *The Lesser Writings of Samuel Hahnemann*, (New Delhi: B. Jain, Reprint 1999).

sequently, he insisted that his patients change the harmful conditions of their lives whenever possible. As an example, the prevailing medical opinion was that exercise was unhealthy. Hahnemann argued otherwise. To his detractors, one of the proofs of Hahnemann's ignorance was his family's practice of going on long walks for health. Hahnemann emphasized the important contribution of environment and lifestyle to health, including concerns about emotional stress and "mental overexertion" that would sound quite familiar today.

Hahnemann held to his belief in the prime importance of a healthy lifestyle throughout his lengthy medical career. Also in his seminal work, he wrote,

> If someone complains of one or more trifling symptoms that he has noticed only recently, the physician should not consider this a full-fledged disease requiring serious medical attention. A slight adjustment in the mode of living usually suffices to remove this indisposition.[101]

Today's homeopathic practitioners are truly Hahnemann's descendants in their staunch advocacy of lifestyle modification over the use of prescription medication. As Goldstein demonstrated, not only do homeopaths advocate lifestyle change, but they are extraordinarily successful at helping their patients implement these health habits.[102]

In 1792 Hahnemann was placed in charge of an asylum for the insane. Perhaps as a consequence of this experience, he was among the very first European or American physicians to speak out against the violent "treatment" directed against patients with mental illness.

> It is impossible not to marvel at the hard-heartedness and indiscretion of the medical men in many establishments for [the insane], who...content themselves with torturing these most pitiable of all human beings with the most violent blows and other painful torments. By this unconscientious and revolting procedure, they debase themselves beneath the level of the turnkeys in a house of correction, for the latter inflict such chastisements as the duty devolving on their office, and on criminals only.[103]

101 Hahnemann, *Organon of Medicine*, 6th ed., trans. Jost Kunzli, Alain Naude, and Peter Pendleton, (Los Angeles: Tarcher, 1982). Aphorism 150.
102 Goldstein and Glik, "Use of and Satisfaction with Homeopathy in a Patient Population," *Altern Ther Health Med* 4 (1998):60-5.
103 Hahnemann, *Organon of Medicine*, 6th ed., trans. William Boericke. (New Delhi:

It isn't just today's homeopathic physicians who agree with Hahnemann. Conventional physicians now widely accept many of his then-controversial opinions. It is safe to say that nearly any modern physician who awoke to find his or her colleagues poisoning their patients by administering arsenic, bloodletting, inducing vomiting and diarrhea, torturing the mentally ill, and urging their patients to avoid exercise at all cost would be just as outraged as Hahnemann was two hundred years ago.

Hahnemann's Experiments with Quinine

Perhaps Hahnemann would have faded entirely from medical history were it not for an incidental discovery he made regarding the clinical effects of quinine. Malaria was an important health problem in Europe during Hahnemann's lifetime, and quinine was the mainstay of conventional treatment. In 1790, while translating one of the most highly regarded medical texts of the time, Cullen's *Materia Medica*, Hahnemann was infuriated by the text. Cullen's claim that quinine was an effective treatment for malaria because it was bitter and astringent was the cause for Hahnemann's anger. Cullen's belief was coherent with the precepts of Galenic Greek medicine, which, though nearly two millennia old, were still generally accepted to be correct. Hahnemann rejected Cullen's claim, and medical tradition, on the basis of his experience that many other substances, even more bitter and astringent, had no effect at all on malaria. Unlike other physicians, Hahnemann learned from his own experience, critiquing the wisdom of the ancients.

Ever the inquisitive scientist, Hahnemann, apparently in a fit of pique, ingested a dose of quinine to assess its actions. He was surprised to discover that he developed a headache, fever, diarrhea, and chills. He was surprised because he recognized a paradox—that is, these symptoms quinine created were the characteristic symptoms of malaria, the very disease quinine supposedly treated so effectively.

Hahnemann reflected on this experience and searched the classical medical literature for similar information about parallels between toxic and beneficial effects of medicines. He also recognized the conventional treatment of tertiary syphilis, which used the likes-to-cure-likes principle. While syphilis was well known for bone destruction, gingivitis, and copious salivation, the standard conventional treatment was mercury.

B. Jain, 1921). Aphorism 228, note 125.

Mercury induced the same physiological responses. Physicians used the patient's copious salivation to gauge whether they had administered an adequate dose of mercury. Not only was this another example of the effectiveness of likes to cure likes, but this treatment appeared to consciously exemplify the approach.

Implications and Applications

The implications of this principle gradually became evident to Hahnemann. Over the following several years, Hahnemann slowly transformed his clinical practice and the content of his writings (most notably his *Essay on a New Principle for Ascertaining the Curative Power of Drugs with a Few Glances at Those Hitherto Employed*), and he founded the medical system called homeopathy.

Considering Hahnemann's pivotal experience, in which he recognize the *similia* principle in the action of quinine, it is interesting to note that the homeopathic explanation of quinine's anti-malarial effects is as good as any other we have two centuries later. Quinine appears not to exert any effect directly on the malarial organism. Instead it acts to alter the function of the immune system, altering its response to the malarial infection. It is also intriguing that both malaria and overdoses of quinine can lead to a disease called blackwater fever, which is often fatal. In other words, an overdose of an effective treatment for a certain disease can cause what appears to be the same disease.

Homeopathic Principles

Certainly homeopathic medicine is so different from conventional medicine that they could seldom be confused for each other. However, arguments over which features are essential to a homeopathic definition have raged for nearly two hundred years.

Hahnemann knew nothing of modern practices of injecting diluted substances into acupuncture points or using electronic devices to guide remedy selection. Presented with these newfangled methods, Hahnemann would certainly have asked, as do many modern classical homeopaths, "What do these methods have to do with homeopathy?" Asking this question isn't based on a judgment of merit or efficacy. Simply, these approaches, good or ill, are the closest to, or very distant relations or offshoots of, homeopathic medicine.

Making sense of the later iterations requires grounding in the foundational concepts of homeopathy. That classical perspective will guide this discussion.

Homeopathy, in its classical form, is founded on four principles. They are the following:

1. Likes cure likes
2. Provings
3. Single medicine
4. Minimal dose

Likes Cure Likes

Considering the paradoxical therapeutic action of quinine and mercury, Hahnemann recalled the admonition to "let likes cure likes" from the writings attributed to Hippocrates as well as the archaic master Paracelsus's correlate "Doctrine of Similars." Hahnemann's experience, coupled with the writings of two of the grandfathers of the Western medical tradition, encouraged him to develop this approach for use in clinical practice. *This method of using a substance that creates certain symptoms to treat a patient suffering the same symptoms is the defining principle of homeopathic medicine.* It is the cornerstone of homeopathy. This importance is reflected in the system's name "homeopathy"—literally, "similar to suffering."

Hahnemann didn't invent the use of likes to cure likes, and this method isn't unique to homeopathy. On the other hand, unlike the other traditions, which selectively apply "likes to treat likes," homeopathic medicine is unique in the uniform application of the homeopathic principle to every patient in every clinical encounter.

A certain measure of debate enters considerations of homeopathy regarding the matter of what exactly does "like" mean. Which elements of the patient's makeup are open to selection as homeopathic characteristics, and how alike must "like" be? How might that "likeness" be assessed?

Some health-care practitioners connect their patients to various electrical devices as a means of determining which homeopathic medicine they need. Anthroposophical practitioners use diluted medicinal agents and prescribe them to patients based on general characteristics of each patient's personality. Nearly five hundred years ago, Paracelsus wrote that a plant, which was growing in the moist darkness hidden among other plants, was a source of medicine for a person who was shy and withdrawn. Although classical homeopaths don't view any of these approaches as purely homeopathic, Paracelsus's intuitive perception of similarity is one with which they feel a great deal of sympathy.

Provings

Medicine's ignorance of the effects of medicinal substances on the human organism initially stymied Hahnemann's intention to use a homeopathic approach. He needed much more information, most specifically detailed indications as to when to give a certain medicine to a certain patient. Obviously, it is impossible to discover the similarity between patient and treatment without familiarity with both sides of the likes-cure-likes equation. Carefully taking the patient's case is crucially important, but at best it can provide only one side, one-half of the required information. Science lacked the other side of the equation. What does the drug do to the human organism? What are the symptoms the drug creates? The practitioner must have fully developed information about the drug side of the equation.

To develop this requisite knowledge base, Hahnemann began testing the commonly used medicines of the time and other promising substances in hopes of using their "homeopathic" characteristics to treat patients. Hahnemann recruited his family, friends, and colleagues to ingest each tested substance and record the symptoms they experienced. These symptoms were compiled and became the initial pool of homeopathic pharmacological knowledge.

In German, these experiments were called "*Pruefung*" (literally, "test"). Today we use the term "*proving.*" This testing process is very much akin to phase-one drug trials currently performed in conventional medicine. The intention of a phase-one trial is to reveal the damaging effects of a study medication. Instead of learning the limitations, the harmful effects of a medication, homeopaths are seeking those adverse effects, hoping to use them to heal their patients. Although Galen, one of Western medicine's great progenitors, had suggested testing medicines on healthy people, Hahnemann appears to have been the first to systematically employ this method. Consequently, most medical historians recognize this testing process, which Hahnemann created, as the beginning of clinical pharmacological research.

This systematic, experimental approach to medicine was absolutely vital to Hahnemann and the establishment of this approach to patient care. Homeopaths claimed their methods were superior, partly because of this carefully analytical approach to clinical medicine. That level of scientific rigor and systematic method was lacking in conventional medical practice. Hahnemann believed that careful scientific experimentation was most important and that theoretical speculations (such as the conventional practice of divining the action of a drug by its color, taste, and smell) were, at best, second rate in comparison. In the preface to his *Materia Medica Pura*, he wrote a passage which should earn him credit as a founder of a truly science-based approach to medicine,

> The day of the true knowledge of medicines and of the true healing art will dawn when men cease to act so unnaturally as to give drugs to which some purely imaginary virtues have been ascribed, or which have been vaguely recommended, and of whose real qualities they are *utterly* ignorant; and which they give mixed up together in all sorts of combinations...By this method no experience whatever can be gained of the helpful or hurtful qualities of each medicinal ingredient of the mixture, nor can any knowledge be obtained of the curative properties of each individual drug.[104]

The guidelines for the homeopathic provings were quite specific and carefully considered.

> As regards my own experiments and those of my disciples every possible care was taken to insure their purity, in order that the true powers of each medicinal substance might be clearly expressed in the observed effects. They were performed on persons as healthy as possible and under regulated external conditions as nearly as possible alike.[105]

If the subjects intentionally or accidentally violated these disciplined experimental conditions (injury, overindulgence, vexation, fright, and so forth), to avoid contaminating the data, no further symptoms were recorded. If some lesser insult suggested the possibility of interference, the subsequent symptoms were marked as of potentially questionable origination.

Hahnemann and his students discovered that each medicine (or "remedy," as the homeopaths call them) created a large number of reactions.

104 Hahnemann, *Materia Medica Pura*, trans. R. E. Dudgeon, (New Delhi: B. Jain, Reprint 1988). Author's Preface, Page 1.

105 Hahnemann, *Materia Medica Pura*, trans. R. E. Dudgeon, (New Delhi: B. Jain, Reprint 1988). Author's Preface, Page 2.

Many of these are familiar to conventional physicians as commonly recognized disease characteristics, such as cough, headache, or back pain. As there were idiosyncratic responses—each person proving a remedy (*provers*, they were called) would respond somewhat differently from the others—the responses were precisely recorded. Equally important was comparing the responses of the provers to ascertain the most fundamental and characteristic healing qualities of each substance. Unique reactions might be useful, but the most common responses indicated the most widespread applications of the remedy.

Similar to the precise symptomatic distinctions between remedies, Hahnemann quickly learned that people responded in their own unique manners to every disease. Although the general pathological changes would be the same (a pneumonia is a pneumonia), careful observation revealed distinct differences between patients. Some patients with pneumonia would have a painful cough. Some patients would have coughs that paradoxically improved when they lay down. Some would be chilly. Many would experience a tremendous variety of associated symptoms.

These individual peculiarities led the homeopath to *different remedies for different patients with the same conventional diagnosis*, as the more precise the match, the better the clinical response to the treatment. The range of individual variability between different patients and different remedies has far-reaching consequences in the clinical practice of homeopathy and for researchers investigating its effectiveness. Fortunately for the patients, but unfortunately for the homeopaths, each patient produces only a fraction of the fully developed complex of homeopathic symptoms the remedy that will help them is known to engender. Some of the symptoms the proving subjects develop are rarely, if ever, seen in clinical practice. The art of homeopathic clinical practice comes in eliciting the symptoms from the patient and then recognizing the same pattern among the palette of over fifteen hundred homeopathic remedies. The clinician must know the remedies well enough to recognize the pattern, even when parts of the pattern are missing.

In addition to provings, there are other sources of indications for homeopathic remedies. For example, the symptoms of poisonings can suggest clinical applications of the diluted substance to the homeopath. Undoubtedly, the most important source of additional information about homeopathic remedies comes from records of symptoms cured in the clinical use of the remedy. Some argue that this information is even more reliable and more important than symptoms learned from provings.

Single Medicine

It would be very difficult to find a health food store in the United States that doesn't sell homeopathic medicines. It is nearly as difficult to find a health food store that sells individual homeopathic remedies but doesn't sell homeopathic combination remedies. These combinations are mixtures of several different homeopathic medicines. As these combinations are rarely tested by traditional provings, they are the focus of controversy within the professional homeopathic community.

Hahnemann reviled the customary practice of mixing several medicinal agents because of the uncertain effects and potential danger to the patient. It is ironic that so much of homeopathic medicine is this type of polypharmacy. Modern homeopaths practicing in the classical homeopathic tradition criticize this mixed approach for essentially the same reasons. While it is difficult or impossible to gauge the style of self-care practices two centuries ago, too many laypeople using homeopathy today seem to operate by the anti-homeopathic belief: "If a little bit is good, more must be better." So they run the risk of overmedicating themselves with homeopathic remedies. Although in my own clinical experience, adverse effects of this approach are uncommon, they do seem to occur, so a more cautious approach appears warranted.

Minimum Dose

Homeopathic use of microdoses is not only controversial, but its historical development is shrouded in mystery. Homeopathic remedies are made from an incredible variety of substances. Plants, minerals, and animal poisons make up the largest groups of remedies. These substances are then diluted and shaken (*succussed* is the term used in homeopathy) serially, so that at each successive step along the way, there is less and less of the original material. After even a short production process, many homeopathic remedies pass a certain dilution that represents an insurmountable barrier to medical minds.

Avogadro's number (or Avogadro's constant) is an important concept in physical sciences. Simplistically, it is the number of atoms or molecules in a set amount of any material. That number ($6.02 \times 1,023$) is always the same. It is connected to the weight of the atom or molecule. Hydrogen has a molecular weight of 1, so 1 gram of hydrogen has 6.02 x 1,023 atoms of hydrogen. Carbon has a molecular weight of 12, so 12 grams of carbon is made up of 6.02 x 1023 atoms of carbon. Statistically, this means there is unlikely to be even one molecule of the original substance remaining in very many of the tubes of homeopathic remedies sold in the United States (see "Commonly Sold Homeopathic Dilutions Relative to Avogadro's Number" on this page).

(Hahnemann didn't have to confront the discovery of Avogadro, because Avogadro's law and number didn't gain acceptance until well after Hahnemann's death in 1843. Since Avogadro, homeopaths contend that the effects of the remedies are the consequence of changes in the diluent, usually water, rather than a primary effect of the source material.)

When Hahnemann began to test his method, he administered the medicines in the same dosages conventional physicians used. Problems

Commonly Sold Homeopathic Dilutions Relative to Avogadro's Number

1X = 1 part in 10

3X = 1 part in 1,000

6X = 1 part in 1,000,000

12X (or 6C) = 1 part in 1,000,000,000,000

-------Avogadran limit here----------

12C = 1 part in 1,000,000,000,000,000,000,000,000

30X = 1,000,000,000,000,000,000,000,000,000,000

30C = 1,000,000,000,000,000,000,000,000,000,000,000,000,0 00,000,000,000,000,000,000,000

In clinical practice, professional homeopaths often use 200C (that is 1 followed by 400 zeros), 1M (that is 1 followed by 2,000 zeros) or "higher" potencies.

ensued. Hahnemann found that conventional dosages of homeopathic remedies often temporarily intensified patients' symptoms. In addition, patients would transiently develop symptoms of the remedy from which they hadn't previously suffered. His patients, much like the provers, would develop the full range of the toxic symptoms of the medicines. To quash this unwanted tendency toward needless, adverse effects, Hahnemann began diluting the medicines he administered.

The homeopathic process of dilution and succussion is carried to such a remarkable degree that many cannot think clearly about the system of homeopathy beyond this issue. They ignore the other principles, most notably the *similia* doctrine, and erroneously view the entire system as a simple matter of diluting medicinal substances beyond the possibility of pharmacological action. This gross error is not only true of detractors. Some health-care practitioners now inject acupuncture points with diluted substances of all sorts and call it homeopathy, even though they completely ignore the fundamental doctrine of "likes cure likes" in their process.

Hahnemann recorded his experiments and patient notes in great detail. Reading his meticulous records of his patient visits, their complaints and his treatment provides fascinating glimpses into the lives of the early 19th century, even if you have no interest in homeopathy. Shockingly, no one has uncovered any record explaining the rationale behind the mechanics of Hahnemann's very specific process of dilution and succussion. Many have theorized that Hahnemann's Masonic affiliation taught him about alchemical principles and then led him to develop this alchemical-like process. However, there is no direct evidence in support of this claim. In view of the great deal of information we possess regarding Hahnemann's thinking and his patient records, our ignorance on this very important matter is remarkable and suggests that Hahnemann intended secrecy.

Homeopathic View of Health and Disease

Homeopaths since Hahnemann have viewed the symptoms of illness a bit differently than conventional physicians. Homeopaths emphasize the importance of the precise characteristics of each patient's symptoms. That is because that precision is the means by which the homeopath ascertains the pattern of each individual's *unique* response to his or her illness. The specific features help the homeopath distinguish the patient in front of him or her from all others with the same disease condition.

Homeopaths also view symptoms as signposts indicating the manner in which the organism is working to restore itself to health. In other words, symptoms are not the problem in themselves; nor are they the disease. Symptoms are a consequence of the body's work to regain health, specifically reflecting the characteristics of that healing process. In that view, treatment then should be directed at improving healthy responses and addressing underlying imbalances.

Furthermore, there is a hierarchy of symptoms in homeopathy. Some symptoms are more important than others. For example, generally speaking, mental and emotional disturbances are more important than dermatologic complaints. A positive response to treatment is reflected in the progression of the disorder from deeper (more important) to more superficial. Interpreting the pattern of symptoms following treatment tells the homeopath whether the treatment was beneficial or harmful. The homeopath must use the analysis framework provided by homeopathic theory to correctly evaluate clinical information and determine the subsequent course of treatment. The answer to the question "Was my treatment effective?" must meet very specific criteria recognized throughout the world's homeopathic community. As a result, two homeopaths will rarely disagree in their evaluation of the changes in a patient's health over the course of time.

In many ways homeopathic principles create a formalized process leading to a determination very much in harmony with the common-sense perspective of laymen.

Here are other examples:

- A patient who is emotionally disturbed is sicker than another patient with a disfiguring skin rash.
- A lively, energetic, and socially involved paraplegic is healthier than an "able bodied" person who is "crippled" by anxiety or depression.

Disturbances in the deepest aspects of a patient's being are reflected in the patient's mind and body. This is disease. Pursuing this line of thought to its logical conclusion, some homeopaths (including Hahnemann) have identified spiritual dysfunction as the primal origin of disease. Few have gone so far as to claim it as the exclusive disease-generating force, generally allowing that external forces (for example, lifestyle and exposures to health-damaging influences) also play a part. In fact,

Hahnemann was infamous for his espousal of the importance of external causes. Philosophy clearly plays a more significant role in homeopathy than it does in conventional medicine. As a highly structured approach to healing, compared to the empirical bent of conventional medicine, this difference isn't surprising.

Homeopathic Survival

One way of answering the question "What is homeopathy?" is to borrow from pop psychology with the answer: "Homeopathy is a survivor." Given the controversy surrounding and even encouraged by Hahnemann and his therapy, the fact that this medical system survived and even came to flourish in the early nineteenth century is intriguing. The principal reason for the rise of homeopathy is a familiar and important one: effectiveness. Homeopathic treatment was at least as successful as conventional medical treatment. There is strongly suggestive evidence that homeopathy was clearly superior to conventional therapies in the treatment of epidemic diseases. The first major advance in homeopathy's popularity was consequent to the success homeopaths achieved treating the typhoid and cholera epidemics that swept through early nineteenth-century Europe. Patients conventional physicians treated didn't do as well.

While the ability to alleviate suffering is the most attractive feature to the largest constituency, philosophy is important as well. The current homeopathic resurgence is fueled partly by enthusiasm for its philosophy and identity as a "natural" form of healing. To some the philosophical perspectives of homeopathy on the nature of health and disease are controversial, but those medically unorthodox views are very appealing to others. Individuals who highly value emotional and/or spiritual principles often find appealingly familiar echoes of the same ideals in homeopathic medicine. Choosing homeopathy gives them a way to incorporate their deepest beliefs into their daily lives.

Homeopathy has always been a minority perspective in medicine. As a dissenting minority, homeopathy and the homeopathic community have forged a contrarian identity. This alternative identity attracts individuals who, for whatever reasons, reject orthodox opinions, medical and otherwise. In this sense, the homeopathic community sometimes provides a comfortable home for people who find themselves at odds with the larger society. This segment of the homeopathic community was proportionately larger in the past when homeopathy was further out on the fringe that it is today. Despite this rapprochement, homeopathic principles simply don't allow complete compatibility between this round system of medicine and the square hole of conventional medicine.

Homeopathy survives because it provides certain elements missing in conventional medicine. It is another option—sometimes complementary to conventional medicine and sometimes alternative to it. Sometimes homeopathy is even hidden within the practice of conventional medicine.

Although it is not a formally established principle of homeopathy, Hahnemann's revolt against the toxicity of conventional medicine is an essential element of the homeopathic heritage. In my view, that resistance to overmedication is the most obvious benefit of homeopathy today. For many years, a large portion of my patients were young children, who had become my patients because their parents were disturbed by the frequency with which their children had been prescribed antibiotics for ear infections. In the great majority of these cases, the antibiotics initially seemed to help the episodes but set off a recurring cycle of increasingly frequent infections. The kids weren't getting healthier, and their parents sensed that the treatment their children were receiving was ineffective and often harmful.

After joining my practice these "worst of the worst" recurrent ear-infection patients literally almost never truly needed antibiotics. With hundreds of such children as my patients, I prescribed antibiotics for an ear infection once every couple of years. I don't mean for each child. I mean for all of them together. I calculated that simply by altering the management of ear infections among those children, I had prevented hundreds of antibiotic prescriptions each year. That not only saved money, but more importantly, the children got better, *and* in the future antibiotics would be more likely to help them if they developed a serious infection. They were less likely to be infested with antibiotic resistant bacteria. That is good for all of us.

Doctors want to help patients, and patients want to feel better. A dangerous consequence of this admirable impulse is the needless use of harmful medications. The overuse of medications has very serious individual and societal repercussions. Using a homeopathic remedy instead of falling into the routine of prescribing unnecessary antibiotics *saves* lives in the long term. Reexamining knee-jerk prescribing and other health practices is absolutely essential for the health of medicine. Because of its critical voice, homeopathy is good medicine *for* medicine.

What Is Homeopathy Good For?

The answer to this question does not come from research. For the reasons described earlier, conducting meaningful homeopathic research is perhaps the greatest challenge in our attempts to scientifically study alternative therapies. Classical homeopathy, which requires such extremely individualized prescriptions, is spectacularly ill-suited to randomized double-blinded trials. Still, there are a number of well-designed studies which have found significant effects.[106, 107, 108, 109, 110, 111, 112, 113] However, the sum of the scientific investigation does not demonstrate which illnesses are most likely to respond.

The most important question for any patient is whether help of any specific sort is likely to lead to better health. For a classical homeopath, the correct answer to such a question is frustrating.

The frustration arises from the seemingly evasive (but entirely correct) response: "Homeopathy doesn't treat diseases. Homeopathy treats people."

As I wrote earlier, the remedy is chosen based on the patient's symptomatic response to the illness. With each person responding somewhat differently, those individual quirks are the principal clues to discovering

---

106 Frenkel et al., "Cytotoxic Effects of Ultra-diluted Remedies on Breast Cancer Cells," *Int J Oncol* 36 (2010):395-403.

107 Jonas et al., "A Critical Overview of Homeopathy," *Ann Intern Med* 138 (2003):393–399.

108 Cucherat et al, "Evidence of clinical efficacy of homeopathy: a meta-analysis of clinical trials," *Eur J Clin Pharmacol* 56 (2000):27–33.

109 Consensus statement: The Commonweal Conference on Homeopathy in Human and Veterinary Medicine, *Hom Int* 2 (1998):24-25.

110 Kleijnen et al., "Clinical Trials of Homeopathy," *BMJ* 302 (1991):316-23.

111 Linde K et al., "Are the Clinical Effects of Homeopathy Placebo Effects? A Meta-analysis of Placebo-controlled Trials," *Lancet* 350(9081):834-843, 1997 (published erratum appears in *Lancet* 351[9097]:220).

112 Taylor MA et al., "Randomised Controlled Trial of Homeopathy versus Placebo in Perennial Allergic Rhinitis with Overview of Four Trial Series," *BMJ* 321:471-476, 2000.

113 Altunç et al., "Homeopathy for Childhood and Adolescence Ailments: Systematic Review of Randomized Clinical Trials," *Mayo Clin Proc* 82 (2007):69-75.

the *best* remedy for that particular person. Observing each patient so carefully and eliciting the required information can be a bedeviling task. The devil isn't merely in the details; the diagnosis is in the details.

When the target of the hunt is a remedy for chronic problems, the match with that remedy must be very close, down to minutiae such as behavioral quirks and dietary preferences. That chronic remedy (some call it a *constitutional* remedy) can be a touchstone for the person. When that individual develops other health problems later in his or her life, there is a high likelihood that the very same remedy, or another that is closely related, might be the proper homeopathic prescription for that entirely different disease.

Such individual, even idiosyncratic, treatment elevates the importance of the homeopath. Her correct determination of the homeopathic prescription is of overwhelming importance. Ignoring the actual homeopathic remedy itself, such careful attention from the homeopath can help the patient by uncovering missed conventional diagnoses. Homeopaths are constitutionally insistent on addressing the entirety of the patient's well-being. The consequence is that homeopathic patients are prompted to overhaul their health strategies and behaviors.

Almost all (90 percent) patients who seek professional homeopathic treatment have tried conventional medicine previously for the same condition. The clinical conditions for which Americans most often seek homeopathic professional care are chronic ones, such as allergies, chronic pain, anxiety, back pain, headaches, chronic fatigue syndrome, and arthritis. I would add digestive complaints, depression, hormonal disturbances, and insomnia to the list.

Regardless of the diagnoses, patients seem to like homeopathic care. Goldstein's study found that patients responded well, preferred the homeopathic approach over conventional, and were much more likely to follow the recommendations of the homeopathic professional than they were their conventional physician.

Optimal Use of Homeopathy for Self-Care

The great majority of homeopathy used in America, about 70 to 80 percent, is by untrained persons treating themselves, friends, or family. Almost the entirety of that usage consists of treating short-term conditions, with colds and influenza leading the way. Ear infections, headaches, menstrual cramps, seasonal allergies, acute injuries, and teething are the most common and most effective applications of homeopathic self-care. Homeopathy gives people safe self-treatment options in those cases, easing their reliance on needless prescription medications.

Summary

- Homeopathy means using likes to treat likes.
- The approach has been used for thousands of years.
- The four homeopathic principles are the following:
  - Using likes to treat likes
  - Provings
  - Single medicine
  - Minimum dose
- Homeopathic self-care is common.
- Treatment of chronic and serious conditions requires a professional.

Further Information

See "A Taste of Homeopathy" on page 310 in Chapter 22.

Michael Carlston, *Classical Homeopathy* (London: Churchill Livingstone, 2002).

As the great majority of homeopathy consists of self-care, the following books are guides to self-care.

- Maesimund B. Panos and Jane Heimlich, *Homeopathic Medicine at Home* (Los Angeles: Tarcher, 1981).
- Dana Ulman, *Homeopathic Medicine for Infants and Children* (Los Angeles: Tarcher, 1982).
- Stephen Cummings and Dana Ullman, *Everybody's Guide to Homeopathy* (Los Angeles: Tarcher, 1997).

Chapter 20

Acupuncture

Acupuncture is the iconic alternative system of healing, or at least it is from a conventional American perspective. It is the most familiar of the distinctively "other" approaches to healing. At some time you have probably seen one of the charts of the human body, overlaid by a map of acupuncture points. The body looks the same as any other body, but the points change the impression entirely. These exotic images exemplify the very interesting otherness of the therapy. Acupuncture has been used in the Far East for thousands of years. Originally, the needles were made of stone, supplanted by metal as technology advanced in the first millennium BCE.

History

The earliest and most comprehensive acupuncture book was *The Yellow Emperor's Internal Classic*. Much like writings ascribed to Hippocrates in the West, in reality a number of authors compiled this book over a very long period of time. As with any ancient tradition, there are many different versions today, with differing emphases on specific techniques and methods of diagnosis. Consequently the following discussion comes nowhere near a full elaboration of the breadth of acupuncture practiced today.

The central therapeutic concept of acupuncture is that illnesses are due to disordered energy flows in the body. Energy is believed to flow along certain channels. In English these channels are most often referred to as "meridians." There are eighteen meridians, which are considered the most important ones, and another fifty-four minor ones. Acupuncture points (roughly three hundred to seven hundred, depending on the system) are usually located along the meridians. Needing to adjust energy flows selectively stimulates these points.

The diagnostic assessments used in acupuncture overlap somewhat with other traditions, the Indian system of Ayurveda most notably. Careful assessment of the patient's pulse, facial characteristics, tongue, and breath as well as personal habits and tastes all come into play. Conventional Western medicine, of course, includes such features, but with barely a fraction of the subtlety. Enamored of higher tech methods, recent generations of conventional Western physicians increasingly ignore the subtleties of physical diagnosis. The sophistication required to achieve the acumen necessary for accurate acupuncture diagnosis is developed over the course of considerable experience. Pulse diagnosis, for example, is dependent on assessing the pulse at three different locations at three different depths. It isn't simply a matter of counting or assessing whether the heart is beating regularly.

Most broadly conceived, the balance of qualities sought as the pinnacle of health in acupuncture is familiar even to those who have very little awareness of acupuncture. The balance of energies, the yin and yang, expressed as the visual symbol of their harmony, has long been iconic. This symbol is iconic not only for traditional Chinese medicine but as *the* image of oriental culture, as seen by the West.

More Than Just Needles

Affiliated practices include moxibustion, which requires heating acupuncture points with burned mugwort either directly on the skin or by heating acupuncture needles. Cupping is similar and typically uses a small bit of a burnable substance (such as an alcohol-soaked cotton ball) on the skin, extinguished by the overlaid cup, which creates a vacuum to stimulate the underlying point or meridian.

Other means of stimulating acupuncture points have become popular in recent years. Among those methods are acupressure, in which the points are stimulated by manual pressure, and electroacupuncture, which uses electrical currents to stimulate points. Those who are needle phobic especially appreciate acupressure. It is often recommended for children and can be used for self-care.

Acupuncture in the West

In America, acupuncture's big breakthrough came with President Nixon's trip to China. This cultural visit opened many new doors, as it marked the end of decades of self-imposed Maoist isolation. Anticipating Nixon's appearance, journalists visited China to learn more about the country and its culture. One of those journalists, *New York Times* writer James Reston, suffered appendicitis while visiting. He was treated with acupuncture and wrote glowingly of the experience in an article published in the *New York Times* on July 26, 1971. These events created both the opportunity for Americans to study acupuncture and the eagerness to do so.

Long before the 1970s shattered cultural barriers, Sir William Osler (1849–1919), a founding professor at Johns Hopkins and a seminal figure in modern Western medicine, extolled the virtues of acupuncture and even used it himself to treat patients with lower back pain.

Osler, so highly regarded as a medical scientist, recognized scientific limitations and recommended a balance of science and experience. "To study the phenomenon of disease without books is to sail an uncharted sea, while to study books without patients is not to go to sea at all."[113]

In recognition of the need for immediate, on-the-spot treatment, a simplified form of acupuncture called *battlefield acupuncture* has become established in the US military, particularly in the United States Air Force.[114, 115] Battlefield acupuncture is a set of even simpler protocols derived from auricular acupuncture, which was developed in France during the 1950s based on the observations of Raphael Nogier, a neurologist. Since 2008, military physicians and other health-care personnel have been receiving elective training in battlefield acupuncture. The

---

113 Sir William Osler, "Of Books and Men," in *Aequanimitas with Other Addresses to Medical Students, Nurses, and Practitioners of Medicine.* (Philadelphia: P. Blakiston's Son & Co., 1904).

114 "Battlefield Acupuncture Fights Pain, Skepticism," Air Force Materiel Command website, http://www.afmc.af.mil/news/story.asp?id=123402789.

115 "AOM Flying High with the Air Force," *Acupuncture Today* website, http://www.acupuncturetoday.com/mpacms/at/article.php?id=31882.

training was initially given only to staff who were about to be deployed into combat zones in Iraq and Afghanistan, targeting pain relief.

Adverse Effects

Like any other healing intervention, acupuncture can harm. Studies find that serious adverse effects are extremely rare (one in twenty thousand to three million), with minor adverse reactions occurring no more than once in every one thousand patient visits.[116] What kinds of adverse reactions are unique to acupuncture? Needles break. Needles pierce unintended body parts. As needles break the skin's protective barrier, local and systemic infections are the most prevalent and significant adverse effect. The risk of hepatitis caused by acupuncture has dropped precipitously since the problem came to light, and acupuncturists *en masse* moved to disposable, single-use needles. Joint infections, collapsed lungs, and peripheral nerve injuries are the most likely, though vanishingly rare, adverse effects of acupuncture treatment.

Effectiveness

Clinical research of the effectiveness of acupuncture has focused predominantly on pain, representing over one-third of the thirty-five hundred acupuncture clinical trials cited on PUBMED (the most comprehensive listing of medical research publications). The evidence, while not incontestable, is strongly supportive in favor of acupuncture's effectiveness for pain. Research also suggests that acupuncture is useful for nausea, infertility, and recovery of neurologic function following stroke.

Growing Popularity

The numbers of individuals possessing the skills required to apply its techniques limit the usage of acupuncture in many countries, including the United States. Despite this obstacle to growth, recent national surveys identified a 50 percent increase in the number of Americans receiving acupuncture treatment, reaching over three million adult patients.

---

116 Xu et al., "Adverse Events of Acupuncture: A Systematic Review of Case Reports," Evidence-Based Complementary and Alternative Medicine 2013 (2013). doi.org/10.1155/2013/581203.

Because they have witnessed its effectiveness, American physicians are also becoming quite comfortable sharing patients with acupuncturists.

Another reality limiting acupuncture's popularity is the fear of needles. That fear is common, and so it is a major impediment to the broadened usage of acupuncture.

My Recommendations for Use

Like so many other physicians, I have seen many of my patients benefit from acupuncture treatments. Much of the research on acupuncture has been on its effectiveness as a treatment for painful conditions. This research popularity matches its clinical popularity. The most likely reason one my patients has sought out an acupuncturist on his or her own has been for pain, especially back pain.

Acupuncture is a much more versatile therapy, however. It should be used more than it is for conditions other than pain. In my experience it is often helpful for nausea and other digestive complaints, as well as insomnia, hormonal symptoms, and injuries.

Like other healing traditions, some acupuncturists achieve better results, with greater consistency than others. It is good then to be choosy when you look for an acupuncturist. Ask around for recommendations.

Summary

- Acupuncture is an alternative system of healing.
- Science and experience show it is effective and not just for pain.
- Seeing a skilled practitioner is necessary.

Further Reading

Books

- Harriet Beinfield and Efrem Korngold, *Between Heaven and Earth: A Guide to Chinese Medicine* (New York: Ballantine, 1992).
- Michael Reed Gach, *Acupressure's Potent Points: A Guide to Self-Care for Common Ailments* (New York: Bantam, 1990).
- Ted Kaptchuk, *The Web That Has No Weaver: Understanding Chinese Medicine* (New York: Rosettabooks, 2010).
- *The Yellow Emperor's Classic of Medicine*

Articles

- Reston, "Now, about My Operation in Peking," *New York Times*, July 26, 1971.
- Vieth, "Sir William Osler, Acupuncturist," *Bull N Y Acad Med.* 51 1975: 393–399.

Chapter 21

CAM as an Essential Health Habit

In a certain way, CAM is the eleventh essential health habit. For sure, the underlying self-determination that leads a person to look for something better is *the* most important health habit. Taking control of your health, being responsible for your choices, making demands, asking questions, insisting on answers to those questions, and being active instead of passive are necessary steps if you want the best for you and your family. Considering other treatments is essential to good health.

There are a number of CAM treatments or approaches I would really hate to lose.

From the perspective of a physician, I'm grateful to have more treatment options for my patients that those I learned in medical school. I still want more, but the additions have been really helpful. Besides the additions, CAM has helped me become a better doctor in several other ways as well.

To feel better, we can't just add. Subtraction is every bit as important. Identifying when and how to avoid normally healthy foods (gluten, lactose, or milk) is a big deal. If you just drop everything that *might* cause you trouble, you will be much sicker very quickly.

A CAM bias to my nutrition studies has taught me about allergy families, not human families—botanically related foods like cashews, mangos, pistachios, and poison oak, for example. Often when people know they are sensitive to something, they don't know that other things in our environment are connected. Similarly, odd things like salicylates or cinnamon, for examples, can hugely impact some few people. In other words, CAM can improve our detective skills.

CAM is "old school." I have learned the value of old-time physical exam techniques that help me make diagnoses other physicians usually miss.

One of the "old school" values, customary in many CAM practices, is spending time with patients. That makes CAM an essential health habit for all of us, patients as well as health-care providers.

Any teacher will tell you that you can't get your diploma if you leave every class after just five minutes. Patient visits are classes for physicians even more so than for patients. We can't learn from our patients if we don't take the time to listen and carefully observe. As a patient, I can't explain what my concerns are when the doctor has his or her hand on the doorknob, ready to leave. Even if I can talk fast, I'm not going to say what I should if I'm fretting about the fleeting seconds. Communication takes time.

Some of My Favorites

- L-Theanine
- Body work (in its infinite varieties)
- Homeopathy
- Acupuncture
- Vitamin D
- Red yeast rice
- CoQ10
- St John's wort
- Gotu kola
- Hypnosis and imagery
- Kava

Chapter 22

Resources

This chapter is a hodgepodge of ancillary material. Most of it, in fact all but the final section, is nuts and bolts, practical information for you to use. The last part is also "practical" and applicable, but only in an educational sense. That portion of this chapter will teach you skills you can apply to critically evaluate scientific information. It is fodder for healthy skepticism.

- Concentrated dietary sources of
  - Protein
  - Calcium
- Essentials for healthy body composition
- Ideal sports and recovery drinks
- A taste of homeopathy
- Research: Lies, damned lies and statistics

Concentrated Dietary Sources of Protein

Legumes

Black beans (dry)	15 g/cup cooked
Garbanzo (chickpeas) (dry)	41 g/cup
Pinto beans (cooked)	44 g/cup
Soybeans (cooked)	20 g/cup
Lentils (cooked)	16 g/cup
Split peas (cooked)	16 g/cup
Kidney beans (cooked)	14 g/cup
Peanuts	38 g/cup

Nuts

Almonds	26 g/cup
Cashews	24 g/cup
Pistachios	26 g/cup
Walnuts	15 g/cup
Pumpkin seeds	40 g/cup
Sunflower seeds	35 g/cup

Grains

Wheat gluten	58 g/cup
Wild rice	23 g/cup (uncooked)
Millet	23 g/cup (uncooked)

Dairy

Cottage cheese	25 g/cup
Yogurt, nonfat	13 g/cup
Yogurt, plain	8 g/cup
Milk	8 g/cup
Cheese	5–7 g/1 oz. (not cream)
Eggs	6 g/egg

Fish

15–18 g/3 oz.

Tuna	49 g/can

Meat

Beef	20 g/4 oz.
Lamb	15 g/4 oz.
Pork	
Bacon	10 g/4 oz.
Ham	20 g/4 oz.
Venison	24 g/4 oz.
Chicken	22 g/4 oz.
Turkey	25 g/4 oz.

Concentrated Dietary Sources of Calcium

(Make your own choices)

Dairy products

Yogurt

Nonfat	452 mg/cup
Low fat	415 mg/cup
Regular	274 mg/cup

Milk

Cow	300 mg/cup
Goat	326 mg/cup

Cheese

Soft

Brie	52 mg/oz.
Cottage	150/cup
Hard cheese	150–200 mg/oz.

Beans

Black	270 mg/cup dry beans
Garbanzo (chickpeas)	300 mg/cup dry beans
Pinto	257 mg/cup cooked
Soybeans	131 mg/cup cooked
Soy milk	48 mg/cup
Tofu	220 mg/cup
Nigari tofu	500 mg/cup
Soy flour	143 mg/cup

Nuts and seeds

Almonds	332 mg/cup
Brazil nuts	260 mg/cup
Hazelnuts	282 mg/cup
Pistachios	173 mg/cup
Cashews	104 mg/cup
Sunflower seeds	174 mg/cup
Sesame seeds	165 mg/cup

Dark green veggies

Collard greens	218 mg/cup
Seaweed (generally)	4–800 mg/ 100 gm (3.3 oz.)
Extremes below:	
Hijiki and wakame	1,400 mg/ 100 gm (3.3 oz.)
Nori	260 mg/ 100 gm (3.3 oz.)
Turnip greens	105 mg/cup
Chard, kale, spinach	less than 100 mg/cup)

Blackstrap molasses

137 mg/tablespoon

Sardines with bones

240 mg/2 oz.

Essentials for Healthy Body Composition

Building muscle

- Exercise at least ten thousand steps (sixty to ninety minutes of moderate intensity daily).
- Consume recovery drink within thirty minutes of exercise, 1:1 carbohydrate to protein (whey is ideal).
- 0.3-0.4 g of protein/kg (20–30 gm for 150 lbs).
- Avoid sweets and high-fructose corn syrup (read labels).
- Drink enough water (keep your urine clear).
- Nutrient timing—avoid famine-feast cycle.
- Eat small portions five to six times per day.
- Eat whole grains only (limit even those).
- Start meals with bulky, nondense foods (veggies).
- Get enough protein and calcium.
- When you are hungry, think protein.
- Target 150 g of protein or more.
- Eat when you eat (not while watching TV, driving, reading, and so forth) slowly and attentively.
- Take a good multiple vitamin.
- Get enough sleep; control stress.

Strength training

Concepts
  1 RM (maximum weight you can lift only once).
  Set = a block of repetitions.
  Eccentric vs. concentric.
Essentials
  Adapt training by your history.
  Stop short of failure.
  Variability is important or essential.
  Don't worry about speed.
  Gradually build all, especially eccentric.

Recommendations for beginners (untrained)

    Start at 50 percent 1 RM.

    1 set of eight to ten reps for each major muscle group, first few weeks to near failure.

    Progress to four sets.

    Progress to mean intensity of 60 percent 1 RM.

    Progress to three per week.

Recommendations for trained

    Progress to mean volume of four sets per muscle group.

    Progress to intensity of 80 percent of 1 RM.

    Progress to frequency of twice per week.

Recommendations for highly trained

    Progress to mean training volume of eight sets per muscle group.

    Progress to mean intensity of 85 percent of 1 RM.

    Progress to frequency of twice per week.

Ideal Sports and Recovery Drinks

Ideal Recovery Drink
Recovery drinks maximize training effects and prevent injury.
These have less fluid and are more concentrated than sports
drinks.
PRO (Protein)
0.3-0.4 g of protein/kg (20–30 g for 150 lbs).
Whey is better than soy. Isolated whey is better than con-
centrate. Hydrolyzed is best.
CARB (Carbohydrate)
High glycemic index (unless targeting weight loss) malto-
dextrin.
Rapidly digested.
CARB:PRO Ratio 3:1 (strength/weight loss 1:1, endurance up to
4:1)
Rapidly digested.
Electrolytes
Antioxidants
Other options (see below)
Drink within twenty to forty minutes of completing exercise.
Chocolate milk is easy, although not ideal, partly because the
lactose it contains commonly bothers people.

The Ideal Sports Drink
- Use only if exercising more than one hour, exercising in hot
  weather, or exercising to gain weight.
- It should be cool. Drink as dictated by thirst or experience.
  Don't overhydrate!
- Carbohydrate (CHO) 4-8 g/100 ml.
  Glucose, maltodextrin, or sucrose (fructose okay with an-
  other CHO, but not by itself).
- Protein (PRO) 1.5-2.2 g/100 ml   (3:1 to 4:1 ratio CARB:PRO)
  Complete protein (whey is best).

- Electrolytes
Sodium	40–80 mg/100 ml
Potassium	20–40 mg/100 ml
Magnesium	10–40 mg/100 ml
- Antioxidants
Vitamin C	30–40 mg/100 ml
Vitamin E	20–30 mg/100 ml

Additional options

- Caffeine: 25 mg/100 ml in sports drink
- Amino acids: Creatine, beta-alanine, branched chain (BCAA), essential (EAA), beta-hydroxymethyl butyrate (HMB)
- Miscellaneous: Betaine, Schisandra, Ashwagandha, Siberian ginseng, glucosamine sulfate

A Taste of Homeopathy

Experience trumps theory. Following are a few examples of simple usages of homeopathy. Going through the process of remedy selection is a means to better understand how the approach is applied. Of course, an experience of effective treatment is the most compelling.

Aphthae (Canker Sores)

In acute episodes, particularly when the origin is infectious (for example, herpes stomatitis), *mercurius vivus* can be useful. These patients usually drool quite a lot, have bad breath, and feel worse during the night.

Croup

There are three homeopathic remedies most commonly used to treat croup. When fear is a defining characteristic, *aconitum napellus* given hourly is the first choice. If it isn't helping after two doses, either *spongia tosta* or *hepar sulphuris calcareum* is likely to help. *Hepar* is the better choice if the child is chilly and quite irritable.

Ear Infections—Otitis Media

The sicker the patient, the more rapid should be the response. A child with a high fever and crying with ear pain should be significantly improved in less than one and a half hours. Give the medicine indicated by pain from once every hour, when the picture is as intense as described below, to once a day when the child is nearly well and spontaneously complains of momentary ear pain only occasionally. It is quite important to avoid giving the remedy when the patient is symptom free, because if given without regard for the patient's clinical improvement, the remedy will cause the patient to become sick again. If there is no improvement after two doses of the medicine, change the prescription.

Although the most certain way to end the recurrent cycle of acute otitis media is with the child's chronic medicine, finding that medicine requires a good deal of training. Unlike other chronic complaints, curing the patient of the tendency toward recurrence is often accomplished by the successful homeopathic treatment of a single episode of acute otitis media.

Belladonna—Symptoms are sudden in onset with high fever and much pain, flushed cheeks, and cold feet with hot body during the fever. Problems tend to be on the right side. Noises and light bother the patient.

Chamomilla—Patient is very irritable. Capricious mood. Wants to be carried around (but nothing satisfies). This is often needed when the ear infection occurs during teething.

Hepar sulph—Patient is very chilly and irritable. Ear is worse with any touch or cool air. Problem is often associated with sore throats. Ear infection is often associated with hard dry cough (for example, croup).

Mercurius vivus—Ear infection with very bad breath, sore throats, and drooling. The condition is often worse at night. It can be associated with mouth sores.

Pulsatilla—The patient is clingy but sweet. He or he desires attention, but there is little (or no) irritability. Ear infection occurs at the end of a cold with thick nasal discharge. There is little thirst (otitis probably due in part to dehydration). This is as slow in onset as the *belladonna* type is fast. Symptoms are on the right side. Symptoms of upper respiratory infection include cough that might make the patient retch. The patient feels better with open air.

Silica—This is difficult to prescribe, because the patient and the clinical picture are mild and typically unexpressive. The problem is a slowly developing ear infection. Patients are often chilly but have a sweaty head and/or feet. They have prominent swollen glands.

Acute Emotional Distress

Aconitum napellus is indicated for patients in a state of hysterical fear. It is often useful following a traffic accident or disaster (for example, earthquake) when the patient is convinced death is imminent. (It is also often needed in croup when the child wakes in a similar state of panic.)

Arsenicum album—The patient is fearful like aconite, but this fear is associated with extreme restlessness. This remedy is often needed with food poisoning. Symptoms are worse from midnight to 2:00 a.m. The patient is very chilly.

Gelsemium is a common homeopathic prescription for stage fright. Its characteristic symptoms are familiar to most people—weakness (especially felt in the knees or abdomen) with trembling. This fear state usually comes about in anticipation of, rather than in response to, a frightening event. *Gelsemium* is also often used in acute influenza because the pattern of symptoms is quite similar—weakness and trembling.

Ignatia amara can be very useful for patients who have recently suffered a significant personal loss. Common symptoms include weeping easily (often the tears will appear at unexpected times), tightness in the throat (*globus hystericus*), sighing, and myoclonic jerks when falling asleep.

Gastroenteritis

Although homeopathic medicine doesn't obviate the need for proper rehydration feeding practices, research confirms the experience of two centuries that remedies can assist this process.

Arsenicum album is undoubtedly one of the most common remedies for this variety of problems, particularly when food poisoning is the cause. The patient is chilly, is restless, and has profuse watery, acrid diarrhea. Nausea can be quite pronounced with ineffectual retching. The patient can be quite weak and is often fearful. Although the pains are burning, warmth (drinks or environmental heat) often makes the patient feel better. The patient tends to be worse during the night from midnight to 2:00 a.m.

Carbo vegetabilis is for conditions characterized by abdominal distention and burping with a rumbling in the abdomen and nausea. It is as if something is rotting in the digestive tract. Food poisoning often creates a *carbo vegetabilis* state. Although they are chilly, these patients strongly desire open air and the loosening of their clothing.

Phosphorus is very similar to *arsenicum*. These patients experience profuse watery diarrhea, which can be acrid or even bloody at times. Symptoms come on or are greatly aggravated right after eating. A classic *phosphorus* symptom is that of the digestive upset triggered after drinks warm up in the stomach. An unusual but memorable characteristic (like *veratrum album*) is simultaneous vomiting and diarrhea. These patients crave cold drinks and salty foods. Like *arsenicum,* fear is common, particularly when alone, but *phosphorus* patients are easily reassured and pleasant company.

Phosphoricum acidum is much like *phosphorus,* but these patients are considerably more debilitated and feel weak immediately after an episode of diarrhea. They crave moist fruits.

Podophyllum's hallmark is painless, yellow diarrhea at 4:00 a.m. The illness most often comes on after eating fruit and in hot weather. Eating often triggers a loose stool.

Mercurius vivus diarrhea is very acrid, creating a good deal of irritation and discomfort occasionally including rectal spasms. Bad breath is common, and these patients are worse during the night; symptoms include profuse night sweats. These patients tend to be very thirsty for cold drinks.

Nux vomica is indicated for stomach pain and indigestion brought on by excesses—overwork or overindulgence. These patients are chilly, irritable, and sensitive to noises, lights, and odors. They find their abdominal pains difficult to relieve because of ineffectual retching and rectal urging. They desire spicy foods, cold drinks, and alcohol. Food poisoning can be another causative factor.

Sulphur, as perhaps the most common homeopathic remedy, inevitably has a role to play in digestive complaints. An irritable, perhaps fearful, patient with acrid, excoriating diarrhea that drives him or her out of bed at 5:00 a.m. is the classic symptom picture. These patients feel hot and dislike warm foods or environments.

Sepia's principal digestive indications are nausea and sensitivity to odors. Homeopaths often use it for nausea of pregnancy in addition to gastroenteritis when the characteristics match.

Veratrum album patients are similar to those of *phosphorus* but they are not fearful. They have copious painless, watery diarrhea, sometimes at precisely the same unfortunate moment that they vomit. The vomiting can be painful. They have an unquenchable thirst for cold drinks, which aggravate the vomiting. Extreme restlessness is particularly represented in their mental state.

Headaches

Belladonna patients have headaches, often pounding, on the right side with a flushed, hot face. They are very sensitive to noises and lights.

Bryonia alba should be considered when motion markedly intensifies the headache and firm pressure relieves the pain.

Nux vomica is indicated when the headache comes on following a time of overwork or overindulgence (alcohol or food). Often the patient needing this remedy for a headache will suffer from concurrent gastrointestinal distress of some sort.

Injuries

Homeopathic remedies are expected to alleviate discomfort and accelerate healing. As with all other conditions, the remedies are taken as indicated based on the severity of the injury (for example, for the pain of a broken leg—from every fifteen minutes to three times a day).

For injuries with bruising, think *arnica montana*. The classic indication for *arnica* is such sensitivity that the bed feels too hard. For good or ill, *arnica* is often given routinely for injuries without consideration of more specific features. If it doesn't help, further consideration regarding the precise quality of the symptoms is necessary.

Bryonia alba is used for sprains or injuries aggravated by motion. The patient wants to hold the area quite still. Better from pressure. They are often irritable when spoken to. The patient could bring the image of a cranky hibernating bear to mind.

Rhus toxicodendron is indicated for sprains or other injuries that feel better with motion. Patients are worse on beginning to move but better from continued motion (like a rusty hinge). They also feel better from warmth. (Don't ignore the conventional use of cold to treat acute injuries. Although these patients might feel better immediately with warm applications, like everyone else, cold is still better to treat acute injuries.) *Rhus tox* patients are often remarkably restless.

Ruta graveolens can be useful for sprains and stiffness of tendons. These patients feel bruised and lame in limbs and joints. These patients feel worse in cold and wet conditions and when beginning to move. Like those who need *Rhus tox,* they feel better from continued motion, although heat doesn't make them feel so much better as it does for *Rhus tox* patients.

Menstrual Cramps

Although dysmenorrhea is a chronic condition and rightfully the province of a professional homeopathic consultation and constitutional prescription, many patients can gain short-term relief simply with the use of *magnesia phosphorica*. The principal relevant indications for this remedy are cramping pains that respond well to pressure and heat.

Motion Sickness

When the primary symptom is dizziness, treat with *cocculus*; when the primary symptom is nausea, use *tabaccum*.

Teething

Sleepless nights caused by teething may be the most common and powerful inducement for parents of young children to try homeopathy. Although the popular over-the-counter homeopathic combinations for teething have earned a following, selecting the precisely indicated remedy should generate the most optimal response.

Chamomilla is the homeopathic teeth remedy par excellence. The indications are the same regardless of the diagnosis for which it is used (also see "Ear Infections"). The child is restless, changeable, and quite irritable. He or she wants to be carried but then wants to get back down, only to demand to get picked up again. When you give the favorite toy, for which the child has been crying, he or she throws it across the room. This is *chamomilla*. The child often experiences diarrhea appearing like chopped spinach (a sign of gastrointestinal distress).

Calcarea phosphorica can be useful for teething when the child isn't so irritable as when he or she needs *chamomilla*. These children spit up a great deal, and the vomitus is often sour smelling.

Things to Know about Homeopathy

Administration

Because the sense of taste can interfere with the action of homeopathic medicine, patients shouldn't taste food or toothpaste when they take the homeopathic remedy, nor should they smell strong odors in the room. The patient shouldn't touch the remedy. Using the bottle cap or a clean metal spoon is customary. Some manufacturers have specifically designed their bottles to allow easy administration of any desired number of pellets. The patient should allow the remedy to dissolve under the tongue and then wait a minimum of fifteen minutes before eating or drinking anything other than water. The remedies must be stored carefully, away from heat (over 110 degrees Fahrenheit) and sunlight. As with any medicinal substance, keeping homeopathic remedies out of the reach of inquisitive children is always a good idea.

Dosages

Potency issues are complicated and controversial. The simplest course is probably to use 12C, 30C, or 30X potencies to limit the frequency of repetition and eliminate any possibility of adverse effects from the crude source material. A few guiding principles will assist you:

1. Always administer homeopathic remedies with an eye on the patient. Adjust potency and dosage regimen accordingly. The frequency of doses is determined by the severity of the illness or injury and the patient's response.
2. Potency is based on the following factors:
   a. Availability: The correct remedy will work regardless of potency, although the frequency of administration may need alteration.
   b. Prescription certainty/remedy fit: A remedy that is an excellent fit will create a healing response in the patient in an extremely diluted or potentized dosage. A mediocre fit requires a lower dose.
   c. Physicality: Many homeopaths believe mental and emotional problems (for example, anxiety or depressive states) require higher potencies (for example, 1M, 200C) to be effective.
3. Dosage regimen
   a. As a *very* crude measure, for a problem of average severity, use one of the following doses: 30C three times per day; 12C (or 30X) four times per day; or 6C (or 12X) four to five times per day.
   b. Wean treatment as symptoms abate.
   c. Two to five pills is an adequate dosage for anyone, infant or adult.

Response

The speed of the patient's response to treatment is proportional to the speed and intensity of the illness. Mouth sores developed in an illness go away over days (the pain should dissipate in hours), whereas a teething child will be better, either sleeping or in a significantly improved mood, in five to thirty minutes.

Research: Lies, Damned Lies, and Statistics

Research is very important. Careful, critical evaluation of health-care interventions is essential, but "the latest study" is just another piece of the puzzle and not the final word. The newness of the study isn't the sole gauge of its importance or the accuracy of its findings. In fact, the latest study is seldom the best one. Unfortunately the media, with its economic incentive to whip up excitement and its attention span of a butterfly, seldom critiques the latest study by looking for faults and or even relating the study findings to prior studies. Since "the latest study" is usually the test of a drug or supplement, some manufacturer hopes to gain from the attention and encourages the media frenzy. Quite often touting "the latest study" becomes yet another example of the worst of Disraeli's triad of lies—lies, damned lies, and statistics.

How can you be healthily skeptical? How can you keep "the latest study" or other seemingly scientific claims about some product from confusing you? The bottom line is all about meaning. What does this research really mean?

First, the existence of any research at all is favorable. Unfortunately, as I wrote earlier, good research is very expensive, so unless there is a product to be sold or money to be somehow made, no private party is willing to spend the money needed to perform the research. That would be a bad investment. Fortunately, governments do fund research without the prospect of financial gain. If the study is well designed and well performed, and if the data is analyzed properly, the conclusions are likely to be meaningful, at least in the context of the study conditions.

Sadly, if the study is poorly done, it can lead to the wrong conclusion. Worse still, if there are only a few studies, just one showing the intervention to be ineffective will unduly slant opinion against the intervention. This error will have a disproportionate influence and stifle further inquiry. That's a big problem.

Our skepticism should extend to our methods of analysis as well.

To begin with, we need to consider what kinds of research there are. Basic sciences research includes studies from the smallest subatomic particles to samples of cellular tissues and living animals. Basic sciences research is considered "pure" science and the best way to understand precisely how things work at an elementary level. There is a huge gulf between the basic sciences and clinical medicine, because the simple purity of basic sciences doesn't encompass the realities and complexities of human life. The approach of basic science investigations is to break things down to smaller parts, carefully investigating those parts. When all the parts are assembled, they often don't fit together quite as expected or predicted. Understanding bits and pieces isn't at all the same as understanding the functioning of the entire complex living organism.

Clinical research involves human subjects and can be observational or interventional. Clinical research is the best way to learn, with the greatest degree of certainty, in regard to what works and what doesn't for patients, not just their parts. The answers we get from clinical research are much closer to the answers we, patients, and health-care providers want, answers that help us make the best choices.

Just like other types of research, clinical research is also imperfect. It inevitably involves undiscovered or uncontrollable factors, which can easily confuse our interpretation of the study findings. Additionally, the circumstances of clinical research are usually markedly different from the daily lives of average people, and so the results might also be misleading. Studies of clinical interventions, particularly randomized and controlled trials, are the most meaningful. That is because they most clearly demonstrate the clinical effects of a specific treatment, what really happens to a patient. However, the best clinical trials, those that are most carefully designed and controlled, still end up being very unlike the messy real world. Learning that an intervention of some sort has a statistically significant impact when applied in ideal circumstances with certain patients is useful information. If the intervention doesn't have the same impact in less-than-perfect circumstances, the intervention is less likely to be helpful.

Along the same lines, we can get too excited about a study finding that a treatment achieves statistical significance. In reality, statistical evidence of a difference between a treatment and a placebo can actually be only faint support for the intervention. Statistical superiority of some treatment might be irrelevant to a patient if the difference isn't enough to significantly improve the patient's life. Statistical significance means that a statistician can see a meaningful difference in the data. *That statistical difference doesn't mean that a patient notices the difference.* Statistics are not people. An asthma study might show that a drug improves patients' breathing, but the effect may be so small that patients don't notice it. Detecting such a clinically irrelevant, minor effect is especially likely to occur in large studies.

If a cancer treatment prolongs the lives of individuals treated for a short time, is that a compelling finding? If the difference is statistically significant, it is only statistically meaningful. What about the patient?

If the adverse effects of the therapy are intolerable, even if it is effective, many patients might elect to forgo such a treatment. If a drug for high blood pressure lowers blood pressure but makes the patient feel unwell, how many patients will actually take the drug? Should they, or should they take it only under certain circumstances?

What we choose to measure is a vital consideration. Studies of cancer treatments, where adverse effects are notoriously unpleasant, now usually include some measurement of the patients' quality of life. That information helps physicians better counsel patients about their choices while helping them make decisions in keeping with their own priorities.

How to Study a Study

The first rule for examining any study is to be skeptical. Every time you read about some medical research, ask yourself what could be wrong with the study. Often the mistakes are surprisingly obvious. What factors could confuse the result? Crucially important, and the source of the biggest misinterpretations of any study, is the question "What is missing?" What did they forget to consider? What don't you know about the study from what you read? Is there something that just doesn't make sense? Who paid for the study? Did those who paid for the study or those who did the research have something to gain from the outcome?

Key questions about medical studies
- Who is being studied?
- What is the intervention?
- How was the study designed?
- What about the data analysis?
- Does the interpretation make sense?
- Making sense out of nonsense.

Who Is Being Studied?

Was the research conducted on humans, animals, or cells? Studies showing that rats taking CLA (conjugated linoleic acid) lose a tremendous amount of weight are great news, but only for overweight rats, as human studies haven't shown similar effects.

Were the right subjects chosen for the study? The health history of the study subjects commonly creates confusion. The primary conclusion of an investigation showing that a drug didn't lower the risk of heart attacks in healthy twenty-year-old college students should be that the company should hire smarter researchers for their next study.

Were the subjects like you? If your interest is personal, the subjects should be like you or the person you are concerned about. If you are middle aged and exercise daily for over an hour, findings from a study of inactive teenagers probably won't teach you much about your health concerns.

What Is the Intervention?

Is the treatment clearly described? For example, if an herb was used, how was it prepared and administered? Was the herb standardized so that we might be able to use the same product with patients? If it was, to what component or components was it standardized? Was it tested to confirm that the herb tested is what it is supposed to be? How much was given, and how often? When was it given? Research evidence that careless or improper use of a treatment doesn't work teaches us only that using it incorrectly isn't a good idea. The treatment might be wonderfully effective when used in the right way, or it might also be a complete waste for all concerned. A poorly designed study cannot tell us one way or the other.

A group of elderly patients received a supplement containing calcium and vitamin D. Headlines about the study shouted that it showed that calcium and vitamin D didn't lower the rate of broken bones. The data did show that there was no reduction in their risk of fractures caused by thin, vulnerable bones (osteoporotic fractures). There were more than few problems with the study, though. The dose of vitamin D they were given was below the recommended daily dose; it was one-half as much as used in several prior studies that *did* show a lower rate of fractures and only a small fraction of the vitamin D dose needed to raise their blood to the optimal level for bone production. Those who read past the "vitamin D failure" headline also learned that subjects who were the most compliant (in other words, they actually took the supplement consistently) were, in fact, less likely to suffer an osteoporotic fracture. In direct opposition to the headlines and the interpretation of the investigators, the study was very positive. It actually showed that even taking suboptimal doses of calcium and vitamin D worked to lower the risk of osteoporotic fractures.

How Was the Study Designed?

The perfect clinical study, the "gold standard," is one in which subjects are randomly assigned to different treatment groups and in which the subjects and investigators are unaware of the subjects' group assignment (in other words, their treatment). Such studies are called randomized, controlled, and double-blinded trials, often abbreviated as RCT. Because the intervention is so tightly controlled, the confusion created by other unknown factors is minimized. When the subjects don't know which treatment group they are in, the potentially powerful effects of placebo (their expectations about the treatment effects) will be evenly distributed between different treatment groups, eliminating that issue as a source of confusion.

How big was the study? Statistical analysis should tell us the likelihood that the research findings weren't just an accident. Most of us don't know enough about statistics to perform the calculations ourselves. Even if you do have a good grasp of statistics, ferreting out sufficient information to do the calculations and confirm or refute the investigators' conclusions can be very difficult or even impossible. Such detailed information is sometimes missing from medical journal articles and is essentially never in the newspaper or online articles. The size of the study can provide some reassurance. Although very large studies can be misleading because of the tendency to make clinically trivial differences appear meaningful, generally larger trials are more meaningful.

Was the study designed so that the treatment was applied correctly? Incorrectly applying the treatment is a common error when the treatment is complex or unfamiliar to the investigators. Such fundamental mistakes often taint studies of complementary and alternative therapies. For example, a clinical trial was conducted in England using the homeopathic remedy *Rhus tox* as a treatment for arthritis.[117] Classical use of homeopathy requires individualized treatment adjusted to an individual response over many months. Homeopaths often expect a worsening of symptoms early in the course of treatment, followed by long-term amelioration. Ignoring the fundamental principles of homeopathy, the investigators made a huge number of errors in their study design. There were so many that following the criticism greeting the publication of

---

117 Shipley, et al, "Controlled Trial of Homoeopathic Treatment of Osteoarthritis," *Lancet* 321 (1983): 97-8.

their trial, one of the study authors wrote an apology, acknowledging that it was impossible to draw any conclusions except that their study was an example of how homeopathic treatment shouldn't be investigated.[118]

What About the Data Analysis?

Wait! Don't go yet. Before you skip this section, fearing that I'm going to launch into a discussion of statistics, please stick around for just one minute (or two?). Although the mathematics of statistical analysis is important, the usual reason there is a problem is because an experienced group of researchers chose the wrong methods. In this book we cannot hope to reach an understanding of statistical methods superior to those experts, so just remember that this can be an issue; and if you have that knowledge, use it to critique the study yourself. There are a few more obvious issues you *can* expect to identify.

The first of these is effect size. As we discussed earlier, the amount of effect determines the clinical impact of a treatment. The amount of effect, the effect size, also determines how easy or difficult it is to measure the influence of the treatment intervention. Studies of larger numbers of subjects and instruments that measure smaller changes make it easier to reach statistical significance. However, statistical evidence of a difference between a treatment and placebo can be faint support for the intervention. Statistical superiority over a conventional prescription medication might be irrelevant to a patient *if the difference isn't enough to significantly improve the patient's life.* In a clinical study, as in a physician's office, it is the patient's experience that ultimately determines whether the treatment is successful or a failure.

Obviously then, the measurement used is pivotally important and underlies all other analysis considerations.

There are many ways to measure the impact of a treatment. Some ways are objective, such as blood tests, x-rays, or quantifying a patient's abilities, such as how well he or she performs a physical task (walking a certain distance) or a mental one (written test performance). Others are more subjective, such as patients rating how well they feel on a scale of one to ten. The accuracy of the measurement influences our ability to detect differences.

---

118 Kennedy et al, "Homeopathy," *Lancet* 321 (1983):482.

For the researcher, choosing a good measurement to assess the outcome of the treatment is a crucial decision. I feel that a good study should almost always include some subjective measurement of the patient's opinion. While objective measurements seem clearer, the founder of the Cochrane Collaboration, Sir Iain Chalmers, commented that the patient's opinion is the ultimate measure of a treatment's success. The goal is to help the patient feel better, not merely to change a laboratory test number, which might possibly be misleading or ill chosen. While we all agree that any laboratory tests selected for use in a study must be meaningfully related to the disease in question, the treatment simply *must* have a meaningful impact on the patients.

Most studies use a number of outcome measurements. This volume of assessment criteria can provide additional information, but it can also mislead. The most prevalent statistical standards of significance are p values or confidence intervals. The targets are a p value of less than 0.05 and/or confidence intervals that don't include 1.0.

A p value of less than 0.05 means there is a less-than-one-in-twenty chance that this result was an accident. Consequently, if twenty or more individual measurements are used, the odds are that one of them will show a p value of less than 0.05. Therefore, the primary outcome measurement must be identified before conducting the study. Any other statistically significant positive outcomes discovered after the study is completed, so called post hoc data, must be viewed skeptically.

A confidence interval (CI) is a range of reliable estimates of possible results. If the number 1 is within the range, it means that both sides might be the same. In other words, a study is looking for a difference. If the CI ranges from 1.2 to 1.4, there is a statistically significant difference. Taking it a step further, if the CI ranges from 1.2 to 7.0, there is a statistically significant difference, and because it might be as much as 7.0, that difference might be very big. On the other hand, a CI that ranges from 0.95 to 20.0 isn't significant. That 20.0 looks quite impressive, but its overinflated apparent importance withers with the recognition that it is just part of a group of results overlapping 1.0. This group is therefore not different.

Although they aren't direct measurements of health outcomes, other considerations can be more than germane and indirectly affect the health of patients, even powerfully so. Differences in cost, accessibility to treatment, adverse effect rates, and severity are some of the factors that can make one treatment better than another, even if the measured health outcomes are no better. In other words, a treatment that doesn't improve patients' health significantly more than another treatment might be clearly better for the patient for other reasons. The less difference there is between the effectiveness of competing treatments, the more salient other factors become.

Does the Interpretation Make Sense?

After concluding a study, the investigators write a research paper for publication, describing the study and drawing their conclusions. Their interpretation of the meaning of the study's findings defines the "bottom line" points readers are to glean from this work. This interpretation should be considered the essence, the essential knowledge gained. The sheer volume of information can be difficult to distill succinctly. Also, the biases of the researchers or of those funding the research often taint the conclusions, sometimes transforming what should be carefully restrained conclusions into well-hidden opinion pieces.

Most people learn about medical research from the media. The media usually simply recycle the opinions of the researchers, whether erroneous or not. Those writing for the mass media rarely have the experience to ask the correct critical questions or know the medical literature well enough to recall previous studies contradicting this new study. The media echo chamber tends to compound or at least obscure errors.

All these twists and distortions lead readers further and further away from any truth the study has revealed.

In my research training and as a reviewer of research articles submitted to medical journals for publication, I learned to watch out for several common mistakes investigators made. First, consider whether the study data reasonably justifies the authors' conclusions. That is often not the case.

Sometimes the interpretation overreaches the findings. If other studies have contradicted this outcome, it is wise to give a careful, tempered judgment. Most commonly an overreaching conclusion is a product of being overly optimistic. The study authors forget that there are good reasons to believe the results they observed in a specific study population won't apply to a more average group of patients. For example, it is unreasonable to assume that an unenthusiastic and unsupervised large population will experience the same benefits achieved by a small group of individuals who were highly motivated to comply with a difficult therapy regimen by personal contact with the investigative team.

At other times the interpretation can be entirely incorrect when the authors overlook a vital flaw in their study design, an unrecognized confounding factor, or make a statistical error. Years ago there was a study showing that taking oral doses of fluoride made bones thicker. The obvious conclusion then was that taking fluoride would be a good way to prevent fractures caused by thin, osteoporotic bones. Hurrah! Actually it turned out that these thicker bones were *more likely, not less likely, to break.* Fluoride made the bones thicker but more brittle. Healthy bones need to bend just a little bit. Darn.

A quite disturbing study researchers at the University of Minnesota conducted was published in *Nature* in 2005.[119] They found that *one out of every three American scientific researchers anonymously admitted to violating ethical protocols.* Most troubling was the finding that 15 percent admitted to altering study design, methods, or results because of pressure from a financial sponsor. Less than 2 percent admitted to falsifying data, the ultimate research lie. Although other confessed unethical activities weren't so venal, many of these improprieties led to equally false conclusions, potentially endangering patients.

Like any of us, a media writer can hear what he or she wants to hear. When United States Track and Field (USTF) issued an advisory cautioning that a small group of athletes (middle-aged women and military recruits doing basic training and participating in lengthy sporting events [four hours or more]) were endangering themselves by drinking huge quantities of water, a writer for the *New York Times* used this statement to advocate against the concern many have about chronic dehydration. Unfortunately this writer misled readers by ignoring the fact that the same USTF statement included an acknowledgment that chronic underhydration was an even more widespread problem, excluding that from her article. She reported the truth but a distorted truth.

Making Sense out of Nonsense

If the findings of a study are surprising, if they contradict our expectations or what we already thought we knew from other studies, should we be more cautious about accepting them at face value?

---

119 Martinson et al., "Scientists Behaving Badly," *Nature* 435 (2005):737-8.

In one way, the answer is no. Science is science, and, barring mistakes, the results should be meaningful.

On the other hand, the answer is yes; we should be more cautious. If we're surprised because other well-designed studies reached opposing conclusions, we need to think harder. Such a situation can provide a fantastic opportunity for learning, because our thinking about this matter might have become completely blind to something important. Shining a light in the gap between these two seemingly contradictory studies might reveal something useful hidden in that blind spot. I'm much more excited by a new study that doesn't appear to fit with what we already know than another one that just adds to the already overwhelming weight of evidence on a particular topic.

It is apparent that all studies are flawed, but they all still have something to teach. Reading the study title and the web article headline are not enough. Reading the posted abstract of the scientific article isn't enough. To really understand the weakness and strength of any study, to learn its true lessons, we must read further into the study, asking questions and looking for holes in the logic. If the answers aren't there, if the results or methods don't make sense, your confusion on reading it is probably because the investigators made improper assumptions. If you develop the habit of asking yourself why the conclusions of a study might not be right, you will uncover many mistakes. You will be a step ahead of those who write the media articles about the research and at least two steps ahead of those who read the articles uncritically; you are in a much better position to make better health decisions for you and your family.

Index

A

about this book 5
acesulfame K 172
aconitum napellus
  acute emotional distress and 311
  croup and 310
  fear and 311
  traffic accidents and 311
acrylamides, formation in foods 86
acupressure 294. *See also* acupuncture
  needle phobia and 295
acupuncture 293–298
  acupressure and 294
  adverse effects of 296
  Asian peoples' use of 230
  Ayurveda and 294
  battlefield 295
  conditions treated by 297
  cupping and 294
  effectiveness of 296
  electroacupuncture 294
  for specific medical conditions 251
  history and theory 293–294
  James Reston's appendicitis and 295
  meridians 293
  moxibustion and 294
  needle phobia and 294
  needles 293
  popularity of 296
  research on 296
  Sir William Osler and 295
  usage in the US 233
  US Military use of 295
  yin and yang symbol and 294
acute emotional distress
  homeopathic remedies for 311

addictions 184
adverse drug effects
  as a leading cause of death 21
  painkilling medications and.
       See painkilling medications
  rate of 21
  steroids and 24
Advil 180
aerobic activities 53
  definition of 53
  high-intensity interval training 53
  Kenneth Cooper and 53
aflatoxin 156
African Traditional Medicine 251
Agent Orange 144
aging
  dioxins and 144
  herbal medicines for 257
air pollution (indoor) 152–156
  assessing effects of 153
  automobiles and 153
  furnaces, fireplaces, and ovens and
     154
  HEPA filters and 155
  radon gas and 152, 154
  sick buildings 183
  smoking and 152
air pollution (outdoor) 151–152
  adverse effects of 151
  as a source of mercury exposure 99
alachlor, water filtration of 164
alcohol addiction, social connections
  and 194
alcohol consumption, health pros and
  cons of 184
Alexander technique 252

allergies
  allergen families 299
  butterbur and 260
  homeopathy and 291
alpha-linolenic acid (ALA).
    See omega-3 oils
alpha lipoic acid 130
  recommendations 130
alternative medicine.
    See complementary and alternative
    medicine (CAM)
altruism 194
Alzheimer's disease
  folates and 118
  sleep and 188
American Botanical Council 233
American diet 76
    sugar consumption in 76
    vitamin and mineral deficiencies in 77
amphibians, decline in populations,
    atrazine and 140
anaerobic activities 53
anchovies, EPA and DHA and 98
anemia, iron-deficiency 123
anesthesia, infants and 28
angiotensin-receptor blockers, cancer
    risk 181
anthocyanosides 263
antibacterial soaps 156
  triclosan in 156
antibiotics
  breast cancer and 180
  ear infections and 23, 289
  overuse in American farm animals 92
  resistant bacteria and 92, 93
  risks in human use of 94
antidepressants
  adverse effects of 178
  breast cancer and 180
antioxidants, death rate and 119
anxiety, homeopathy and 291
aphthae (canker sores), homeopathic
    remedy for 310
Apitherapy 253
applied kinesiology 252

aquatic animals, decline in populations,
    atrazine and 140
arabinogalactans, benefits of 78
Aristolochia 261
arnica montana, injuries and 314
arsenic 161
  fertilizers and 161
  in drinking water 161
    removing 164
  in herbal supplements 262
arsenicum album
  fear and 311
  food poisoning and 311, 312
arthritis 253
  homeopathy and 291
artificial flavors, colors, and
    preservatives 172
artificial sweeteners. *See* sugars and
    sweeteners
artificial turf, lead in 148
art therapy for specific medical
    conditions 249
Asian diets 107
asparagine and acrylamides 86
aspartame 172
asthma
  air pollution and 151
  butterbur and 260
  chlorinated water and 158
  mold and 156
  sulfites and 172
atheists, prayer for 214
athletic injuries
  static stretching and 58
  strength training and 55
athletic performance
  dehydration and 46
  ferritin and 123
Atlas, Charles 55
atrazine 140
  decline in aquatic animal populations
    and 140
  human birth defects and 140
  water filtration of 140, 164

attention-deficit/hyperactivity disorder (ADHD)
food additives and 85
Aude sapere 273
autism, Roundup and 141
automobiles, air pollution inside of 153
Avogadro's constant 284
Ayurvedic medicine 251
acupuncture and 294

B
babies. *See* infants
back problems
acupuncture for 239
CAM and 231, 252
flexibility and 56
homeopathy and 291
bacteria
antibiotic resistant, American deaths and 92
intestinal, human health and 79
balance training 61
Ballentine, Rudolph B. 11
ballistic stretching. *See* stretching
barefoot running 72
basic human needs and our health 31
battlefield acupuncture 295
beef, ALA and 98
bee venom therapy 253
behavioral problems in children.
See attention-deficit/hyperactivity disorder (ADHD)
food additives and 85
belladonna (homeopathic remedy)
ear infections and 311
headaches and 313
benzene 164
berries as a source of polyphenols 78
beta-amyloid and Alzheimer's disease 188
beta-glucans and cancer 78
Better Than Medicines
about the series 4
Workbook 6
Bhopal Disaster 161

bilberry 263
bioelectromagnetic applications in medicine 237
for specific medical conditions 250
biofeedback
for relaxation 239
for specific medical conditions 249
biological age, telomeres and 126
biological therapies 235
biotin recommendations 130
birds of prey and environmental toxins 80
birth defects
atrazine and 140
folates and 118
folic acid and 115
bisphenol A (BPA) 145–147
adverse health effects of 146
Down syndrome and 145
in humans 136
plastic recycling code for 147
reproductive health and 145
sources of 146
carbonless sales receipts 146
bisphenol S (BPS) 147
bitter-tasting plants, benefits of 78
bladder cancer, chlorinated water and 158
bladder infections. *See* urinary tract
Blake, William 67
blame 211
blindness, zinc and 113
blood, omega-3 levels in 102
blood pressure. *See* high blood pressure; low blood pressure
blood sugar levels, regulating, St. John's wort and 260
body fat and your health 219
body sculpting, fat burning activities and 66
bones
density of, calcium supplements and 32
fluoride and 159, 325
vitamin D and 111

borage oil, seizures and 102
bottled water. *See* water
BPA. *See* bisphenol A (BPA)
BPS (bisphenol S) 147
brain chemistry and structure 50
  exercise and 50
  habits of thought and 202
  learning and 51
Brainerd Diarrhea 159
Brainerd, Minnesota
  water fluoridation and resident health
      159
breakfast
  health and 36
  importance of 106
breast cancer
  antibiotics and 180
  antidepressants and 180
  breast self-examination and 35
  Iscador/mistletoe and 253
  mammograms and 35
  nighttime shift work and 106
  nuts and seeds and 98
  survival rates
      social connections and 193
breast milk
  PBDEs in 169
  perchlorates in 142
breast self-examination
  breast cancer and 35
breathing techniques for specific
    medical conditions 249
bromomethane 150
Bryant, Dorothy 189
bryonia alba
  headaches and 313
  injuries and 314
butterbur 260
B vitamins. *See also* the names of
    individual B vitamins
  recommendations 129, 130

C

cadmium 150
  in herbal supplements 262

calcarea phosphorica, teething and 315
calcium and calcium supplements
  colon cancer and 32
  dietary sources of calcium 304
  insomnia and 32
  muscles and 111
  positive effects of 32
  recommendations 130
California
  perchlorate standards 144
  unsafe mercury levels in residents 98
CAM. *See* complementary and
    alternative medicine (CAM)
cancer. *See also* specific types of cancer
  acrylamides in our food and 86
  alcohol and 184
  beta-glucans and 78
  blood pressure medications and 181
  CAM treatments for 253
  caused by cosmetic ingredients 174
  cell phones and 171
  chemotherapy's adverse effects and
      CAM 251
  dioxins and 144
  eating patterns and 106
  environmental chemicals and 138,
      139
  fluoride and 160
  folates and 118
  folic acid and 116, 128
  immune system destruction of 139
  methyl iodide and 150
  patients' use of CAM 234
  President's Panel on Cancer 134
  Roundup and 141
  statin drugs and 180
  sweeteners and 172
  telomeres and 127
  turmeric and cinnamon and 78
  ultraviolet light water purification and
      163
  vegetarian and vegan diets and 80
  vitamins C and E and 117
  VOCs and 165

canker sores, homeopathic remedy for 310

carbohydrates and marathon running 66

carbon blocks for water filtration 164

carbonless sales receipts, BPA in 146

carbo vegetabilis
gastroenteritis and 312

Carlston, Michael
favored CAM approaches 300
history and experiences 9–17
Hmong refugees and 13
introduction to homeopathy 11
years of experience 3

carotenoids, recommendations 130

Carson, Rachel 84

cast-iron cookware 168

cataracts
high blood sugar and 42
statin drugs and 180
vegetarian and vegan diets and 81

cell phones 171
recommendations 171
specific absorption rate (SAR) 171

Chalmers, Sir Iain 323

chamomilla
ear infections and 311
teething and 315

chelated nutrients 130

chemicals in food 84

chemotherapy's adverse effects and CAM 251

chicken, food poisoning and 93

children
behavioral problems, food additives and 85
eating breakfast and 106
flame retardants and 169
lead and 148
premature puberty in girls 92, 145
strength training benefits for 55

Children's Health Protection Advisory Committee, perchlorate standards and 144

Chinese herbal medicines
adulteration of 263

chiropractic medicine 252
usage in the US 233

chloramine, water filtration of 164

chlordane in freshwater fish 98

chlorine
gas 84
purifying water with 157
threshold of harm 158
toxic effects of 158
water filtration of 164

chocolate
as a source of polyphenols 78
dark, heart health and 36

cholera, water quality and 157

cholesterol, high levels of
lowering naturally 42
red yeast rice for 239

chromium, water filtration of 164

chromosomes, BPA and 145

chronic fatigue syndrome, homeopathy and 291

chronic health conditions
effectiveness of homeopathy for 239
social connections and 193

chronic pain, homeopathy and 291

cigarette smoking. *See* smoking

cinnamon
benefits of 78
sensitivity to 173

circulatory problems, sexual function in males and 199

cleaning products in the home, safety information 165

climate change and loss of plant species 271

clinical research. *See* scientific research

cocculus, motion sickness and 314

Cochrane Collaboration 323

coffee, polyphenols in 78

cognitive behavior therapy, sleep and 189

colds, social connections and 193

colic, butterbur and 260
colon cancer
  calcium and 32
  nighttime shift work and 106
Colorado River, perchlorates in 142
Colorado, unsafe mercury levels in
    residents 98
colorectal cancer and use of CAM 234
communication, evening family meal
    and 107
community. *See* social connections
complementary and alternative
    medicine (CAM). *See also* specific
    names of medical approaches
  approaches favored by Michael
      Carlston 300
  as an essential health habit 299–300
  attitudes in the alternative community
      14
  back trouble and 231
  definition of 226–228
  five categories of 235
  in US medical schools 226
  list of types 237–238
  practitioners, evaluating 242–256
  reasons for using 230
  self-care and 245
  usage in the US 30, 228, 232
  using 239–256
      importance of medical diagnosis
          240
  worldwide use 229
compliance of patients 246
concentric muscle strengthening 59
confidence interval 323
constitutional remedy 291
Consumer Products Safety
    Commission (CPSC) 148
contact dermatitis, cosmetics and
    personal care items and 173
conventional medicine
  chronic health problems and 239
  herbs and 24, 26, 260
  in the 1800s 227

medical interventions
    lack of research support for 26
  patient compliance 246
  practitioners' attitudes 15
      toward CAM 235
  strengths 241
  use of herbal medicines 234
cookware
  cast-iron 168
  nonstick 166
Cooper, Kenneth, aerobics and 53
coping skills. *See also* stress
    management
  flexible coping 207
  improving 205
  positive reappraisal 209
  quality of life and 204
  social interactions 207
copper
  in herbal supplements 262
  zinc and 113
CoQ10 130
cosmetics and personal care items
  cinnamon in 173
  health risks of 173
  information resources 175
  phthalates in 199
counseling
  effect on brain 202
  value of 217
Counterstrain 252
cows, grass-fed, ALA and 98
craniosacral therapy 252
croup, homeopathic remedies for 310
cryptosporidium 157, 164
cupping and acupuncture 294
Curanderismo 251
Curie, Marie 170
cursed bread 155

D

daily value percentage of nutrients 129
dance therapy for specific medical
    conditions 249

DDT 84
  in freshwater fish 98
  malaria and 85
dead zones in the environment
  nitrogen fertilizers and 84
death fogs 151
death rate
  antioxidants and 119
  due to radon gas 152
  from medications 177
  lowering through strength training 56
  social connections and 193
dehydration. *See also* water
  athletic performance and 46
  calculating your fluid levels and 46
  color of urine and 47
  distortions about in media 325
  health effects of 46, 47
  thirst and 46
dental amalgam as a source of mercury
    exposure 99
dental fluorosis 160
depression
  CAM and 251
  changes in brains with treatment 203
  homeopathy and 291
  social connections and 193
DES. *See* diethylstilbestrol (DES)
dextrose. *See* sugars and sweeteners
diabetes
  BPA and 146
  chelation therapy and 253
  dioxins and 144
  eating breakfast and 106
  link to starvation in grandparents 140
  treating naturally 42
  turmeric and cinnamon and 78
  vegetarian and vegan diets and 80
diagnosis, importance of 240
diarrhea
  Brainerd 159
  homeopathic remedies for 312–313
  sulfites and 172
dichlorodiphenyltrichloroethane.
    See DDT

diet. *See also* food
  Asian 107
  benefits of variety in 78
  bitter-tasting plants and 78
  deficiencies in. causes of 82
  eating low on the food chain 80
  fermented foods in 78
  Latin American 107
  Mediterranean 107
  vegetarian and vegan. *See* vegetarian
    and vegan diets
Dietary Reference Intake
  nutrient deficiencies and 110
diethylstilbestrol (DES) 145
digestion
  eating slowly and 106
  meal timing and 105
digestive upsets
  homeopathic remedies for 312–313
  homeopathy and 291
dioxin 144. *See also* polychlorinated
    biphenyls (PCBs)
  exposure to
    reducing 145
    sources of 144
  health effects of 144
  in breast milk 144
  in freshwater fish 98
disaster-related fear, homeopathic
    remedy for 311
diseases. *See also* specific diseases
  blame and 211
  chronic
    effect of social connections on 193
    omega-3 deficiency and 97
  essential health habits and 42
  exercise and 49
  homeopathic treatment of 291
  infectious, antibiotic-resistant bacteria
    and 92
  risk of, omega-3 oils and 102
  spiritual dysfunction and 287
Disraeli, Benjamin 317
DNA
  chromosomes. BPA and 145

environmental damage of 139
related to diseases 139
viral 79
docosahexaenoic acid (DHA).
    See omega-3 oils
Doctrine of Signatures 280
Down syndrome, BPA and 145
drinking water. *See* water
drinks, recovery and sports.
    See recovery and sports drinks
drug addiction, social connections and
    194
dry macular degeneration, zinc and
    113
dynamic stretching. *See* stretching
dysmenorrhea 314

E

ear infections
    antibiotics and 23, 289
    homeopathic remedies for 310
eating 105–107
    breakfast, importance of 106
    evening family meal, importance of
        107
    meal timing 105
    portion size 105
    slowly 106
eating low on the food chain 80
eccentric muscle strengthening 59
    as a cure for tennis elbow 59
echinacea
    contamination of 262
    echinacoside 263
    popularity of 257
    purity concerns 261
Eclectic tradition in herbal medicine
    230
E. coli. See Escherichia coli
eicosapentaenoic acid (EPA).
    See omega-3 oils
eight glasses of water a day 47
Eisenberg, David 232
elderly individuals
    benefits of strength training for 55

community-based exercise programs
    and 193
supplements and 109
electric fans 171
electroacupuncture 294
electromagnetic radiation (EMR)
    169–171
    cell phones and 171
    microwave ovens and 170
ElliptiGO 73
Emerson, Ralph Waldo 258
emotional bonds
    evening family meal and 107
endocrine disruption
    flame retardant chemicals and 169
    PFOA and 167
    Roundup and 141
    scientific studies on 137
The Endocrine Society's report on
    environmental chemicals 138
endometriosis, BPA and 145
endurance runners. *See* marathon
    runners
energetic healing 235
enteric coatings, phthalates and 130
environment 133–186
    Hippocrates and 133
    pesticides, herbicides, and fertilizers
        and 84
    prescription medications in 181
environmental chemicals 135–151. *See
    also* individual chemical names
    cancer and 139
    delayed effect of 139
    found in humans 136
    human hormones and 138
    reproductive health and 138
environmental health resources 137
environmental toxins
    diet and 80
    predators and 80
Environmental Working Group
    as a resource for water information
        165

eosinophilic myalgia, genetically
    modified L-tryptophan and 89
EPA. *See* omega-3 oils; US
    Environmental Protection Agency
    (US EPA)
epigenetic effects 139
Escherichia coli
  in supermarket meats 92
  O157:H7 strain
    kidney failure and 93
escin 263
essential health habits
  #1: drink enough water 45–48
  #2: exercise almost every day 49–74
  #3: eat well 75–108
  #4: take your supplements 109–132
  #5: avoid the things that make you sick
    133–186
  #6: get enough sleep 187–190
  #7: be involved in your community
    191–196
  #8: create a healthy sex life 197–200
  #9: remember that attitude is
    important 201–212
  #10: develop a purpose or spirituality
    213–216
  as treatment for diseases 42
  CAM and 299
  introduction to 41–44
  longevity and 42
  putting into practice 217–222
estrogen
  BPA and DES and 145
  phthalates and 142
evening family meal, importance of
    107
evening primrose oil (EPO)
  seizures and 102
exercise. *See also* specific types of
    exercise
  adjusting workouts 62
    talk test and 63
  aerobics. *See* aerobic activity
  brain cells and 50
  flexibility. *See* flexibility

gadgets for. *See* gadgets for exercise
  guidelines 53
  heart health and 28, 34
  heart rate and 63
  importance of 49
  meal timing and 105
  optimal activities 67
  principles of 61
    overload 62–66
    recovery 67–68
    variability 66–67
  problem-solving abilities and 51
  programs. *See* exercise programs
  recommended number of hours 50
  recovery drinks and 68
  social connections and 195
  strength training. *See* strength training
  ten thousand steps a day 52
exercise programs
  community based
    and the elderly 193
  creating 68
  importance of recovery and 68
  importance of starting slowly 70
  planning 70
  starting 220
explosive physical activities, ballistic
    stretching and 60
explosive stretching. *See* stretching
extract ratios in herbal medicines 269
eye health
  dry macular degeneration 113
  vegetarian and vegan diets and 81

F
farm-raised fish, health hazards of 87
fat in food 77
FDA. *See* Food and Drug
    Administration (FDA)
fear, homeopathic remedies for 311
Feldenkrais healing touch 252
fermented foods 78
ferritin. *See* iron
fertilizers. *See* pesticides, herbicides,
    and fertilizers

fetal malformations, Roundup and 141
filters
    air, importance of replacing 155
    water. *See* water purification
FindNano app 176
fireplaces, indoor air pollution and 154
fish
    consumption guidelines
        from Michael Carlston 100
        from the FDA 99
    EPA and DHA and 98
    farm-raised, health hazards of 87
    freshwater, toxins in 98
    risks of eating 98
fitness. *See* exercise
flame retardants 168
    adverse health effects of 168
    in humans 136
flax seeds, omega-3 oils and 98
flexibility 56–61
    back problems and 56
    ballistic stretching and 60
    drinking water and 57
    effect of diet on 57
    stretching and 57, 58
flexible coping 207
Florida, unsafe mercury levels in
    residents 98
fluoride
    bone brittleness and 159, 325
    in drinking water 158
        removing by water filtration 164
folic acid and folates
    cancer risk and 116, 128
    genetic inability to metabolize 118,
        128
        form of folate to take for 118
    health benefits of folates 118
    heart disease and 116, 128
    neural tube birth defects and 115
    recommendations 130
    vitamin B12 deficiency testing and
        122

food. *See also* diet; specific types of food
    bacterial contamination of 93
    chemicals in 84, 86
    domesticated, nutrients in 89, 114
    fat in 77
    fermented, benefits of 78
    flame retardant chemicals in 169
    fortification 115
    genetically modified. *See* genetically
        modified foods (GMOs)
    industrial farming and 91
    local, advantages of 95
    nutrients in (list of sources) 302
    organic. *See* organic foods
    poisoning. *See* food poisoning
    processed
        disadvantages of 80, 82, 114
        obesity and 80
        salt in 172
    quality of, industrial farming and 91
    raw 83
    shopping for 103, 104
    wild
        benefits of 87
        vitamin and mineral levels in 89
food additives 172
    ADHD and 85
    artificial flavors, colors, and
        preservatives 172
    health effects of 85
    sulfites 172
food allergies and intolerances
    dietary deficiencies and 82
Food and Drug Administration (FDA)
    fish-consumption advisories 98
    fish consumption guidelines 99
food-borne illnesses. *See* food
    poisoning
food industry, intentions of 80
food plants
    genetic diversity of
        industrial farming and 91
food poisoning 93
    chicken and 93
    homeopathic remedy for 311

food supplementation. *See
also* supplements
national programs 116
forgiveness 209
and injustice 210
and our health 210
fortification of foods 115
fragrances, sensitivity to 173
fructose. *See* sugars and sweeteners
fruit juice 76
fruits and vegetables
sugar levels in 114
fungi. *See* molds and yeast
furnaces in the home
importance of maintaining 154
indoor air pollution and 154

G

gadgets for exercise 70
ElliptiGO 73
heart rate monitors 71
MP3 players and smart phones 72
pedometers 71
shoes 72
special equipment 73
trekking poles 72
gamma linolenic acid (GLA)
seizures and 102
garlic, popularity of 257
gasoline, MBTE and 141
gastroenteritis, homeopathic remedies
for 312–313
gastrointestinal infections, probiotics
and 239
gelsemium, stage fright and 311
genes
environmental damage of 139
related to diseases 139
genetically modified foods (GMOs) 87
concerns about 88
eosinophilic myalgia and 89
increase of herbicide use and 141
National Research Council report on
90
ProdiGene incident 90

rice, human genes in 87
risk-benefit ratio of 91
Roundup and 140
genetic diversity of plants
industrial farming and 91
giardia 164
ginkgo, popularity of 257
ginseng
ginsenosides 263
hairs on, use of 262
Panax 263
popularity of 257
rhodiola and 258
Siberian 263
globus hystericus, personal loss and 312
glucose. *See* sugars and sweeteners
gluten sensitivity, Roundup and 141
glyphosate. *See* Roundup
GMP-certified herbs 267
goals, setting 218–220
goiter, iodine and 115
grapes as a source of polyphenols 78
grass-fed cows, ALA and 98
Great Fear (French Revolution),
mycotoxins and 155
grehlin, obesity and 113
groundwater, MBTE and 141
growth hormones in meat
premature puberty in girls and 92
gynecologic cancer and use of CAM
234

H

Haber, Fritz, chemical legacy 84
habits of thought
and our health 201–212
as a biological process 201
optimism and pessimism 203
Type A personalities 201
Hahnemann, Samuel 228. *See
also* homeopathy
development of homeopathic
principles 280–292
history of 275–279
insane asylums and 277

Masons and 286
motto for homeopathy 273
physician's duty and 16
quinine experiments 278
hair growth, ferritin and 123
HBCD (hexabromocyclododecane) 169
HDPE (plastic recycling code) 147
headaches 252
homeopathic remedies for 313
migraine, butterbur and 260
head trauma 252
healing touch 252
heart disease
air pollution and 151
BPA and 146
drinking water and 48
eating breakfast and 106
exercise and 28
folates and 118
folic acid and 116, 128
polyphenols and 78
social connections and 193
vegetarian and vegan diets and 80
vitamins C and E and 117
heart health
effect of dehydration on 47
exercise and 34
foods for improving health of 36
heart rate
as affected by different activities 65
exercising and 63
Karvonen (Heart Rate Reserve)
formula and 72
maximal 64
calculating 64
resting 64
training zones 65
heart rate monitors 71
Heart Rate Reserve formula 72
heart rate variability (HRV) 153
heavy metals 147–149. See also specific
names of heavy metals
in freshwater fish 98
in herbal supplements 262

Heisenberg, David
alternative medical usage surveys 30
HEPA filters 155
hepar sulphuris calcareum
croup and 310
ear infections and 311
herbal medicines 251, 257–272. See
also specific names of herbs
adulteration of 263
ancient wisdom and 271
animal use of 257
best forms of 262
certification of 266
Chinese origin, cautions 267
Chinese (traditional)
contamination of 263
climate change and 271
conventional medications and 24
Eclectic and Thomsonian traditions 230
ethnic minorities and 230
extracts
cautions 263
ratios 269
herb-drug interactions 265
how to read labels 269
marker compounds 262
Native American healers and 230
prescription medications and 257
proprietary blends 267
purity concerns 260, 262
safety 265
guidelines 268
scientific research and 259
usage in the US 233
use in conventional medicine 234
herb-drug interactions 265
herbicides. See pesticides, herbicides,
and fertilizers
Hering, Constantine 230
herring, EPA and DHA and 98
hexabromocyclododecane (HBCD) 169
high blood pressure
lead poisoning and 148

lowering naturally 42
medications, cancer risk of 181
meditation and 239
processed foods and 82
sexual function in males and 199
vegetarian and vegan diets and 80
vitamin D and 126
high blood sugar, cataracts and 42
high-fructose corn syrup (HFCS) 76,
172
high-intensity interval training (HIIT)
53
highway patrol officers, automobile
interior air quality and 153
Hippocrates 20
environment and 133
Hippocratic Oath, other medical
traditions and 20
Hmong people 13
iron-deficiency anemia and 112
holistic medicine. *See* complementary
and alternative medicine (CAM)
homeopathy 273–292. *See
also* Hahnemann, Samuel
applications of 290, 291
Avogadro's constant and 284
chronic health conditions and 239
constitutional remedy 291
definitions 275
dilution of remedies 284
mystery behind 286
table 285
effectiveness of 288
for specific medical conditions
251. *See also* specific medical
conditions
information resources 292
lifestyle changes and 277
misconceptions about 274
patient compliance 246
patient preference for 291
principles 280
likes cure likes 279, 280
minimum dose 284
provings 281–284

single medicine 284
remedies 310–315
administering 315
dosages 315
process of selecting 283, 290
responses to 316
scientific method and 15, 281
self-care and 291
short-term conditions and 291
succussion 284
usage in the US 233
view of illness 286
spiritual dysfunction and 287
hormones
dioxins and 144
disturbances, homeopathy and 291
horse chestnut 263
household products
cookware
cast iron 168
nonstick 166
safety information 167
HRV (heart rate variability) 153
human genes in GMO rice 87
Human Genome Project, identifying
genes related to diseases 139
human hormones
atrazine and 140
environmental chemicals and 138
human physical development
running and 50
humans, social nature of 191
hydration. *See* dehydration
hyperbaric oxygen 253
hypericin and hyperforin 263
hyperparathyroidism
vitamin D and 125
hypnosis for specific medical
conditions 249

I

ibuprofen 180
ignatia amara, personal loss and 312
imagery for specific medical conditions
249

immune system
  destruction of cancer cells 139
  dioxins and 145
  intestinal bacteria and 79
  PFOAs and 168
  stimulants of 78
indoor air pollution. See air pollution
  (indoor)
industrial farming, food quality and 91
infant formula, contaminants in 142
infants
  anesthesia and 28
  fluoridated water and 160
  stillborn, trihalomethanes and 158
infections, social connections and 193
infectious diseases
  antibiotic-resistant bacteria and 92
infertility. See reproductive health
ingredient labels, benefits of reading 79
injuries, homeopathic remedies for 314
injustice and forgiveness 210
insect repellents, alternatives 166
insomnia
  calcium supplements and 32
  homeopathy and 291
insulin, obesity and 113
insulin sensitivity
  St. John's wort and 260
integrative medicine.
    See complementary and alternative
    medicine (CAM)
Internet, using for medical information
  245
interventional screenings 35
  risks of 34
intestinal bacteria
  human health and 79
iodine, thyroid disease and 115
ionizing radiation 170
iPod, exercise and 72
IQ
  fluoridated water and 160
  lead and 148
iron
  cast-iron cookware and 168

deficiency 123
  anemia 123
  organic foods and 116
ferritin form 123
  athletic performance and 123
  hair growth and 123
  restless leg syndrome and 123
recommendations 130
usefulness of 123
zinc and 112
Iscador (mistletoe) 253
Ivy, John 106

J
junk food 76
  obesity and 80

K
Karvonen formula, heart rate and 72
kava
  lactones 263
  liver damage and 265
  noble cultivar 266
Keflezighi, Meb 73
kidneys
  damage
    cadmium and 150
    statin drugs and 180
    sweeteners and 172
  disease
    PFOAs and 167
    vitamin D and 125
  failure of
    drinking water and 48
    E. coli O157:H7 and 94
    painkilling medications and 22
knees
  leg muscles and 56
  problems
    strength training and 69

L
labels on herbal medicines, reading
  269
lab testing resources 126

LaLanne, Jack 55
Latin American diets 107
LDPE (plastic recycling code) 147
lead (heavy metal) 147–149
    adverse health effects of 148
    exposure to
        reducing 147–149
        sources of 148–149
    Herbert Needleman and 148
    in artificial turf 148
    in herbal supplements 262
    water filtration of 164
learning, brain cells and 51
leg muscles, knee health and 56
leptin, obesity and 113
life changes, stress and 192
lifestyle, changes in
    homeopathic practitioners and 277
    improvements in health and 32
    nonmedicinal 36
likes cure likes homeopathic principle
        279, 280
liver
    damage
        dioxins and 144
        from cosmetics 174
        kava and 265
        sweeteners and 172
    toxicity
        BPA and 146
local food, advantages of 95
London death fogs 134
longevity
    essential health habits and 42
    purposeful life and 214
    telomeres and 42, 126
Los Angeles, medications in water 182
low blood pressure, salt and 83
Lown, Bernard 232
LSD, food molds and 155
L-tryptophan, genetically modified
    as a cause of eosinophilic myalgia 89
lung cancer
    air pollution and 151
    blood pressure medications and 181
    use of CAM and 234
lungs, methyl bromide and methyl
        iodide and 150
Luskin, Fred 210
lymphedema, strength training and 28

M
macadamia nuts, omega-3 oils and
        98
macronutrients
    vegetarian and vegan diets and 82
macular degeneration, dry
    zinc and 113
magnesia phosphorica
    menstrual cramps and 314
malaria and DDT 85
maltose. See sugars and sweeteners
mammograms, risks of 35
manipulation and body work 235, 238
    for specific medical conditions 252
    types of 252
marathon runners
    carbohydrates and 66
    strength training and 54
marker compounds in herbs 262
masks, safety 183
Masons and Samuel Hahnemann 286
Massachusetts' perchlorate standards
        144
massage therapy 252
maximal heart rate 64
    calculating 64
meal timing 105
    exercise and 105
    sleep and 105
meats
    antibiotics and 92
    E. coli in 92
medical diagnosis, importance of 240
medical journals
    pharmaceutical industry and 25
medical oaths 20
medical screenings. See interventional
        screenings
medical supplies, phthalates in 142

medical treatments, critical evaluation of 16
medications 177
  adverse effects of 178
  advice for using 181
  alternative medicine and 179
  blood pressure medications and breast cancer 180
  deaths related to 177
  effectiveness of alternatives to 22
  found as adulterants in herbal medicines 263
  herbal medicines and 257
  increase in number of prescriptions for 21
  information resources 182
  in the environment 181
  painkilling. See painkilling medications
  proliferation of 178
  safe disposal of 182
meditation/relaxation for specific medical conditions 249
Mediterranean diet 107
memory, ginkgo and 257
men
  importance of relationships to 193
  sexual function and circulatory problems 199
menstrual cramps, homeopathic remedies for 314
mental healing 249
mentally ill patients and Samuel Hahnemann 277
mercurius vivus
  canker sores and 310
  ear infections and 311
  gastroenteritis and 313
mercury 149–150
  in fish 98
  in herbal supplements 262
  in humans 98
  sources of exposure to 99, 150
  testing for in yourself 103
  toxicity, symptoms of 99, 149
meridians in acupuncture 293

methyl bromide (bromomethane) 150
methylcobalamin 129, 130
methylfolate 129, 130
methyl iodide (iodomethane) 150–151
  adverse health effects of 150
methyl mercury. See mercury
methyl tertiary butyl ether. See MTBE
Michaels, Marina 210
micronutrients
  obesity and 113
  vegetarian and vegan diets and 82
microwave ovens 170
migraine headaches. See also headaches
  butterbur and 260
milk, vitamin D and 115
Minamata, Japan 149
mind-body interventions 235, 237
  for specific medical conditions 249
minerals, dietary. See vitamins and minerals
minimum dose (homeopathic principle) 284
Minneapolis, caffeine in drinking water 182
mistletoe (Iscador) 253
MK7 (vitamin K) 130
modern life and basic human needs 31
molds and yeast 155–156
  adverse effects of 155
  aflatoxin 156
  managing exposure to 156
  mycotoxins 155
  respiratory problems and 156
  usefulness of 155
Monsanto and Roundup 140
mortality rate. See death rate
mothers, depression in, and social connections 193
motion sickness, homeopathic remedies for 314
moxibustion and acupuncture 294
MP3 players and exercise 72
MRIs, health concerns about 171
MTBE 141
  groundwater contamination and 141

in humans 136
municipal water systems and 141
water filtration of 142
multiple vitamin mineral supplements.
    See supplements
muscles
    ballistic strengthening and 60
    building 306
    concentric strengthening and 59
    cramps and spasms
        calcium and 111
    eccentric strengthening and 59
    leg, knees and 56
    stiff and cold, stretching and 60
    tightness
        tendons and 59
        value of 56
music therapy for specific medical
    conditions 249
MVMs. *See* supplements
mycotoxins, negative effects of 155

N

nanotechnology 174–176
    dangers of nano-sized particles 175
    FindNano app 176
naproxen 180
National Academy of Sciences (NAS)
    study on fluoridated water 160
National Research Council's report on
    GMOs 90
nationwide food supplementation
    programs 115
    organic foods and 116
Native Americans
    health-care practices 251
    use of CAM 229
Naturopathic medicine 251
nausea
    B vitamins and 129
    homeopathic remedies for 312–313
nectar. *See* sugars and sweeteners
Needleman, Herbert, lead toxicity and
    148
needle phobia and acupressure 294

nervous system
    damage to
        from artificial sweeteners 172
        from cosmetic ingredients 174
        methyl bromide and methyl iodide
            and 150
        Roundup and 141
    development of
        perchlorates and 143
Nestle, Marion 89
neural tube defects, folic acid and 115
New Orleans, medications in water 182
New York, unsafe mercury levels in
    residents 98
niacin, pellagra and 115
nighttime shift work, cancer risk and
    106
nitrates and nitrites, water filtration of
    164
nitrogen fertilizers. *See also* pesticides,
    herbicides, and fertilizers
    effects on environment 84
noble cultivars 266
Nogier, Raphael 295
nonstick cookware 166
    alternatives to 168
NSAIDs, breast cancer risk and 180
nutrients. *See also* supplements and
        specific nutrients
    sources of in food 302
nutritional studies
    challenges of 116
nuts and seeds
    nuts as a source of polyphenols 78
    omega-3 oils and 98
nux vomica
    gastroenteritis and 313
    headaches and 313

O

O157:H7. *See* Escherichia coli
obesity
    eating breakfast and 106
    hormones and 113
    micronutrients 113

physical fitness and 219
processed foods and 80
strength training for weight loss 55
vegetarian and vegan diets and 80
vitamin D and 113
omega-3 oils 97–103
  ALA, EPA, and DHA and 97
  deficiency in, chronic diseases and 97
  disease risk and 102
  farm-raised fish and 87
  measuring blood levels of 102
  nuts and seeds and 98
  recommendations 130
  supplements 100–102
  vegetarian and vegan diets and 82
    supplements for 101
  wild game and grass-fed cows and 98
omega-6 oils 97
  seizures and 102
omega-9 oils 97
optimism and our health 203
organic foods
  advantages of 83
  chemicals and 84
  contaminated 86, 142
  food supplementation programs and
    116
  pesticides, herbicides, and fertilizers
    and 84
  vitamin and mineral deficiencies and
    116
  wild foods and 87
organ transplants, St. John's wort and
  265
Osler, Sir William 295
osteopathic medicine 252
osteoporosis 32
  fluoride and 159
  vitamin D and 124
osteosarcoma, fluoride and 160
other (plastic recycling code) 147
otitis media. See ear infections
our thinking. See habits of thought
ovens (for cooking)
  indoor air pollution and 154

overload in exercise 62
ovo-lacto vegetarian. See vegetarian
  and vegan diets
OxyContin 21
ozone (ground-level) 152
ozone layer, methyl bromide and 150
ozone water purification 164

P

painkilling medications. See
  also medications
  adverse effects of 22
  fatalities from 22
  increase in prescriptions for 21
  kidney failure and 22
  OxyContin 21
  Vicodin 21
pain management 252
  acupuncture treatment for 296
  St. John's wort and 260
paint (household), safety information
  165
Panax ginseng 263
Paracelsus' Doctrine of Similars 280
pasteurization and fermented foods 79
patient compliance and responsibility
  246
Pauling, Linus 113
PBDEs (polybrominated diphenyl
  esters)
  adverse health effects of 168
  in breast milk 169
PC-SPES 264
pedometers 71
pellagra 115
perchlorates
  in breast milk 142
  in drinking water 86, 142
    removing 144
  inhibition of thyroid function 143
  in human bodies 136
  in organic foods 86, 142
  reproductive health and 143
  standards 144
  US EPA and 143

water filtration of 164
perfluorooctanoic acid (PFOA) 167
personal care products. *See* cosmetics
    and personal care items
personality and health 201
pessimism and health 203
pesticides, herbicides, and fertilizers.
    See also specific names
    arsenic and 161
    DDT 84
    effects on nutrients in plants 85
    GMOs and 141
    health hazards of 84
    household pesticides
        safety information 165
    industrial farming and 91
    in herbal supplements 262
    methyl iodide 151
    Roundup 89
    water contamination and 161
    Zyklon B 84
PETE or PET (plastic recycling code)
    147
PFOAs 167
pharmaceutical industry
    criminal penalties and 25
    deceptiveness of 25
    medical journals and 25
phosphoricum acidum
    gastroenteritis and 312
phosphorus (homeopathic remedy)
    gastroenteritis and 312
phthalates 142
    enteric coatings and 130
    in cosmetics 173
    plastic recycling code for 147
    sources of 142
physical activity. *See* exercise
physicians
    asking questions and 28
    CAM as an additional option for 299
    duty of, Samuel Hahnemann and
        16
    errors in treatments 10

evaluating CAM practitioner referrals
    254
religion and spirituality and 215
phytosterols, health benefits of 98
pig farming, use of antibiotics and 92
Pilates 252
plant estrogens, health benefits of 98
plastic food wrap, phthalates in 142
plastic recycling codes and safety 147
pneumonia, rickets and 112
podophyllum, gastroenteritis and 313
polybrominated diphenyl esters
    (PBDEs) 168
polycarbonate water bottles, BPA and
    146
polychlorinated biphenyls (PCBs). *See
    also* dioxin
    in farm-raised salmon 87
    in fish oil supplements 101
    in freshwater fish 98
the polymeal and the polypill 36
polyphenols 130
    benefits of 78
    recommendations 130
    sources of 78
polyurethane foam, PBDEs and 169
Pong Research cell phone products 171
Pope, Alexander 209
portion size 105
positive reappraisal 209
postural reeducation therapies 252
PP (plastic recycling code) 147
prayer and mental healing 249
prayer for atheists 214
predators, environmental toxins and
    80
premature puberty, growth hormones
    in meat and 92
pre-methylated folate 118
prescription medications.
    See medications
President's Panel on Cancer 134
pressure point therapies 252
preventive activities 36
    effect on health 41

primary prevention 34
probiotics
 benefits of 79
 GI infections and 239
 oral, tooth health and 161
problem-solving abilities
 exercise and 51
processed food. *See* food, processed
ProdiGene incident 90
proprietary blends of herbs 267
proprioception, static stretching and
 58
prostate
 BPA and 145
 cancer 35
  nuts and seeds and 98
  PC-SPES and 264
protein
 dietary sources of 302
 vegetarian and vegan diets and 82
provings (homeopathic principle)
 281–284
Pruefung (homeopathic provings) 281
PS (plastic recycling code) 147
psychosis
 religion and spirituality and 214
psychotherapy for specific medical
 conditions 249
PTFE in nonstick cookware 166
purposeful life, life expectancy and 214
p value 323
PVC (plastic recycling code) 147

Q

qigong for specific medical conditions
 251
quinine, Samuel Hahnemann's
 experiments with 278

R

radiation 169
radium 164
radon gas
 death rate due to 152
 testing for in your home 154

water filtration of 164
Rating of Perceived Exertion (RPE) 62
raw food 83
reactions to medical drugs. *See* adverse
 drug effects
recommended daily allowance (RDA)
 of vitamin C 120
recovery and sports drinks
 after exercise 68
 ideal 308
 milk and 68
 when to consume 306
recovery in exercise 67
recreational activities as stress
 management 210
red yeast rice for high cholesterol 239
regular soap's usefulness 156
relationships. *See also* social
 connections
 importance of 191
 men and women and 193
 sexuality and 198
 stress and 192
religion and spirituality 213–216
 importance of 213
 physicians and their patients and 215
 psychoses and 214
 purposeful life and 214
remedies, homeopathic.
 See homeopathy
reproductive health
 BPA and 145
 environmental chemicals and 138
 lead and 148
 PDBEs and 169
 perchlorates and 143
 PFOAs and 167
research, scientific. *See* scientific
 research
respirator masks 183
respiratory health
 chlorine and 158
 mold and 156
resting heart rate 64
restless leg syndrome, ferritin and 123

Reston, James 295
resveratrol 78
reverse osmosis systems 163, 164
rhodiola, ginseng and 258
rhus toxicodendron
  injuries and 314
rickets 111
  pneumonia and 112
  vitamin D and 124
risk-benefit ratio 23
  eating and vitamin supplementation
    and 90
  of GMOs 91
Rolfing 252
Roundup 140–141
  GMOs and 140
  health problems linked to 141
  ill effects of 89
  Monsanto and 140
running
  barefoot 72
  human capacity for 50
  human physical development and 50
  marathon. *See* marathon runners
  shoes and 72
ruta graveolens
  injuries and 314

S

saccharin 172
safety goggles and safety masks 183
Salem witch trials, mycotoxins and 155
salmon
  EPA and DHA and 98
  farm-raised, PCBs in 87
  salmon oil supplements 101
salt
  high blood pressure and 82
  in processed foods 172
  iodine and 115
  low blood pressure and 83
San Francisco Bay Area
  medications in water 182
  mercury and fish consumption and 98

Santa Monica municipal water system,
    MTBE and 142
Santeria 251
sarcoidosis, vitamin D and 125
Schwarzenegger, Arnold 55
scientific research
  clinical
    advantages of 318
    beginnings in homeopathic testing
      281
    problems with 318
  errors in 117
  ethical concerns 325
  evaluating 316–326
    data analysis 322
    questions to ask 319
  mass media and 324
secondary prevention 34
sedentary athletes 52
seizures, evening primrose and borage
    oils and 102
selenium, recommendations 130
self-assessment 217
self care 245
  dangers of 231
  homeopathy and 291
self-evaluation 206
sepia (homeopathic remedy) 313
Seralini Affair, Roundup and 89
serotonin syndrome 179
sexuality 197–200
  attitudes toward 197
  definition of healthy sex 198
  health problems affecting 199
  improving your sex life 199
  relationships and 198
  suppressing 197
Shakespeare, William 20
shamanic healing, use of 230
shamanism 251
sharks, environmental toxins and 80
shoes for exercising 72
shopping for food 103
short-term conditions
  homeopathy and 291

Siberian ginseng 263
sick buildings 183
silica (homeopathic remedy)
    ear infections and 311
similia (likes cure likes) homeopathic
    principle 279
Sinclair, Upton 92
single medicine (homeopathic
    principle) 284
skeletal muscles. *See also* muscles
    importance of exercise for 55
skin
    CAM treatments for 253
    cancer, sunlight and
        125
    cinnamon sensitivity 173
    color, vitamin D and 112
    cosmetics and personal care items and
        173
sleep 187–190
    Alzheimer's disease and 188
    deprivation and our health 188
    healing power of 188
    hygiene 190
    importance of 187
    improving 189, 190
        cognitive behavior therapy and 189
        sleeping medications and 189
    whales and dolphins and 187
sleep apnea 188–189
smart phones
    exercise and 72
    safety, SAR and 171
smoking
    cadmium exposure and 150
    dioxins and 144
    importance of quitting 133, 184
    indoor air pollution and 152
soap, usefulness of 156
social connections 191–196. *See
    also* relationships
    aging and 194
    altruism and 194
    and the elderly 193
    creating and building 194

drug or alcohol addiction and 194
    exercise and 195
    health and 193
    value of 191, 207
social nature of humans 191
social networks. *See* social connections
soil
    depletion, nutrient deficiencies and
        111
    organisms in, pesticides, herbicides,
        and fertilizers and 84
sorbitol 172
specific absorption rate (SAR)
    cell phones and 171
spiritual dysfunction and disease 287
spirituality. *See* religion and spirituality
spongia tosta, croup and 310
sports drinks. *See* recovery and sports
    drinks
sports medicine, Rating of Perceived
    Exertion (RPE) and 62
sports performance
    strength training and 55
sprains, homeopathic remedies for 314
sprinting, static stretching and 58
stage fright, homeopathic remedy for
    311
Stamets, Paul 155
starvation, diabetes in grandchildren
    and 139
static stretching. *See* stretching
statin drugs, health risks of 180
Stephania 261
steroids, adverse effects of 24
St John's wort
    hypericin and hyperforin and 263
    purity concerns 261
St. John's wort 260
    organ transplant rejection and 265
stomach problems, homeopathic
    remedies for 312–313
strawberries, methyl iodide and 151
strength training 54
    athletic injury reduction and 55
    body building and 55

children and 55
dynamic stretching and 60
elderly individuals and 55
guidelines 306
knee problems and 69
lowering death rate and 56
lymphedema and 28
marathon runners and 54
sports performance and 55
static stretching and 58
weight loss and 55
women and 55
stress management 208. See also coping
skills
CAM and 251
life changes and 192
recreational activities and 210
stretching
ballistic 58
explosive physical activities and 60
flexibility and 60
cold stiff muscles and 60
dynamic 60
strength training and 60
flexibility and 57
static 58
athletic injuries and 58
proprioception and 58
sprinting and 58
weight training and 58
studies of injury rates and 57
tendons and 59
the right way 58
strokes, air pollution and 151
styrene, plastic recycling code for 147
succussion in homeopathy 284
sucralose 172
sucrose. See sugars and sweeteners
sugars and sweeteners
artificial, adverse health effects of 172
consumption of 76
different names for 76
food industry and 76
fruit juice and 76
fruits and vegetables and 114

healthy alternatives 172
high-fructose corn syrup (HFCS) 76,
172
sulfites in food, health effects of 172
sulphur (homeopathic remedy)
gastroenteritis and 313
sun exposure, vitamin D and 112
supplements 109–132. See
also vitamins and minerals;
individual supplement names
chelated 130
criticisms of taking 116
elderly individuals and 109
interactions 112
nationwide supplementation programs
116
recommendations 130
sweeteners. See sugars and sweeteners
syrup. See sugar

T

tabaccum, motion sickness and 314
tai chi as therapy 249
talk test, adjusting workouts and 63
tBBPA (tetrabromobisphenol-A) 169
tea as a source of polyphenols 78
teething, homeopathic remedies for
315
Teflon 167
telomerase. See telomeres
telomeres
biological age and 126
cancer and 127
longevity and 42
testing 126
tendons
stiff, homeopathic remedy for 314
stretching and 59
tendinosis 59
tendonitis 59
tight muscles and 59
tennis elbow, eccentric muscle
strengthening and 59
ten thousand steps a day 52
for building muscles 306

tetrabromobisphenol-A (TBBPA) 169
thallium in herbal supplements 262
therapy, choosing a type of 248
thirst
  dehydration and 46
  importance of 45
Thomsonian tradition in herbal
    medicine 230
thought. *See* habits of thought
thyroid
  cancer and use of CAM 234
  disease, iodine and 115
  perchlorates and 143
  PFOAs and 167
  triclosan and 156
tilapia, farm-raised 98
  saturated fats in 87
tooth decay
  fluoride and 160
  oral probiotics and 161
toxins
  exposure to 134
  in fish 98
  water filtration and 164
traditional Oriental medicine.
    See specific approaches, such as
    acupuncture
traffic-accident-related fear,
    homeopathic remedy for 311
trekking poles 72
trichalomethanes, water filtration of
    164
triclosan 156
trihalomethanes, stillborn babies and
    158
tuning fork test for vitamin B12
    deficiency 123
turmeric, benefits of 78
Type A personalities 201

U

ultraviolet light
  for water purification 163, 164
  vitamin D and 112
unclean water. *See* water

unconventional medicine.
    See complementary and alternative
    medicine (CAM)
United States Pharmacopeia (USP)
  certification 266
United States Track and Field 325
urinary tract
  E. coli and 93
  infections in women
    food-related illness and 93
urine, color of, dehydration and 47
US Air Force's use of acupuncture 295
US Environmental Protection Agency
    (US EPA)
  lead exposure and 149
  perchlorates and 143
USP 37 certification 128, 266
UV-B, vitamin D and 112

V

vaccinations, mercury exposure and 99
variability in exercise 66–68
vegetarian and vegan diets 80. *See
    also* diet
  advantages of 80
  cataracts and 81
  disadvantages of 81
  micronutrient deficiencies in 82
  need for protein in 82
  omega-3 supplements and 82, 101
  zinc and 130
veratrum album
  gastroenteritis and 312, 313
Vicodin 22
viral DNA 79
vitamin A
  caution 129
  interference of vitamin D 101
vitamin B6, vitamin B12 deficiency
    testing and 122
vitamin B9 118
vitamin B12
  deficiency
    organic foods and 116
    testing for 122, 123

recommendations 129, 130
vitamin C
  cancer and heart disease and 117
  chimpanzee study 113
  RDA 120
  recommendations 129, 130
vitamin D 111–112
  benefits of 78
  bone health and 111
  cautions for certain diseases 125
  deficiency as a health crisis 77
  high blood pressure and 126
  interference from vitamin A 101
  milk and 115
  obesity and 113
  osteoporosis and 124
  recommendations 129, 130
  rickets and 111, 124
  sarcoidosis and 125
  skin color and 112
  sunlight and 112, 125
  testing for 124–126
    controversy 124
    timing of 125
    Vitamin D Council and 126
  ultraviolet light and 112
Vitamin D Council 126
vitamin E
  cancer and heart disease and 117
  recommendations 129, 130
vitamin K 130
vitamins and minerals. See
    also supplements; individual names
    of vitamins
  antioxidant vitamins. See antioxidants
  chelated 130
  daily value percentage 129
  deficiencies
    in the American diet 77, 83,
      110–115
    soil depletion and 111
    testing for 120
    worldwide 114
  Dietary Reference Intake 110
  information resources 121

in wild foods versus domesticated 89
pros and cons of taking 88
recommendations 127–129, 130
testing for 110–115
USP 37 certification 128
volatile organic compounds (VOCs)
  in the home 165
  safety masks and goggles and 183
  water filtration of 164

W

walnuts, omega-3 oils and 98
warming up. See stretching, dynamic
water. See also dehydration
  arsenic in 161
  bottled 162
  chlorinated 157
    adverse health effects of 158
  consumption
    physical flexibility and 57
  contamination 141, 157. See
      also specific contaminant names
  cholera and 157
  organic foods and 86
  fluoridated 158
    Brainerd diarrhea and 159
    dental fluorosis and 160
    lower IQ and 160
  guidelines for how much to drink 47
  importance of drinking 45–48
  in wells 162
  prescription medications in 182
  purifying. See water purification
  quality 156
  study on health effects of drinking 45
  toxins in
    exposure levels 164
    removing (table) 164
water bottles, safe materials in 146
water distillers 164
water filtration. See water purification
water purification 163
  Environmental Working Group and
    165
  reverse osmosis systems 163

table of filtration methods 164
ultraviolet light and 163
water softeners 164
wealthy countries
nutrient deficiencies and 114–115
weight gain, dioxins and 144
weight loss
fat burning activities and 66
strength training and 55
weight training. *See* strength training
whales and dolphins, sleep habits of
187
wholistic medicine. *See* complementary
and alternative medicine (CAM)
wild foods
benefits of 87, 113–114
vitamin and mineral levels in 89
wild game, ALA and 98
women
importance of relationships to 193
strength training benefits for 55
working out. *See* exercise
workplace
challenges of 207

health hazards 183
World Health Organization, vitamin
and mineral deficiencies and 114

X

x-rays, risks of 35
xylitol 172

Y

yeast (environmental). *See* molds and
yeast
yin and yang symbol 294
yoga for specific medical conditions
249

Z

zinc
blindness and 113
copper and 113
deficiencies, organic foods and 116
iron and 112
recommendations 130
zoopharmacognosy 257
Zyklon B 84

Made in the USA
San Bernardino, CA
29 September 2016